XIIth I.S.C.E.R.G. Symposium

Documenta Ophthalmologica
Proceedings Series volume 10

Editor H. E. Henkes

Dr. W. Junk by Publishers The Hague 1976

XIIth I. S. C. E. R. G. Symposium
Clermont-Ferrand 20-22 MAY 1974

edited by R. Alfieri & P. Solé

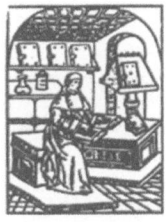

Dr. W. Junk by Publishers The Hague 1976

ISBN 978-90-6193-150-8   ISBN 978-94-010-1575-2 (eBook)
DOI 10.1007.978-94-010-1575-2

CONTENTS

ULTRASTRUCTURE AND
MICRO-ELECTROPHYSIOLOGY OF THE MACULA

L. MISSOTTEN

(Louvain, Belgium)

Mr Chairman
Ladies and Gentlemen,

Ultrastructure, micro-electrophysiology and electro-retinography of the fovea are the subjects of this paper.

The detection, by means of electroretinography, of a potential generated in the fovea, requires two conditions. First: a potential must be created by the separation of charges across a barrier; Second: this barrier should extend along the greatest part of the eye so that the current generated by the potential has to make a detour through the anterior chamber and the tissues around the eye and may be detected by electrodes on the cornea and on the skin. First the anatomy will be studied. Second the potentials they generate are described as recorded by microelectrodes. Third the evidence concerning the electrical barriers, the 'R membrane' according to BRINDLEY, is reviewed.

The dimensions of the fovea are somewhat arbitrary because it has no clear cut margins. The central foveola where the inner layers are absent, measures about 250 microns. The external fovea, this is the area where the photoreceptors are longer than anywhere else in the retina, has a diameter of about 600 microns. This area is rod free.

Their number increases rapidly; at about 500 microns from the center of the fovea rods and cones exist in equal numbers. In the retinal periphery rods outnumber cones 20 to 1.

VISUAL CELLS

The structure of rods and cones probably is familiar to the reader. A picture in STEINBERG's paper (1973) shows the rods and the cones of the frog retina by scanning electron microscopy. It shows the photosensitive outer segment, the connecting cilium, the inner segment, the cell body and the synaptic endbuds. The cones of the fovea are different, however, from these in the retinal periphery. They are very rodlike and in well fixed preparations the difference between a cone and a rod is very hard to see. The better the fixation, the more they resemble each other. Fortunately, well fixed specimens are few and usually artefacts appear, the artefacts are different in rods and in cones.

In rods the saccules swell, in cones they do not, in rods the saccules remain well aligned, in cones they shift, form loops or become completely disoriented. Cones appear to be liquid structures, liquid cristals in aqueous

1

medium. In comparison the fragile rods seem solid and indestructible.

The embryogenesis of rods and cones is similar as is shown in the diagrams by TOKOYASHUS & YAMADA (1959) and NILSON (1969). A cilium grows out of the cell body and invaginations form in the plasma membrane. In the cones of the lower vertebrates these invaginations remain connected to the plasma membrane. In rods the saccules are pinched off. In human retina, however, the saccules appear not to be connected to the plasma membrane, neither in rods nor in cones. The exceptions to this rule are so few that in my opinion they have no functional consequences.

The renewal of rods and cones during life appears to be different, as shown by an experiment of YOUNG (1968). He injected radioactive amino acids into frogs and waited for variable intervals of time in order to allow for the incorporation of the amino acids into proteins. The animals were killed at various times after the injection and the retina was investigated by autoradiography in order to detect the radioactive proteins.

In rods, a layer of labeled proteins has been added to the outer segment. In cones less protein was incorporated and apparently in a diffuse way. A few days later, the band of labeled protein has migrated towards the tip by apposition of newly formed saccules. These saccules have been slightly labeled by the few radioactive aminoacids still available. The upper-most part of the rod remains unlabeled because these saccules have been formed before the injection of radioactive aminoacids. In cones again the labeling is diffuse and less intensive.

The resorption of the added material has been investigated. YOUNG & BOK (1970 have demonstrated that the tips of the growing rods are cut off and digested by the pigment epithelium. This slide shows a rod, its tip against the pigment epithelium cell surrounded by long expansions. I n the cytoplasme of the pigment epithelium cell a piece of rod, pinched off and encapsulated in a phagosome may be seen. It has been suggested that cones are not digested in the same way. However, last year HOGAN studied the foveal area of the human retina and found similar phagosomes in the pigment epithelium cells. We have been able to confirm this finding and have observed phagosomes containing tips of foveal cones. This is not so surprising, since pigment epithelium cells phagocytise everything they can lay their hands on.

Summarising the life cycle of rods and cones: their embryogenesis is similar, their renewal is different, and their resorption may be similar.

It is wel known that visual cells generate potentials: the early receptor potential which has something to do with photochemistry, and the late receptor potential which is an event on the cellular level.

Recently WHITTEN & BROWN (1973) recorded the late receptor potential from the cones of the fovea in the cynomolgus monkey, which has a retina very similar to ours. A micro-electrode has been placed among the photoreceptors of the fovea and the potential recorded for flashes of light of different wavelengths. The late receptor potentials of a cone is a potential with a fast rise, a plateau that lasts as long as the light stimulus, and a rapid decline. In comparison, the late receptor potential of rods builds up and declines slowly. Optimal wavelenghth sensitivity of the rods, as compared to the cones, is shifted towards the shorter wavelenghths, as could be expected.

2

The next question is: are these potentials generated across a barrier that stretches along a major part of the eye fundus. Could the outer limiting membranes act as an R membrane?

A barrier for the late receptor potentials could be composed of the plasma membranes of visual cells and that of Muller cells joined at the outer limiting membrane.

PIGMENT EPITHELIUM

A closer look at the pigment epithelial cells reveals their apical membrane covered with micro villi, seen in a picture from a frog eye studied by scanning electron microscopy (STEINBERG 1973). The basal side of the pigment epithelial cells rests on the Bruchs membrane. Their lateral walls are bound together near the apical border by means of a complex structure: a zonula adherans combined with a zonula occludens. At this level both plasma membranes are close together; the inter cellular space appears to be closed off.

There are many ways to demonstrate that this zonula occludens severely restricts the diffusion through the intercellular space. For example let us consider this micrograph from an experiment by SHIOSE (1973). He injected a foreign protein in the blood stream of a rabbit; six minutes later the animal was killed. The eyes were fixed and the protein detected by a histochemical method which produces a black osmiophylic deposit on this preparation. Bruchs membrane is completely impregnated. The spaces between the infoldings of the basal membrane are filled with the protein and the intercellular space between adjacent pigment epithelial cells contains the protein up to the zonula occludens but never beyond. So the pigment epithelial cells form a tight barrier. Conceivably the barrier is built either by the basal membranes up to the zonulae or by the apical membranes or by both.

Pigment epithelial cells generate potentials upon stimulation by light (STEINBERG et al. (1970). Intracellular recording shows a very slow potential, continuing to increase after the end of the illumination and slowly declining. The time constants of rise and fall are identical to those of the C wave of the electroretinogram. The intracellular response is always opposite in polarity to the C wave and larger than the C wave, indicating that this potential is generated across the apical membrane of the pigment epithelium. However, it could be that this potential is of no use for the study of the center of the fovea. It seems to be generated only by pigment epithelial cells in contact with rods and to be absent in pure cone retinae. For this reason, it may be non existant in the rod free central area of the fovea.

Muller cells

The center of the fovea contains in addition to the photoreceptor cells and pigment epithelium cells only one other component: the Muller cells. Electromicroscopy shows that Muller cells are numerous in the fovea, forming intricate whorls between the cone fibers. Muller cells do generate potentials as has been shown by MILLER & DOWLING (1970) in the retina of an

3

amphibian, Necturus. This slide shows an intracellular recording of Muller cell potentials, while the retina is stimulated by light over a wide range of intensities. The similarity of this potential to the B wave of the electroretinogram is obvious.

The retina might act as a barrier across which this potential is generated. The retina as a whole is a compact structure with few intercellular spaces. Its electrical resistance is superior to that of intercellular fluid. The only cell that stretches across this barrier is the Muller cell with its micro villi on the apical surface and its basal feet on the inner limiting membrane. Therefore any potential generated by the Muller cells will most likely appear on the electroretinogram.

The other cells of the retina: horizontal cells, bipolar cells, amacrine cells and ganglion cells also have electrical activities, but they do not seem to generate this potential across a barrier stretching along a major part of the eye fundus. For this reason the potentials they generate are probably very hard to record by electrodes outside of the eye.

SYNAPTIC RELATIONS OF THE VISUAL CELLS

A light micrograph of the center of the fovea shows only cones and no synapses. We have to move to the next field, where the first synaptic pedicle is seen at a distance of about a 150 microns from the center. The first pedicles are placed at somewhat irregular intervals, but from about 250 microns from the center, there is a continuous layer of pedicles stretching out to about 800 microns from the center, where the first rod spherules appear. This centrifugal displacement of the pedicles from the foveal cones has two consequences: 1. a radical pattern of fibers in the fovea: Henle's fibers, connecting each cone to its pedicle. The 2.500 cones of the central bouquet situated in the black area of this diagram, have their endbuds in this dotted zone. This demonstrates the second consequence: the area of the synapses and neurons is much larger than the corresponding area of the cones.

Divers kinds of neurons of the second echelon are seen in front of the pedicles. Outermost: the horizontal cells, each in contact with several pedicles. A small piece of their axon can often be seen. The next slide shows a diffuse bipolar cell with its cell body, main dendrite and endbuds in contact with several pedicles. The next slide shows a midget bipolar cell with a tiny arborisation just large enough to contact a single pedicle. Its axon can be seen to go on to the inner plexiform layer where it seems to make a synapse with a single midget ganglion cell. The midget bipolar cells and their organisation was discovered by POLYAK and for some time many people forgot about the other types of cells. They got used to thinking in the fovea each pedicle is connected to a single bipolar cell which in turn relayed a single ganglion cell. This opinion, however, is an error.

A diagram and an electromicrograph of the pedicles of a foveal cone show that each pedicle is in contact with each of its neighbours. The synaptic surface is irregular. Some dendrites are invaginated in the pedicle in groups of three: a central one, and two lateral ones. The other dendrites make only superficial contacts with the synaptic surface of the pedicle.

BIPOLAR AND HORIZONTAL CELLS

The origin of the dendrites in contact with the pedicles can not be seen on an ordinary micrograph. Only cross sections of dendrites are apparent. One way to get around this difficulty is to analyse serial sections. This method is well known to you. One collects some 50 consecutive sections, photographs them all, and traces from one section to the next the dendrites throughout the block. Each section of a dendrite is then drawn on a sheet of transparent plastic. The superposition of these sheets reveals the outlines of the dendritic tree. A midget bipolar cell is shown in contact with a single pedicle. All the dendrites are invaginated in the central position of triads at the synaptic surface of this pedicle as can be seen in electron micrographs.

Another method to study the synaptic relationship between neurons is to analyse Golgi stained sections by electron microscopy. An example of a midget bipolar cell is shown. The end branches marked by silver stain are all found in a central psotion in triads at the synaptic surface of one pedicle. As we can see both methods give identical results.

The study of many bipolar cells in the foveal region leads to the following diagram. Pedicles are in contact with each other. Horizontal cells are connected to pedicles by means of dendrites in a lateral position in the triads of several pedicles. Diffuse cone bipolars are connected to several pedicles by means of superficial contacts. There are two varieties of midget bipolar cells (KOLB et al. (1969). One is in contact with a single pedicle by means of dendrites in a central position in triads. The other variety touches one pedicle by means of superficial contacts.

Investigations in electrophysiology have shown that horizontal cells react to illumination with a graded hyperpolarisation potential. Bipolar cells have a more complex behaviour, at least in Necturus where they have been the most thoroughly analysed. Some bipolar cells hyperpolarize by illumination of the center of their receptive fields. However, this reaction disappears when the surrounding region of the retina is also illuminated. Other bipolar cells react with a depolarizing potential that is equally counteracted by illumination of the periphery of their receptive field.

THE INNER PLEXIFORM LAYER AND THE GANGLION CELLS

The organisation of the inner plexiform layer is more complex than that of the other plexiform layer. Dendrites from amacrines cells, endbuds from bipolar cells and dendrites from ganglion cells interact in a very complex way that was most intensively studied by DOWLING and his coworkers. We will not go into details of this organisation, but limit ourselves to a rapid survey of the electrical activity that results from these interactions. Amacrine cells react with graded potentials and some spikes at each variation of the intensity of illumination. Ganglion cell react in many complex ways. Some of them react with a burst of spikes at the start and at the end of the illumination. Others react with a sustained discharge of spikes as long as the center of their receptive fields is illuminated. However, their activity is inhibited by illumination of the periphery of the receptive field. Many ganglion cells react in different ways to light of different wavelenghts.

CONCLUSION

Our conclusion is as follows: First concerning the electroretinograph. All cells of the retina have electrical activities but some of them are positioned in such a way that they generate an electrical potential across a barrier that extends along the major part of the inner wall of the eye. This favors the detection of this electrical activity by means of electrodes positioned outside of the eye, as is done in electroretinography. The visual cells generate the late receptor potential ressembling the 'a' wave of the electroretinogram. The Muller cells generate a potential similar to the 'b' wave. The electrical activity recorded in the pigment epithelial cell is similar to the 'c' wave.

Concerning the function of the neurons of the fovea. Each pedicle is connected to several bipolar cells. Some of them are hyperpolarizing, others depolarizing upon the illumination of this visual cell. The endbuds in the inner plexiform layer are connected in such a way to the ganglion cells that some of them are excited while others are inhibited by the light stimulus. One may object that this schema is impossible because the number of ganglion cells is not higher than that of the pedicles. However, we should keep in mind that the neighbour pedicle is also connected to several bipolar cells some of which are hyperpolarized and other depolarized by the excitation of the cone. They, too, have branches in the inner plexiform layers that may be connected to the same ganglion cells, inhibiting the first and exciting the second cell. In this way, the information about two pedicles may be transmitted by means of two ganglion cells. However, ganglion cells are not paired two by two, but act in complex interconnected groups. The combination of their activity permits to transmit an enormous amount of information about the activity and the illumination of the foveal area.

BIBLIOGRAPHY

DOWLING J.E. & WERBLIN F.S. *Vis. Res. Suppl.* 3: *1-15,* 1971.
KOLB H., BOYCOTT B.B. & DOWLING J.E. *Phil. Trans. B* 255: *177-183,* 1969.
MILLER R.F. & DOWLING J.E. *J. Neurophysiol.* 33: *323-342,* 1970.
NILSON S.E.G. & CRESCITELLI F. *J. Ultrastr. Res.* 27: *45-62,* 1969.
POLYAK S.L. The Retina. Univ. of Chicago Press, 1941.
SHIOSE Y. Electron Microscopic. Atlas in ophthalmology (Ed. YAMADA E. & SHIKANO S.) G Thieme Stuttgart 1973.
STEINBERG R.H. *Z. Zellforsch.* 143: *451-463,* 1973.
STEINBERG R.H., SCHMIDT R. & BROWN K.T. *Nature,* Vol. 227: *728,* 1970.
WHITTEN D.N. & BROWN K.T. *Vision Research,* 13: *107-135,* 1973.
YOUNG R.W. & BOK D. *Invest. Ophtal.* 9: *524-36,* Jul. 70.
YOUNG R.W. & DROZ B. *J. Cell. Biol.* 39: *169-184,* 1968.

NORMAL AND ABNORMAL VISUAL PATHWAYS AND THE CORTICAL REPRESENTATION OF THE VISUAL FIELD[1]

R.W. GUILLERY

(Madison, Wisconsin)

INTRODUCTION

I was asked to present an introductory survey that would deal with the representation of the retina upon the cortex. My request to change the subject from 'the retinal representation' to the 'visual field representation' was not merely a semantic squabble; it was based upon observations that the cortex is not concerned specifically with the order of the retinal representation, but rather with the visual field representation. In this respect the cortex differs from lower brain centers within which the order of the retinal projection is critical, while the visual field representation appears to be irrelevant for establishing connectivity patterns.

In a normal animal, of course, the retinal and visual field representations are mere reversals of each other, and it is not easy to dissociate the two in the developing visual system. However, there are certain congenital abnormalities of the visual pathways in which the two can be dissociated, and these demonstrate that the cortex seeks to establish the visual 'sense' of its inputs while the lateral geniculate nucleus is primarily concerned with the retinal locus.

I want first to review some aspects of the normal retinogeniculo-cortical pathways, briefly comparing knowledge of the human pathways with experimental observations obtained primarily from cats and monkeys. Then I want to consider congenital abnormalities that are best known in cats, and that lead to a partial reversal of the visual field representation in the brain. Finally, I shall argue that a similar abnormality must occur in man, and that a systematic study of the pattern of the human abnormality may prove possible with modern methods.

THE CORTICAL MAP IN MAN

The strongest evidence for an orderly mapping of the visual fields upon the cortical surface in man comes from systematic studies of scotomata produced by brain injuries. Perimetric methods provided some of the earliest evidence that there is an orderly mapping of the visual field upon the cortical surface, and systematic comparisons of visual defects with post-mortem findings (see especially HENSCHEN, '93, '12) have produced remarkably detailed

* The work reported here was supported by Grants EY00962 and RO1 NS06662 from the National Institutes of Health.

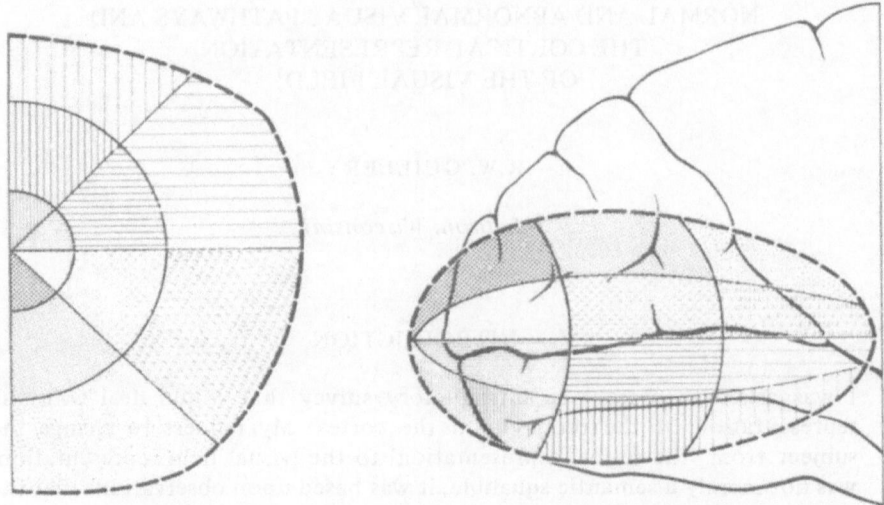

Fig. 1, (Adapted from SPALDING, 1952b). The visual field representation is shown as it would appear if the cortex within the calcarine fissure were flattened out on the surface of the brain. Thus, most of the representation actually lies within the depth of the fissure; the lower fields in the upper banks and the upper fields in the lower banks of the fissure. The representation of the horizontal meridian probably lies near the bottom of the fissure.

maps for man (INOUYE, '09; HOLMES, '19). Unfortunately, it is difficult to use these methods on experimental animals, where one has had to rely primarily on electrophysiological methods.

The basic pattern of visual field representation shown in Figure 1 is well known. Figure 1 is adapted from SPALDING ('52b) and shows that the macula is represented at the occipital pole, with the retinal periphery further anteriorly within the banks of the calcarine fissure; the upper fields below the fissure and most of the lower fields above the fissure.

A number of the features shown in this mapping deserve comment. The first is that the central, macular areas have a disproportionately large cortical representation. As a result of this deformation, one finds that the scotomata produced by suprageniculate lesions are commonly wedge-shaped (POLYAK, '57; TEUBER, et al., '60, KOERNER & TEUBER, '73); that is damage to equal amounts of neural tissue in the geniculo-cortical pathways produces relatively larger defects for peripheral than for central fields. We do not know the precise extent to which the representations of the different parts of the visual field are thus deformed in the cerebral pathways in man, but studies of non-human primates have shown that the 'magnification factor' (that is, the number of mm. of visual cortex per degree of visual field) is roughly proportional to the ganglion cell density in the corresponding portion of the retina (ROLLS & COWEY, '70; WHITTERIDGE, '73). WHITTERIDGE has pointed out that the magnification factor is a linear ratio, whereas ganglion cell density is measured per unit area. Thus, it appears that the disproportionate representation of central areas is only partially accounted for by the relatively high ganglion cell density in the central parts

8

of the retina and that the volume of cortex receiving from a single central ganglion cell is likely to be greater than the volume receiving from one peripheral ganglion cell (see, however, CHOW, et al., '50 for a contrary conclusion).

Although the visual field is distorted in the cortical map, it is not discontinuous. In each hemisphere there is a continuous topographical (point-for-point) representation of the contralateral hemifield, and this representation stops quite abruptly along or close to the midline vertical meridian. This midline break in the visual field representation is only an apparent break; the two representations are joined together by the fibres of the corpus callosum (MYERS, '62, EBNER & MYERS, '65; WILSON, '67; HUBEL & WIESEL, '67). It has been shown that many of the fibres in the posterior part of the corpus callosum connect the border of areas 17 and 18, within which the region immediately adjacent to the midline is represented. GLICKSTEIN & WHITTERIDGE ('74) have shown that many of these fibres arise within a cytoarchitectonically distinct strip, area OBγ of VON ECONOMO ('29), which is characterized by unusually large pyramidal cells. It is the axons of these pyramidal cells that serve to join the two representations into a single continuous whole.

Plots of the scotomata that occur after suprageniculate lesions have repeatedly shown that the area of the macula tends to be spared more commonly than other regions. To some extent this may be because the macular representation is relatively large and because the posterior tip of the occipital lobe, within which the macula is represented may be selectively spared (see SPALDING, '52a, b; TEUBER et al., '60; DUKE-ELDER and SCOTT, '71). However such an explanation does not account for many published observations of macular sparing, and there is at present no good anatomical basis for this phenomenon. Explanations of macular sparing in man that involve a projection from one lateral geniculate nucleus to both hemispheres have been suggested, but there is no evidence for such a projection (see TEUBER, et al., '60; HUBER, '70; DUKE-ELDER & SCOTT, '71). SPALDING ('52a) has pointed out that if there were such a projection one would not expect to see macular splitting with quite small occipital lesions, and this does occasionally occur. Further, in experimental animals no fiber degeneration has generally been traced from a lateral geniculate lesion to the contralateral hemisphere (WILSON & CRAGG, '67; HARTING et al., '73a). Reports of a bilateral projection (GLICKSTEIN, et al., '64, '67) have not been confirmed, although few studies have concerned themselves with this specific point.

It is possible to argue that a differential blood supply to different parts of the visual radiation in man may account for some cases of macular sparing, while anastomotic channels between branches of the middle and posterior cerebral arteries supplying the posterior borders of area 17 may account for others (see FORSTER, '90; SHELLSHEAR, '27; ABBIE, '38; STEPHENS & STILLWELL, '69). However, the evidence is rather tenuous and not enough is known about the variability of the relevant blood vessels.

Suprageniculate lesions in man can produce non-congruent scotomata (TEUBER et al., '60; HARMS, '65; MARINO & RASMUSSEN, '68). In the visual cortex of cats, monkeys and other species the visual field maps for the two eyes are strictly congruent (e.g. HUBEL & WIESEL, '62, '68; ALLMAN & KAAS, '71; HALL et al., '71) and there is no reason for thinking that the human cortex is different. Thus, the non-congruent scotomata must be produced by subcortical damage and must involve the geniculo-cortical fibres in a region where the pathways from the two eyes do not run closely together. A detailed study of the geniculo-striate pathways, designed to show how the axons run from each geniculate lamina to the cortex has never been undertaken. In view of the observations on scotomata one can reasonably expect to find that the pathways concerned with each eye do not join until they are close to the cortex, or in it. It is of some interest that geniculo-cortical axons can generally be seen running through the lowest cortical layers obliquely (CAJAL, '11; COLONNIER & ROSSIGNOL, '69; HUBEL & WIESEL, '72) as though during development their final path to the correct terminal locus in layer 4 of the visual cortex was still being determined as they entered the cortex.

THE CORTICAL MAPS IN EXPERIMENTAL ANIMALS

The most reliable visual field maps have been obtained by electrophysiological microelectrode recordings from individual nerve cells or groups of nerve cells (see e.g. DANIEL & WHITTERIDGE, '61, COWEY, '64; ALLMAN & KAAS, '71, '74; WOOLSEY, '71). A good example of the maps that can be obtained by such methods is to be found in the recent careful and extensive study that ALLMAN & KAAS ('74) have made of cortical visual fields in owl monkeys. Figure 2 shows schematically how the visual field is mapped onto the cortical surface in this species. The mapping onto visual area I (V I or area 17) shows the sharp midline demarcation and the relative central enlargement mentioned above. The deformation of the map is such that a very small cortical zone receives from the periphery of the visual field (shown by triangles). The relatively large zone that receives from the region of the midline is indicated by small circles and extends almost entirely around the borders of area 17.

The cortical region adjacent to area 17 has long been recognized as an architectonically distinct area (area 18; BRODMANN, '09; OTSUKA & HASSLER, '62). Some or all of this region receives a separate visual field map[1] (THOMPSON et al., '50; HUBEL & WIESEL, '65; WOOLSEY, '71; HALL, et al., '71). The pattern of this second representation is also shown in Figure 2 (V II). It is to be noted that central vision is again heavily represented in this area, and that, in contrast to area 17, area 18 or V II does not show a continuous representation of the visual field. The horizontal meridian is split to within about 7° of the center of gaze and most of this meridian is represented twice, once at the top and once at the bottom of the figure. A similar split has also been demonstrated for the macaque by ZEKI ('69) and CRAGG & AINSWORTH ('69).

Beyond area 18[1], area 19 is generally recognized (BRODMANN, '09;

---

1. In the macaque the second visual field map includes only a portion of BROD-MANN's area 18, and further representations of the visual field are found in the rest of area 18 defined by BRODMANN.

10

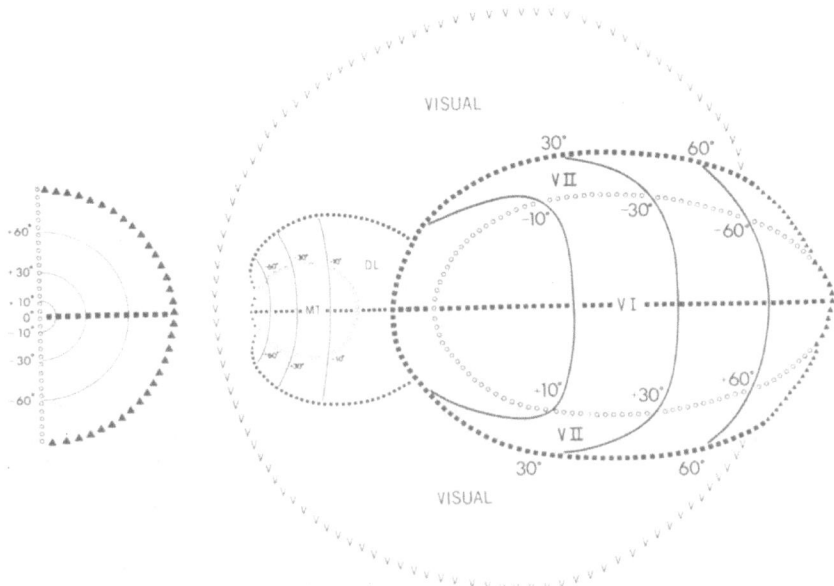

Fig. 2. (From ALLMAN & KAAS, 1974). The representation of the right visual field upon the left visual cortex of the owl monkey. For the lower figure the cortical surface has been unfolded to show the relationships of the visual field representations in VI and VII, and to indicate the region rostral to VII within which are several representations of the visual field, only one of which (MT) is shown. The smaller figure shows the conventions used for identifying the parts of the visual field.

OTSUKA & HASSLER, '62). However, it appears that this may not be a single cortical area and that many details regarding the visual field projections beyond area 18 remain to be studied. ALLMAN & KAAS (see Fig. 2) show a large area beyond 18 and within this several reduplicated versions of VI and VII can be found although only one is shown (see also ZEKI, '69 and '70). It appears that in macaque and owl monkeys, cortex with visual functions extends well into the temporal lobe, that in this region there are several distinct representations of the visual fields, and that quite specific visual functions are associated with each (ZEKI, '73, '74).

Although in cats geniculo-cortical projections go to cortex beyond area 17 (GLICKSTEIN et al., '67; GAREY & POWELL, '67; WILSON & CRAGG, '67; ROSENQUIST & EDWARDS, '73), in primates the lateral geniculate nucleus appears to project exclusively to area 17. Extra-striate visual areas receive afferents from area 17 itself (ZEKI, '69; CRAGG & AINSWORTH, '69; SPATZ et al., '70) and in addition they receive afferents from the superior and inferior pulvinar. The inferior pulvinar in turn receives a major input from the superior colliculus (see MATHERS, '71; HARTING, et al., '73a, b; GLENDENNING et al., '73; WAGOR & LIN, '74). These visual pathways have only recently been demonstrated in primates. Many details remain to be studied, and so far nothing is known about comparable pathways in man. However, it is clear that a long unsuspected

11

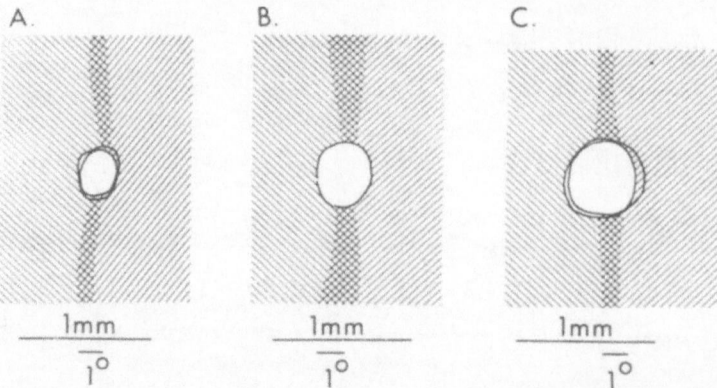

Fig. 3. (From STONE et al., 1973). The distribution of retinal ganglion cells with crossed and uncrossed axons is shown for three individual macaque monkeys. Ganglion cells having crossed axons are shown by one type of hatching, and ganglion cells having uncrossed axons by another. The zone of overlap, about 1° in width, shows the region of the retina that contains some ganglion cells with crossed and some with uncrossed axons. The foveola is shown in white.

and largely independent pathway from the retina to the cortex must be recognized. In addition there is a third pathway that goes through the pretectal nuclei and also reaches extra-striate cortex via a non-geniculate relay (GRAYBIEL, '72). All three systems carry an orderly mapping of the retinal surface.

When one is considering fibre systems that link the thalamus to visually responsive cortex, it is necessary to consider more than just the geniculo-cortical fibres in the optic radiation. The pulvino-cortical fibres are likely to pass somewhat rostral and dorsal to the geniculo-cortical system. Although details of the pulvino-cortical pathway are not known for most species, GRAYBIEL ('72) has shown that in the cat some of the fibres go through the lateral geniculate nucleus (see also ROSENQUIST & EDWARDS, '73). In addition to the fibres that carry visual inputs to the cortex, there is a rich fiber system carrying impulses from visual cortex back to the tectum, pretectum, pulvinar and lateral geniculate nucleus (GUILLERY, '67; GAREY, et al., '68; MATHERS, '72; HOLLÄNDER, '72, '74). These corticofugal axons pass lateral to the geniculo-cortical fibres (FLECHSIG, '96; GUILLERY, '67).

THE LATERAL GENICULATE NUCLEUS

The dorsal lateral geniculate nucleus of all mammals is laminated (KAAS, et al., '72, fig. 4). One set of layers receives afferents from the ipsilateral eye, and a second set receives from the contralateral eye. The visual field is mapped onto each geniculate layer in an orderly manner, and the several layers are arranged so that all the representations are in register (see KAAS et al., '72). That is, single points in the visual field can be represented as lines that pass through all the layers, the lines of projection (see fig. 4).

If the pattern of the visual projection to the cortex is known, the geniculate map can be readily determined by defining the sectors of retrograde degeneration that are produced in the nucleus by cortical lesions. If the cortical map is not known, the visual field map for the lateral geniculate nucleus can be determined by studying the activity of geniculate cells with microelectrodes, and plotting the receptive fields of the cells (SANDERSON, '71; GUILLERY & KAAS, '71).

Each geniculate nucleus carries a set of orderly representations of the contralateral hemifield. The two half maps overlap to only a very limited extent (SANDERSON & SHERMAN, '71). The overlap occurs because there is a narrow vertical strip of retina, which passes through the fovea in monkeys and through the area centralis in cats, and within which there is a mixture of ganglion cells, some with crossed axons, and some with uncrossed axons (see Fig. 3, and see STONE, '66, STONE et al., '73). This overlap zone corresponds approximately to the narrow zone of sparing described in man after large occipital lesions (see HUBER, '70). However, it should be noted that the zone is far too narrow to account for the macular sparing discussed earlier, and also that the zone extends above and below the fovea, while the macular sparing does not.

In owl monkeys central vision is represented in the posterior part of the lateral geniculate nucleus, and the monocular (temporal) crescent of the visual field is represented rostrally (KAAS et al., '72). There are reasons for believing that this is also the condition in other higher primates (see POLYAK, '57; KUPFER, '62). In the posterior part of the nucleus most higher primates have six distinct layers (2 magnocellular and 4 parvocellular), although one commonly finds that in the thickest parts of the nucleus two of the parvocellular layers are duplicated, so that central vision may be represented by eight layers instead of the classical six (LE GROS CLARK & PENMAN, '34; CHACKO, '48). In the peripheral parts of the visual field representation there are only four layers, one magno- and one parvocellular layer innervated from each eye (KAAS, et al., '72), and for the most peripheral, monocular crescent only two layers remain, one small celled and one large celled. It appears that the basic pattern is for each eye to innervate one parvo- and one magnocellular layer, and that the parvocellular layers show a tendency to split, so that a six or even an eight layered structure is found in regions representing central vision. The classical six-layered lateral geniculate nucleus is a convenient but mythical oversimplification.

The lateral geniculate nucleus receives one of its major inputs from the retina. However, in addition to this there are also numerous afferents from the visual cortex (BERESFORD, '62; GUILLERY, '67; HOLLÄNDER, '72, '74). In cat and monkey these cortico-geniculate axons arise in areas 17 and 18 and distribute through all the geniculate layers. A few afferents also reach the lateral geniculate nucleus from the superior colliculus (GRAYBIEL & NAUTA, '71). In a cat the retinal afferents make up only about 15 to 20% of the synaptic terminals in the lateral geniculate nucleus; the number coming from the cortex is not known, but may well be higher than this (GUILLERY, '69b, c), while the tectal input is probably minor. There is no reason for thinking that the figures for primates are strikingly different (see GUILLERY & COLONNIER, '70), although no counts have been made.

13

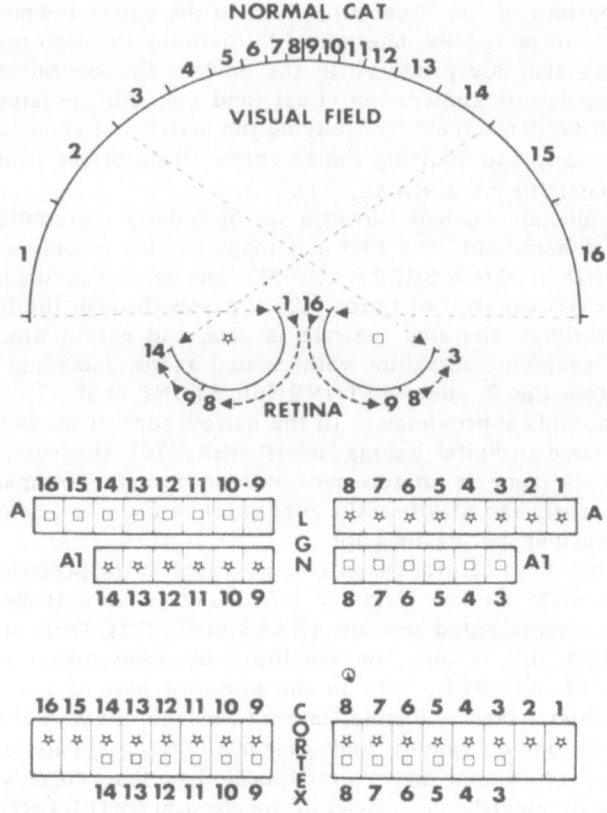

Fig. 4. (From GUILLERY et al., 1974). Schema to show the central, geniculo-cortical projection in a normal cat. The segments of the visual field are numbered sequentially and the corresponding parts of the retina, lateral geniculate nucleus and visual cortex are identified by corresponding numbers. Connections from the left eye are indicated by stars and connections from the right eye by squares. Notice that within the layers of the lateral geniculate nucleus (only two layers are shown for the sake of simplicity) the two representations of the contralateral hemifield are precisely aligned with each other and that the cortex receives its ordered inputs from these aligned, binocular representations of the visual field.

Thus, the impulses travelling through the optic radiation to the visual cortex represent more than a simple 'relaying' of the patterns that pass from the eye to the lateral geniculate nucleus.

CONGENITALLY ABNORMAL PATHWAYS

Retino-geniculate pathways are abnormal in albinos of several different mammalian species. In the abnormal animals some retinogeniculate axons take an inappropriate path through the optic chiasm. Generally the abnormality involves fibres from the temporal retina that cross instead of staying on their own side as they would in a normal animal (LUND, '65; GUIL-

14

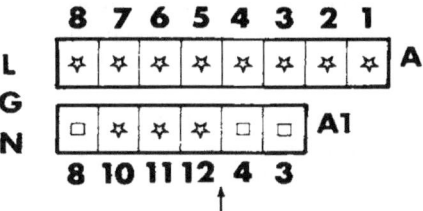

Fig. 5. (From GUILLERY et al., '74). Conventions as in Fig. 4. The sequence of visual field representations that has been found in Siamese cats. Notice that within layer A1 of the lateral geniculate nucleus there is an abnormal input coming from the contralateral eye (10*, 11*, 12*) and that the mediolateral sequence of this input is appropraite for lamina A1 of the opposite side (see Figure 4).

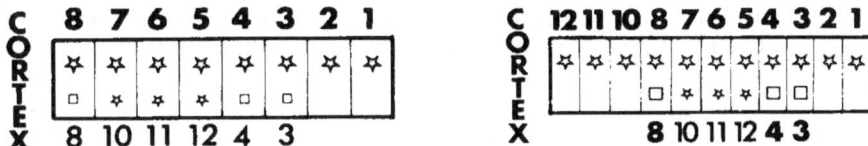

Fig. 6, 7. (From GUILLERY et al., '74). Conventions as in Fig. 4. The representation of the visual field that has been found in the visual cortex of Siamese cats is shown in these figures. In some cats (Fig. 6) the whole of the input coming through layer A1 (see Fig. 5) is supressed at cortical levels (light numbers, small stars and squares) and the cat is effectively blind in the temporal retina. In other cats (Fig. 7) the sequence of the abnormal representation is changed in the geniculo-cortical projection (see upper row of figures) so that a normal sequence of visual field representations is recreated.

LERY, '69a, '71; GUILLERY et al., '71, '73; GIOLLI & CREEL, '73). However, in some animals abnormal fibres appear to arise in the nasal retina and these pass ipsilaterally instead of taking their normal crossed course through the chiasm (SANDERSON et al., '74). A misrouting of fibres from the temporal retina is more common, and if there are abnormal nasal fibres in an animal, there are likely to be an even greater number of abnormal temporal fibres.

The abnormality is found not only in albinos, but in all animals that have significantly low amounts of pigment in the retinal pigment epithelium (SANDERSON et al., '74). The pigment in the chorioid or the iris seems irrelevant, as does the general body pigment. The abnormality is known in most detail for Siamese cats in which there is relatively little pigment in the retina.

If one takes the projection pattern shown in Figure 4 as normal, then the retinogeniculate projections that have been demonstrated for Siamese cats can be summarized by the schema shown in Figure 5. The pattern of the abnormality is relatively constant in these cats (see GUILLERY & KAAS, '71; KALIL et al., '71 HUBEL & WIESEL, '71). The laminae that normally receive a crossed retinal input (lamina A in the figures) are normal. The other layers (shown as A1 in the figures) are broken up. There is generally a

15

medial normally connected segment (8□ in figure 5) and a lateral normally connected segment (3□ and 4□). In between there is an abnormally connected segment that receives crossed inputs instead of the normal uncrossed ones.

The laminar structure of the lateral geniculate nucleus in Siamese cats is recognizably abnormal, even in a routine Nissl preparation, where it is possible to see that some of the geniculate layers are broken up into separate cell islands. Cells that are innervated by one eye tend to form groups distinct from those innervated by the other. Thus, the existence of the abnormality can be recognized from a post-mortem specimen alone (see GUILLERY & KAAS, '73), although one needs to use electrophysiological methods to study the precise pattern of the abnormality.

It is evident from Figure 5 that the axons going to the wrong side of the brain appear to end in the lateral geniculate nucleus in an order that is appropriate for their retinal origin; thus, axons from segments 10, 11 and 12 are arranged in the lateral geniculate nucleus so that those from segment 10 end medial to those from segments 11 and 12, as is normal. Since this retinotopically organized projection is on the wrong side of the brain, however, the visual field representation is quite abnormal. Not only are the visual field representations in adjacent layers not in register, as they would be in a normal animal (see Figure 4), but also, the visual field representation within a single layer is disrupted. This representation runs first in one direction (3 to 4), then in another (12 to 11 to 10), and finally, within segment 8 there is the first (normal) order of representation.

It might appear from the retino-geniculate projection that the visual cortex must be receiving a confusing and ambiguous map of the outside world. However, it can be shown that this does not happen. Cats use one of two quite distinct strategies to overcome the sensory problem (HUBEL & WIESEL, '71; KAAS & GUILLERY, '73). Some cats simply supress the whole of the abnormal sequence that is relayed through the A1 layers. In these cats one finds that little or no cortical activity is elicited by stimulation of the temporal retina, and the cats show no behavioural responses to visual stimuli falling upon the temporal retina (ELEKESSY et al., '73 GUILLERY et al., '74). The cortex does not merely suppress the abnormal inputs to layer A1, but suppresses the whole disrupted sequence (8, 10 to 12, 4 and 3) within the one set of geniculate layers (Fig. 6).

Other cats use a different solution: there is a rearrangement of the geniculo-cortical projection. The geniculate segments that receive an abnormal input (10* to 12*) send their axons to a separate piece of cortex, so that the approximate *order* of the normal visual field representation is recreated in the cortex (see upper row in Figure 7). Thus, some of the geniculo-cortical axons run a quite abnormal course through the visual radiation. Each hemisphere is now looking at more than one visual hemifield, since each hemisphere receives from the total contralateral hemifield and also from a portion of the ipsilateral hemifield.

Each of these two central modifications recreates a continuous, uninterrupted representation of the visual field upon the cortical surface. It would appear that the cortex is concerned with the order of the visual field representation, while the lateral geniculate nucleus is connected in terms of

16

specific retinal loci. The geniculate nucleus can accept nonsense sequences of visual field representation and unlike the cortex it is not concerned with the visual 'sense' of its inputs.

I shall not discuss the mechanisms by which the cortical modifications may be produced, or the possibilities that these abnormalities raise for further experimental studies (see GAZE & KEATING, '72; GUILLERY et al., '74). The points that link the first part of this essay to the second are: first, that even though the representation of the visual field upon the cortex may be produced, or the possibilities that these abnormalities raise for the visual pathways similar to those found in Siamese cats are very likely to occur in man. Since an abnormality has been found in albinos of eight different species (see SANDERSON et al., '74), and since there is already some evidence to suggest that visual evoked responses are abnormal in albino people (CREEL et al., '74), a systematic study of individuals who have low amounts of pigment in their retinal pigment epithelium seems justified.

There are many ways in which such individuals might be studied, since one can expect abnormalities in all parts of the post-chiasmatic visual system. Probably post-mortem specimens could be informative*, and cerebral lesions might lead to unusual defects. The visual evoked response, which is most relevant for this conference, will perhaps provide some of the best clues about the nature of the abnormality, since the geniculocortical projection and the cortical map of the retina will both be abnormal.

If the albino abnormality can be defined in man, it may throw some light on the visual defects (amblyopia and nystagmus) that commonly affect albino people. However, it is also possible that these defects are produced by different abnormalities of the visual pathways; their common occurrence in albino people will certainly make it technically difficult to undertake a systematic study of the pathway abnormality. In view of the interesting effects that the abnormality may have upon the organization of the visual cortex, and upon visual perception as well, it seems reasonable to hope that a thorough knowledge of the normal anatomy of the human visual pathways will provide a basis from which one can carry out detailed studies of the albino abnormality as the material and the techniques become available.

REFERENCES

ABBIE, A.A., The blood supply of the visual pathways. *Med. J. Aust.*, 2: *199-202*, (1938).
ALLMAN, J.M. & J.H. KAAS, Representation of the visual field in striate and adjoining cortex of the owl monkey (*Aotes trivirgatus*). *Brain Res.*, 35: *89-106*, (1971).
ALLMAN, J.M. & J.H. KAAS, The organization of the second visual area (VII) in the owl monkey: a second order transformation of the visual hemifield. *Brain Res.*, 76, *247-265* (1974).
BERESFORD, W.A. & A. NAUTA and gallocyanin study of the corticolateral geniculate projection in the cat and monkey. *J. Hirnforsch.*, 5: *210-228*, (1962).
BRODMANN, K., Vergleichende Lokalisationslehre der Grosshirnrinde in ihren Prinzipien dargestellt auf Grund des Zellenbaues. J.A. Barth, Leipzig, *1-324*, (1909).

* Such a study has now been done (GUILLERY et al., 1975) and it shows that the lateral geniculate nucleus of a human albino has the expected abnormality.

CAJAL, S. RAMON y, Histologie du Système Nerveux de l'Homme et des Vértébrés. Maloine, Paris, (1911).

CHACKO, L.W., The laminar pattern of the lateral geniculate body in the primates. *J. Neurol. Neurosurg. Psychiat.*, 11: *211-219*, (1948).

CHOW, K.L., J.S. BLUM & R.A. BLUM, Cell ratios in the thalamocortical visual system of *Macaca mulatta*. *J. Comp. Neur.*, 92: *227-239*, (1950).

CLARK,, W.E. LE GROS & G.G. PENMANN, The projection of the retina in the lateral geniculate body. *Proc. Roy. Soc. B.*, 114: *291-313*, (1934).

COLONNIER, M. & S. ROSSIGNOL, Heterogeneity of the cerebral cortex. In: H.H. JASPER, A.A. WARD and A. POPE eds., Basic mechanisms of the epilepsies, Boston Little Brown, *29-40*, (1969).

COWEY, A., Projection of the retina on to striate and prestriate cortex in the squirrel monkey *Saimiri sciureus*. *J. Neurophysiol.*, 27: *366-393*, (1964).

CRAGG, B.G. & A. AINSWORTH, The topography of the afferent projections in the circumstriate visual cortex of the monkey studied by the Nauta method. *Vision Res.*, 9: *733-744*, *(1969)*.

CREEL, D., C.J. WITKOP, & R.A. KING, Asymmetric visually evoked potentials in human albinos: evidence for visual system anomaly. *Invest. Ophthalmol.*, 13: *430-440* (1974).

DANIEL, P.M. & D. WHITTERIDGE, The representation of the visual field on the cerebral cortex in monkeys. *J. Physiol.*, 159: *203-221*, (1961).

DUKE-ELDER, S. & SCOTT, G.I., Neuro-ophthalmology. Vol. XII of System of Ophthalmology. Edited by S. DUKE ELDER. C.V. Mosby, pp. *1-994*, (1971).

EBNER, F.F. & R.E. MYERS, Contribution of corpus callosum and anterior commissure in cat and raccoon. *J. Comp. Neurol.*, 124: *353-366*, (1965).

ECONOMO, C. VON, Cytoarchitectonics of human cerebral cortex. Trans. S. Parker, Oxford University Press, (1929).

ELEKESSY, E.I., J.E. CAMPION & G.H. HENRY, Differences between the visual fields of Siamese and common cats. *Vision Res.*, 13: *2533-2547*, (1973).

FLECHSIG, P. VON, Weitere Mittheilungen über den Stabkranz des Menschlichen Gehirns. *Neurol. Centralbl.*, 15: *2-4*, (1896).

FÖRSTER, R.F., Uber Rindenblindheit, *von Graefe's Arch. Ophthalmol.*, 36: *94-108*, (1890).

GAREY, L.J., E.G. JONES & T.P.S. POWELL, Interrelationships of striate and extrastriate cortex with the primary relay sites of the visual pathway. *J. Neurol. Neurosurg. Psychiat.*, 31: *135-157*, (1968).

GAREY, L.J. & T.P.S. POWELL, The projection of the lateral geniculate nucleus upon the cortex in the cat. *Proc. Roy. Soc. B.*, 169: *107-126*, (1967).

GAZE, R.M. & M.J. KEATING, The visual system and 'neuronal specificity'. *Nature (Lond.)*, 237: *375-378*, (1972).

GIOLLI, R.A. & D.J. CREEL, The primary optic projections in pigmented and albino guinea pigs: an experimental degeneration study. *Brain Res.*, 55: *25-39*, (1973).

GLENDENNING, K.K., V. CASAGRANDE, J. HALL & W.C. HALL, An analysis of the connections of the inferior and superior divisions of the pulvinar in the bushbaby (Galago senegalensis). Proc. Soc. Neurosci., San Diego, p. 301, (1973).

GLICKSTEIN, M., R.A. KING, J. MILLER & M. BERKELEY, Cortical projections from the dorsal lateral geniculate nucleus of cats. *J. Comp. Neurol.*, 130: *55-76*, (1967).

GLICKSTEIN, M., J. MILLER, & O.A. SMITH, Lateral geniculate nucleus and cerebral cortex. Evidence for a crossed pathway. *Science*, 145: *159-161*, (1964).

GLICKSTEIN, M. & D. WHITTERIDGE, Degeneration of layer III pyramidal cells in area 18 following destruction of callosal input. *Anat. Rec.*, 178: *362-363*, (1974).

GRAYBIEL, A.M., Some fiber pathways related to the posterior thalamic region in the cat. *Brain Behav. Evol.*, 6: *363-393*, (1972).

GRAYBIEL, A.M. & W.J.H. NAUTA, Some projections of superior colliculus and visual cortex upon the posterior thalamus in the cat. *Anat. Rec.*, 169: *328*, (1971).

GUILLERY, R.W., Patterns of fiber degeneration in the dorsal lateral geniculate nucleus of the cat following lesions in the visual cortex. *J. Comp. Neurol.*, 130: *197-222*, (1967).

18

GUILLERY, R.W., An abnormal retinogeniculate projection in Siamese cats. *Brain Res.*, 14; *739-741*, (1969a).

GUILLERY, R.W., The organization of synaptic interconnections in the laminea of the dorsal lateral geniculate nucleus of the cat. *Z. Zellforsch.*, 96: *1-38*, (1969b).

GUILLERY, R.W., A quantitative study of synaptic interconnections in the dorsal lateral geniculate nucleus of the cat. *Z. Zellforsch.*, 96: *39-48*, (1969c).

GUILLERY, R.W., An abnormal retinogeniculate projection in the albino ferret. (*Mustelo furo*). *Brain Res.*, 33: *482-485*, (1971).

GUILLERY, R.W., V.A. CASAGRANDE & M.D. OBERDORFER, Congenitally abnormal vision in Siamese cats. *Nature* 252, *195-199* (1974).

GUILLERY, R.W. & M. COLONNIER, Synaptic patterns in the dorsal lateral geniculate nucleus of the monkey. *Z. Zellforsch.*, 103: *90-108*, (1970).

GUILLERY, R.W. & J.H. KAAS A study of normal and congenitally abnormal retinogeniculate projections in cats. *J. Comp. Neur.*, 143: *73-100*, (1971).

GUILLERY, R.W. & J.H. KAAS, Genetic abnormality of the visual pathways in a 'white' tiger. *Science*, 180: *1287-1289*, (1973).

GUILLERY R.W., A.N. OKORO & C.J. WITKOP. The visual pathways in the brain of a human albino. *Brain Res.* 96, *373-377* (1975).

GUILLERY, R.W., G.L. SCOTT, B.M. CATTANACH & M.S. DEOL, Genetic mechanisms determining the central visual pathways of mice. *Science*, 179: *1014-1016*, (1973).

GUILLERY, R.W., C. SITTHI-AMORN & B.B. EIGHMY, Mutants with abnormal visual pathways: an explanation of anomalous geniculate laminea. *Science*, 174: *831-832*, (1971).

HALL, W.C., J.H. KAAS, H. KILLACKEY & I.T. DIAMOND, Cortical visual areas in the grey squirrel (*Sciureus carolinensis*): a correlation between cortical evoked potential maps and architectonic subdivisions. *J. Neurophysiol.*, 34: *437-452*, (1971).

HARMS, H., Visuelle und pupillomotorische Störungen bei Veränderungen des Occipitalslappen. *Proc. 8th Internatl. Congr. Neurol.*, Vol. S. *57-78*, (1965).

HARTING, J.K., I.T. DIAMOND & W.C. HALL, Anterograde degeneration study of the cortical projections of the lateral geniculate and pulvinar nuclei in the tree shrew. *J. Comp. Neur.*, 150: *393-440*, (1973a).

HARTING, J.K., K.K. GLENDENNING, I.T. DIAMOND & W.C. HALL, Evolution of the primate visual system: Anterograde degeneration studies of the tecto-pulvinar system. *Am. J. Phys. Anthrop.*, 38: *383-392*, (1973b).

HENSCHEN, S.E. On the visual path and center. *Brain*, 16: *170-180*, (1893).

HENSCHEN, S.E., Spezielle Symptomatologie und Diagnostic der intrakraniellen Sehbahnaffectionen. In: M. LEWANDOWSKY Handbuch der Neurologie, III, 2, *751-810*, (1912).

HOLLÄNDER, H., Autoradiographic evidence for a projection from the striate cortex to the dorsal part of the lateral geniculate nucleus in the cat. *Brain Research*, 41: *464-466*, (1972).

HOLLÄNDER, H., Projections from the striate cortex to the diencephalon in the squirrel monkey (*Saimiri sciureus*). *J. Comp. Neurol.* (In Press), (1974).

HOLMES, G., The cortical localization of vision. *Brit. Med. J.* ii, *193-199*, (1919).

HUBEL, D.H. & T.N. WIESEL, Receptive fields, binocular interaction and functional architecture in the cat's visual cortex. *J. Physiol. (Lond.)*, 160: *106-154*, (1962).

HUBEL, D.H. & T.N. WIESEL, Receptive fields and functional architecture in two non-striate visual areas (18 and 19) of the cat. *J. Neurophysiol.*, 28: *229-289*, (1965).

HUBEL, D.H. & T.N. WIESEL, Cortical and callosal connections concerned with the vertical meridian of visual fields in the cat. *J. Neurophysiol.*, 30: *1561-1573*, (1967).

HUBEL, D.H. & T.N. WIESEL, Receptive fields and functional architecture of monkey striate cortex. *J. Physiol. (Lond.)*, 195: *215-244*, (1968).

HUBEL, D.H. & T.N. WIESEL, Aberrant visual projections in the Siamese cat. *J. Physiol. Lond.*, 218: *33-62*, (1971).

HUBEL, D.H. & T.N. WIESEL, Laminar and columnar distribution of geniculo-cortical fibres in the macaque monkey. *J. Comp. Neurol.*, 146: *421-450*, (1972).

HUBER, A., *Homonymous hemianopsia* after removal of one occipital lobe. Proc. 21st Internat. Cong. Ophthalmol. Mexico, March 1970 Vol. II, *1333-1343*, (1970).

INOUYE, T., Die Sehstörungen bei Schussverletzungen der corticalen Sehspäre. Leipzig. W. Engelman, pp. *1-113*, (1909).

KAAS, J.H. & R.W. GUILLERY, The transfer of abnormal visual field representations from the dorsal lateral geniculate nucleus to the visual cortex in Siamese cats. *Brain Res.*, 59: *61-95*, (1973).

KAAS, J.H., R.W. GUILLERY & J.M. ALLMAN, Some principles of organization in the dorsal lateral geniculate nucleus. *Brain Behav. Evol.*, 6: *253-299*, (1972).

KALIL, R.E., S.R. JHAVERI & W. RICHARDS, Anomalous retinal pathways in the Siamese cat. An inadequate substrate for normal binocular vision. *Science*, 174: *302-305*, (1971).

KOERNER, F. & H.L. TEUBER, Visual field defects after missile injuries to the geniculo-striate pathways in man. *Exp. Brain Res.*, 18: *88-113*, (1973).

KUPFER, C., The projection of the macula in the lateral geniculate nucleus of man. *Am. J. Ophthalmol.*, 54: *597-609*, (1962).

LUND, R.D., Uncrossed visual pathways of hooded and albino rats. *Science*, 149: *1506-1507*, (1965).

MARINO, R. & T. RASMUSSEN, Visual field changes after temporal lobectomy in man. *Neurology*, 18: *825-835*, (1968).

MATHERS, L., Tectal projection to the posterior thalamus in the squirrel monkey. *Brain Res.*, 35: *295-298*, (1971).

MATHERS, L.H., The synaptic organization of the cortical projection to the pulvinar of the squirrel monkey. *J. Comp. Neur.*, 146: *43-59*, (1972).

MYERS, R.E., Commissural connections between occipital lobes of the monkey. *J. Comp. Neurol.*, 118. *1-16*, (1962).

OTSUKA, R. & R. HASSLER, Uber Aufbau und Gliederung der corticalen Sehspäre bei der Katze. *Arch. Psychiat. Nervenkr.*, 203; *212-234*, (1962).

POLYAK, S., The vertebrate visual system, Chicago, University of Chicago Press, (1957).

ROLLS, E.T. & A. COWEY, Topography of the retina and striate cortex and its relationship to visual acuity in rhesus monkeys and squirrel monkeys. *Exp. Brain Res.*, 10: *298-310*, (1970).

ROSENQUIST, A.C. & S.B. EDWARDS, Projections of the lateral geniculate nucleus in the cat as demonstrated by autoradiography. *Anat. Rec.*, 175: *428-429*, (1973).

SANDERSON, K.J., The projection of the visual field to the lateral geniculate and medial interlaminar nuclei in the cat. *J. Comp. Neur.*, 143: *101-117*, (1971).

SANDERSON, K.J., R.W. GUILLERY & R.M. SHACKELFORD, Congenitally abnormal pathways in mink (*Mustela vision*) with reduced retinal pigment. *J. Comp. Neurol.*, 154: *225-248*, (1974).

SANDERSON, K.J. & M.S. SHERMAN, Nasotemporal overlap in the visual field projected to the lateral geniculate nucleus in the cat. *J. Neurophysiol.*, 34: *453-466*, (1971).

SHELLSHEAR, J., A contribution to our knowlegde of the arterial supply of the cerebral cortex in man. *Brain*, 50: *236-253*, (1927).

SPALDING, J.M.K., Wounds of the visual pathway. Part,I. The visual radiation. *J. Neurol. Neurosurg. Psychiat.*, 15: *99-107*, (1952a).

SPALDING, J.M.K., Wounds of the visual pathway. II the striate cortex. *J. Neurol. Neurosurg. Psychiat.*, 15: *169-181*, (1952b).

SPATZ, W.B., J. TIGGES & M. TIGGES, Subcortical projections, cortical associations, and some intrinsic interlaminar connections of the striate cortex in the squirrel monkey (*Saimiri*). *J. Comp. Neur.*, 140: *155-174*, (1970).

STEPHENS, R.B. & D.L. STILWELL, Arteries of the human brain. C.C. Thomas − Springfield, *1-181*, (1969).

STONE, J., A quantitative analysis of the distribution of ganglion cells in the cat's retina. *J. Comp. Neur.*, 124: *337-352*, (1966).

STONE, J., J. LEICESTER & S.M. SHERMAN, The naso-temporal division of the monkey's retina. *J. Comp. Neur.*, 150: *333-348*, (1973).

TEUBER, H.L., W.S. BATTERSBY & M.B. BENDER, Visual field defects after penetrating missile wounds of the brain. Cambridge, Mass. Harvard Univ. Press (1960).

THOMPSON, J.M., C.N. WOOLSEY & S.A. TALBOT, Visual areas I and II of cerebral cortex of rabbit. *J. Neurophysiol.*, 13: *277-288*, (1950).

WAGOR, E.F., & C.S. LIN, A projection from the pulvinar to the middle temporal visual area (MT) of primates. *Anat. Rec.*, 178: *483*, (1974).

WHITTERIDGE, D., Projection of optic pathways to the visual cortex. Handbook of Sensory Physiology, Springer, Berlin, Vol. VII, No. 3, *247-268*, (1973).

WILSON, M.E., Cortico-cortical connections of the cat visual areas. *J. Anat. Lond.*, 102: *375-386*, (1967).

WILSON, M.E. & B.G. CRAGG, Projections from the lateral geniculate nucleus in the cat and monkey. *J. Anat. Lond.*, 101: *677-692*, (1967).

WOOLSEY, C.N., Comparative studies of cortical representation of vision. *Vision Res. Suppl.*, 3: *365-382*, (1971).

ZEKI, S.M., Representation of central visual fields in prestriate cortex of monkey. *Brain Res.*, 14: *271-291*, (1969).

ZEKI, S.M., Interhemispheric connections of prestriate cortex in monkeys. *Brain Res.*, 19: *63-75*, (1970).

ZEKI, S.M., Colour coding in rhesus monkey prestriate cortex. *Brain Res.*, 53: *422-427*, (1973).

ZEKI, S.M., Functional organization of a visual area in the posterior bank of the superior temporal sulcus of the rhesus monkey. *J. Physiol.*, 236: *549-573*, (1974).

DATA ANALYSIS OF ELECTROPHYSIOLOGICAL SIGNALS

J. STRACKEE & L.H. VAN DER TWEEL

(Amsterdam, The Netherlands)

INTRODUCTION

The aim of this contribution is to evaluate the principles that are underlying the quantitative evaluation of, in this case electrophysiological, waveforms. Initially these waveforms have been described not so much in a quantitative way, but with regard to conspicuous patterns. The ECG is one of the most striking examples of this, but also already early in ERG research different waves were described and for the visual evoked responses this lead to the naming of a number of so-called peaks and waves. Although it may seem that in a certain sense this is a primitive way of looking at curves, the clinical success, especially in electrocardiography has been impressive. One of the reasons for this latter is due to the underlying physiological insight in the different shapes encountered. Moreover there is a reasonable independence between different parts of the ECG.

The possibility of modern analysing methods has brought about the attempt to give a quantitative description of electrophysiological curves ranging from a simple measuring of for instance peaks and throughs — we like to call this the mountaineering approach — to the sophisticated application of mathematical techniques only possible by use of a computer. It is of course impossible to go into detail in all the methods but there are a number of fundamental common aspects that will be the main subject of this paper.

DESCRIPTION OF A SIGNAL

In the following we assume in general that we already possess a signal that can be thought to be 'significant enough' i.e. the inherent noise is negligible with regard to the distinctions we want to make on the basis of this signal. This means that either the signal in itself is so large that it does not need to be averaged, or we use an averaging technique.

As already mentioned the clinician uses a highly complicated pattern criterion and beats in that, at least up till now, any computer. As soon as a quantitative statistical procedure is needed, for instance for distinction between normality and abnormality, pattern (Gestalt) as a criterion is not a feasible concept any more and choice of quantifiable aspects — called features — appears. We will elucidate some principles of quantifications on two examples: the ERG with oscillatory potentials (OP's) and the Visual Evoked Response (VER), both to a flash.

Although there are transitions between the methods which will be used for distinction, the following division is used:

23

A. pure description based on the time course of the curve. No explicit hypotheses about the genesis are introduced.

B. the curve is thought to be composed of a comparative small number of 'waves', each having a fundamental physiological meaning. For instance Granit's P1, P2 etc.

C. the curve is represented in another descriptive system i.e. mathematical functions are basically used. Examples of this are the decomposition in Gaussian curves or the often used concept of Fourier Analysis. Although the basic elements (Gaussian curves, sine waves) of the new system are in principle descriptive and do not yield more information, they can sometimes serve for a distinction in a better way than using directly the curve. It should be realised that they do not often have a physiological meaning.

We will give some further discussion of A and C only.

A.1.) Mountaineering Approach

Let us first look at Fig. 1A. This is a well known type of ERG, which the oscillatory potentials (OP's) are clearly seen. We shall direct our attention to these OP's. There have been many attempts to give a quantitative description of such ERG's on the basis of the prominent aspects. This is superficially seen the nearest to the original way of using pattern criteria, but it becomes soon apparent that certain assumptions have always to be made to give a meaning to the features measured. For instance, if as in our case the Op's are on a steep slope of a supposedly other origin, it is difficult to know how an amplitude of such an OP should be measured. Measurements have been done from a supposed zero line, i.e. before the onset of the ERG; others have tried to measure the potentials by taking the diffirence between the peaks and throughs. A first important point is that, as soon as these numbers are obtained and have to be compared with other numbers, the statistical technique will be largely influenced whether the diffirent aspects measured are strongly correlated or not.

It is clear that a number of disadvantages are inherent to this mountaineering method. First of all large deflections attract more attention than small ones, whereas it is not sure that, from the standpoint of pathology – or even normal function –, they are the most important, a problem that we shall also meet when applying Fourier methods. Secondly, as soon as curves are composed of different components, changes in the relative strength or position can deliver quite different curves in which case it is not even any longer possible to apply the measurement system originally started with, as in case of splitting of peaks, etc.

A.2.) All sample technique

It is possible to give a complete representation of curves by samples. The theorem of SHANNON indicates the minimum number of values – i.e. features – for a full description of a curve. Finer structuring of the curve – i.e. taking more samples – does not increase the information. This optimal number is determined by the highest frequency f recorded and amounts to 2f for every second of registration. To compare two sets (groups) of curves

24

techniques exists in which all the data points are used with the inherent advantage that no information is lost. A serious disadvantage is that prior knowlegde can, if at all, only very difficultly be incorporated in the method. Furthermore, the number of curves needed for a reliable statistical evaluation, if patients and normals have to be distinguished, has to be large. In practise this means that if a curve is described by 100 data points the material will have to encompass not less than about 1000 individuals.

C Fourier technique

The basis of Fourier analysis is the decomposition of curves in sine waves. For a description of a practical curve it suffices to present only a finite number of sine waves, each with its own amplitude and phase. This can be compared with the optimal number of features of above. Very often only the amplitudes are given either directly (amplitude spectrum) or as energies (power spectrum or periodogram).

The advantage of Fourier analysis is that the techniques are readily available and that it gives a principally other representation of the recorded curve. A disavantage is that it is an artificial technique which needs not be relevant for the system under study.

The relative magnitude of Fourier components within one curve must be considered carefully with regard to its physiological meaning. A component with a relatively small amplitude for instance may be a more important indicator for a certain problem than a large one. An example is given in Fig. 1b where a Fourier analysis is presented of the curve in Fig. 1a and where due to the scaling it looks as if the high frequencies are just not present! As will elaborated under the heading feature enhancement scaling problems of this kind can be overcome by removing from the signal the

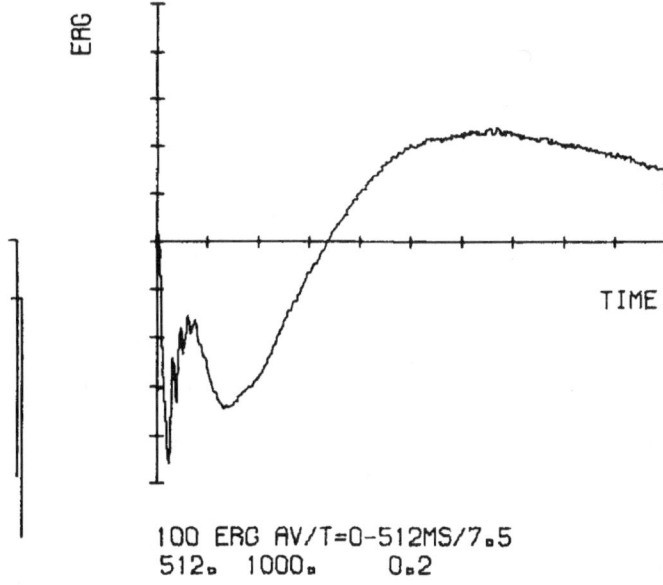

100 ERG AV/T=0-512MS/7.5
512. 1000.   0.2

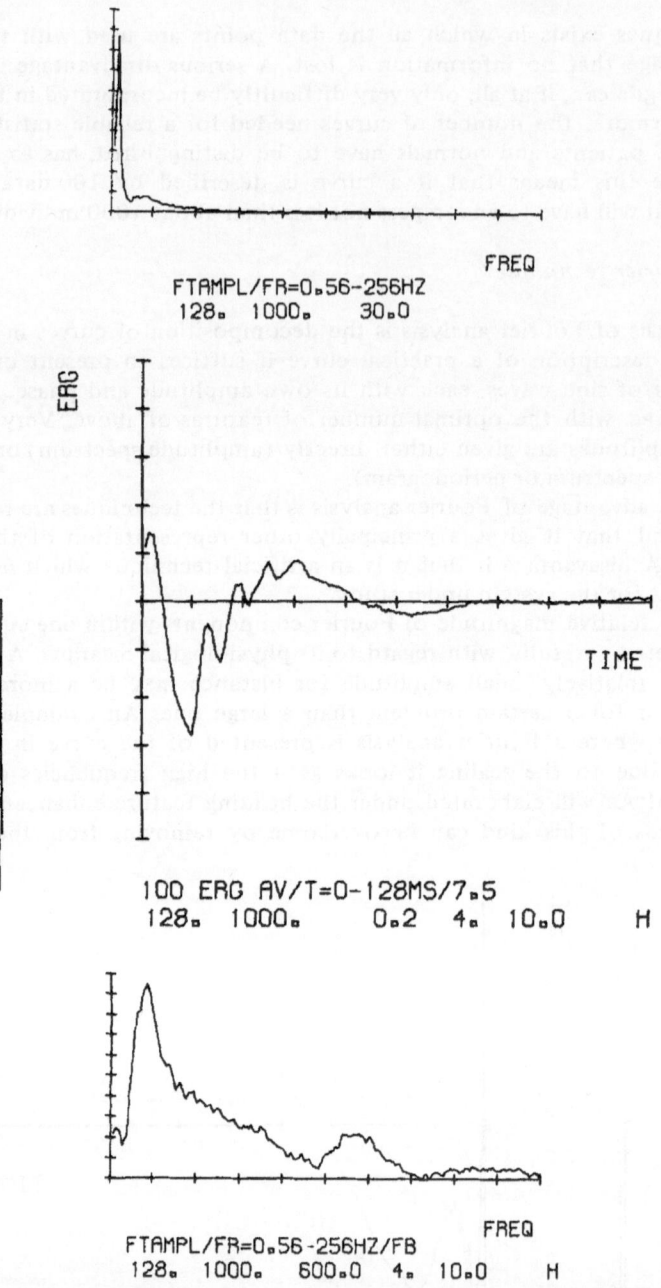

FREQ

FTAMPL/FR=0.56-256HZ
128. 1000.   30.0

ERG

TIME

100 ERG AV/T=0-128MS/7.5
128. 1000.   0.2   4.   10.0   H

FREQ

FTAMPL/FR=0.56-256HZ/FB
128. 1000.   600.0   4.   10.0   H

Fig 1. ERG recorded with a vacuum contact lens, to a Xenon flash. Distance 24 cm. Subtended angle 45°. Flash energy 40 and 80. A Broad bandrecordings of ERG; C. Low frequency cut off 10 Hz, 6 db. Note expanded time base of Fig. 1c; B and D. Fourier analysis of Fig. 1a, 1c. 128 frequency steps are presented. Because of the normalization the frequencies around 150 Hz are only visible in Fig. 1d, but they are of equal absolute magnitude in Fig. 1b.

frequencies which show up with the highest amplitudes. In Fig. 1c we have attenuated the frequencies below 10 cps. In the ensuring ERG in which the expanded time scale should be noted, the OP's become more prominent. Equivalent with that in the Fourier spectrum (Fig. 1d) at 100 cps now a peak emerges.

We would like to underline the following. The Fourier spectrum in elec-

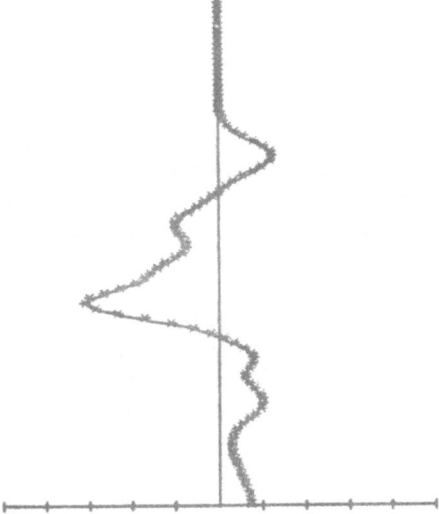

Fig 2a. VEP to a flash. Adapted and digitalized from Lehman & Fender's.

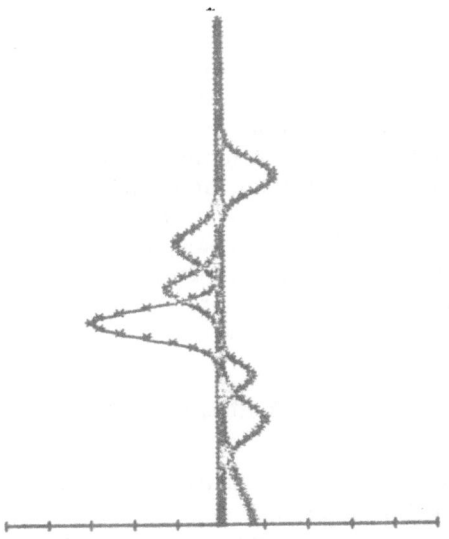

Fig. 2b. Analysis in Gaussians of the VEP of Fig. 2a. The curves are slightly different of those of Lehman & Fender due to a different procedure.

27

trophysiology is presented more and more with the energy as a normative parameter. The 'energy' is in itself a purely — and very useful — physical measure, but its relevance in electrophysiology is, to say the least, doubtful. Moreover, the presentation of the power spectrum may amplify differences in an intolerable way without being meaningful, because the signal to noise ratio is not improved by squaring.

Historically the accent on the application of Fourier techniques has been laid on the amplitude spectrum. The phase plot of the composing sine waves is rarely presented. It will be shown that the phase part can by no means always be neglected.

It should be noted that Fourier analysis in the end gives a set of numbers in the *frequency* domain which for the quantification problem is not different from the set of numbers representative for the original curve. Actually if one notices certain dominant frequencies this is just as descriptive as noticing peaks in the original curve.

Another important point, demonstrated in Fig. 1d, is the following.

The seemingly continuous curve is built up from 128 equally spaced amplitudes, linked by straight lines. As already mentioned a finite set of numbers can give an adequate description of the original data available. The presented curve suggests, however, that in practice a courser division could already be sufficient. The continuity of the curve indicates that adjacent frequencies have a high degree of dependency. The irregularities in the curve must be to a large extent considered as non-relevant noise. For a statistical evaluation this type of dependency must be carefully checked.

Gaussian technique

Literature (LEHMAN & FENDER 19   ) gives also a decomposition in Gaussian curves. We adapted the figures of LEHMAN & FENDER to our computerprograms (Fig. 2a). A decomposition, as is done by the authors, is presented in Fig. 2b. This method seems only indicated if there is enough physiological basis for the assumption of separate Gaussian processes, which then should be not too many. A definite disadvantage of this technique is that the amplitudes and widths of the composing curves are intrinsically if they overlap related. Therefore there are no simple recipies for the treatment of interdependency in this type of representation. This is contrary to Fourier analysis in which the amplitudes and phases of different frequencies are in principle independent, i.e. in practice one can remove low frequencies without affecting distant high frequencies.

ASPECT ENHANCEMENT

It is common practice to try to enhance certain aspects of a curve, which are of special interest. This applies as well to the direct curve as to i.e. Fourier representation. Sometimes this enhancement is disadvantageous to the signal to noise ratio. When, for instance, fast deflections are stressed by means of differentiation the noise contributions will generally be relatively increased.

28

Averaging

Commonly, averaging is used for overcoming noise problems such as the one mentioned above. Two different and important points regarding averaging techniques will be treated.

Amplitude stationarity

In the first place one has to make sure that the stationarity of the system is safeguarded, which may prove difficult especially in the case of VEP's The concept of stationarity is well defined for random (stochastic) signals, but not so easily for responses to stimuli. It is clear that due to, in a way external factors (fixation, attention, eye blinking etc.) subsequent responses will be different even when the inherent noise is negligible.

A basic requirement is that there must no trend with regard to the amplitude of the responses. Even if this is fulfilled and the requirement of latency constancy also holds, some remarks can be made about the quantification of the *result* of the averaging proces. The average response can be built up from totally different statistical distributions. Generally, for instance, the ERG's to the subsequent stimuli will vary much less than the corresponding VEP's. If it is wanted to distinguish between different sets of responses (normal versus abnormal, attention versus non-attention) it depends upon the specific problem set, whether the *average response* is indeed a good measure. It is easily conceived that for certain questions, for instance 'the amplification' between ERG and VEP one should aim at the highest responses that occur. Knowledge of the variability and the noise contribution will then be needed.

Latency connstancy

For any kind of averaging the constancy of latency is an absolute condition. As can be seen in figure 3, a sharp block averaged with a Gaussian spread of latencies, will be smoothed by averaging. The effect is equivalent with that of a very sharp high frequency cut-off filter. One can estimate this cut-off from the following relation:

$$A = A_0 \, e^{-\omega^2 \sigma^2/2}$$

with $\omega = 2\pi f$ and σ the standard deviation of the Gaussian distribution of the latencies. For a frequency of 100 cps this means that for σ equalling about 2 msec the amplitude of the averaged signal has dropped to $e^{-1} = 0.37$; for $2 \times 2 = 4$ msec this would already be $e^{-4} = 0.02$! In VEP's latencies of 40 msec and more are present; therefore inconstancies of the order of 2 msec are by no means impossible and great caution should be exerted in the study of high frequency aspects by means of averaging. Other methods can then be more favourable. For instance the summation of the Fourier amplitude spectra of separate responses, would eliminate latency effects.

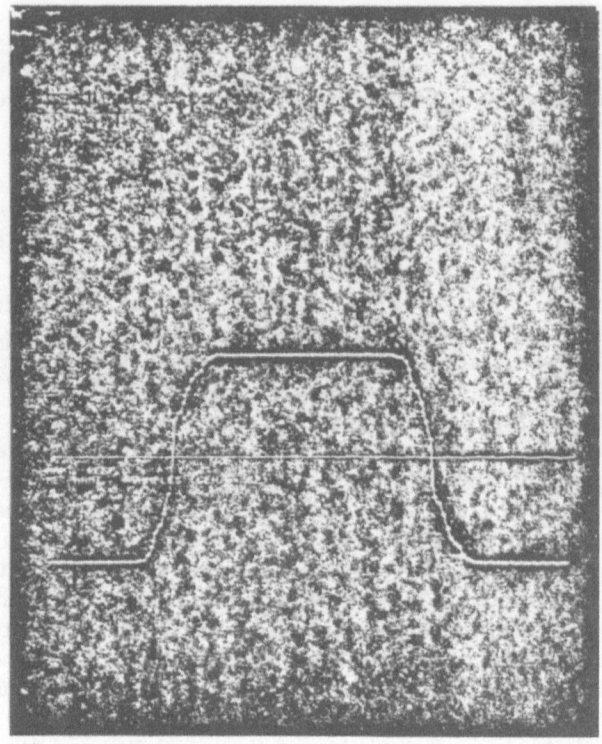

Fig. 3. Smoothing of a sharp block by averaging with a variable delay with a σ of 3 msec. Number of sweeps.

OSCILLATORY POTENTIALS (OP'S)

For ERG purposes it is important to quantify the OP's and to represent them in such a way that already inspection gives reliable information. An established procedure for OP's is electronic filtering in which high frequencies are passed through and low frequencies are relatively attenuated. Filtering, however, will in general change the phase relations of the constituent frequencies (Fourier components). This implies a.o. that the wavelets in the filterrecord may be considerably displaced in time, as can be seen in Fig. 4. Fig. 4a is the 4 times expanded curve of Fig. 1a, the undistorted ERG to a strong flash; Fig. 4b represents the same curve filtered with a simple 10 Hz-3db filter, which does not appreciably affect the OP part. Fig. 4c gives the result when the filtering is performed by conventional techniques in which low frequencies have been attenuated strongly (80 Hz, 24 db/oct). The representation is markedly improved, but it is evident that the first peak (arrow in Fig. 4b) is displaced by ms (arrow in Fig. 4c).

This means that if one compares latencies in different studies full knowledge of the applied filter techniques should be available. Also the apparent latencies will be influenced by the time course of the OP's themselves.

30

Moreover, there are deflections — at the onset of the curve — which are instrumental artefacts. This can be seen from fig. 4d where a technically, correct procedure has been applied. In fact the signal was normally filtered with a 12 db (80 Hz) filter and afterwards the result was time reversed and again filtered in the same manner. In this way the amplitudes in the Fourier representation are identical with those of Fig. 4c, but the unavoidable phase shift in conventional filtering is absent and therefore the peak of the OP's are appearing at their proper times. Whereas these curves were obtained by computer processing, the 'trick' would also be possible with analog tape.

STATISTICAL APPROACHES

In general one should distinguish between descriptive and inference procedures. To the first belong the presentation of the material with help of for instance mean and standard deviation. Depending on the material itself other statistics may be more indicated or even better: percentiles, median (= 50% percentile), range etc.

Inference procedures use the same data but try to draw conclusions from it; for instance comparing different material. Although one often uses this

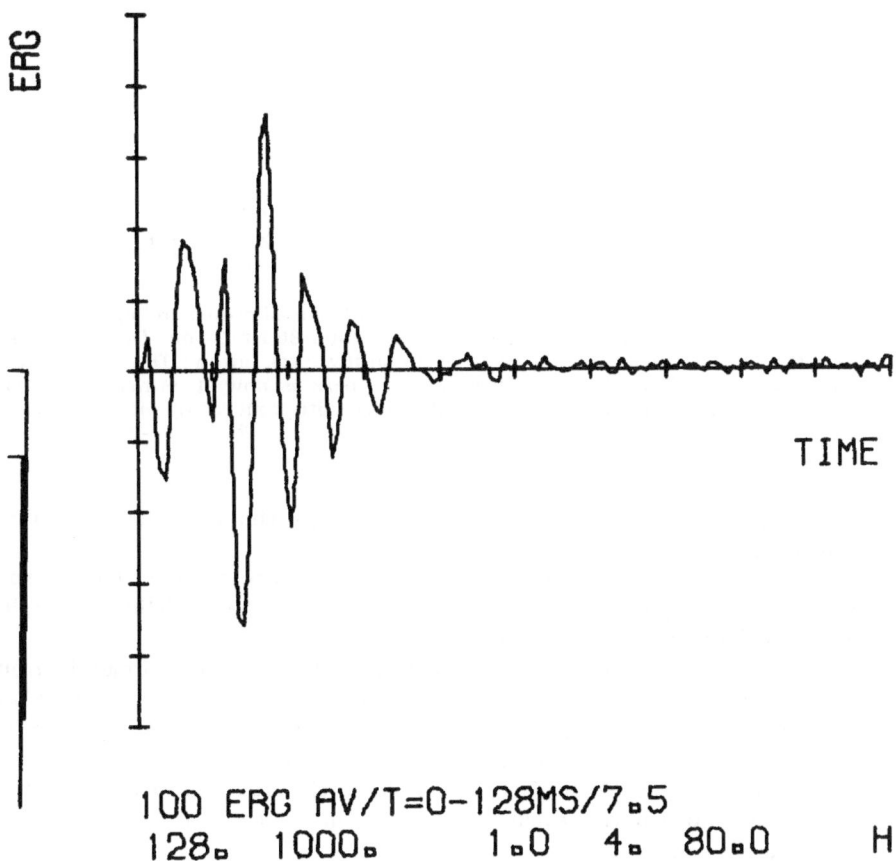

100 ERG AV/T=0-128MS/7.5
128. 1000.   1.0   4.   80.0   H

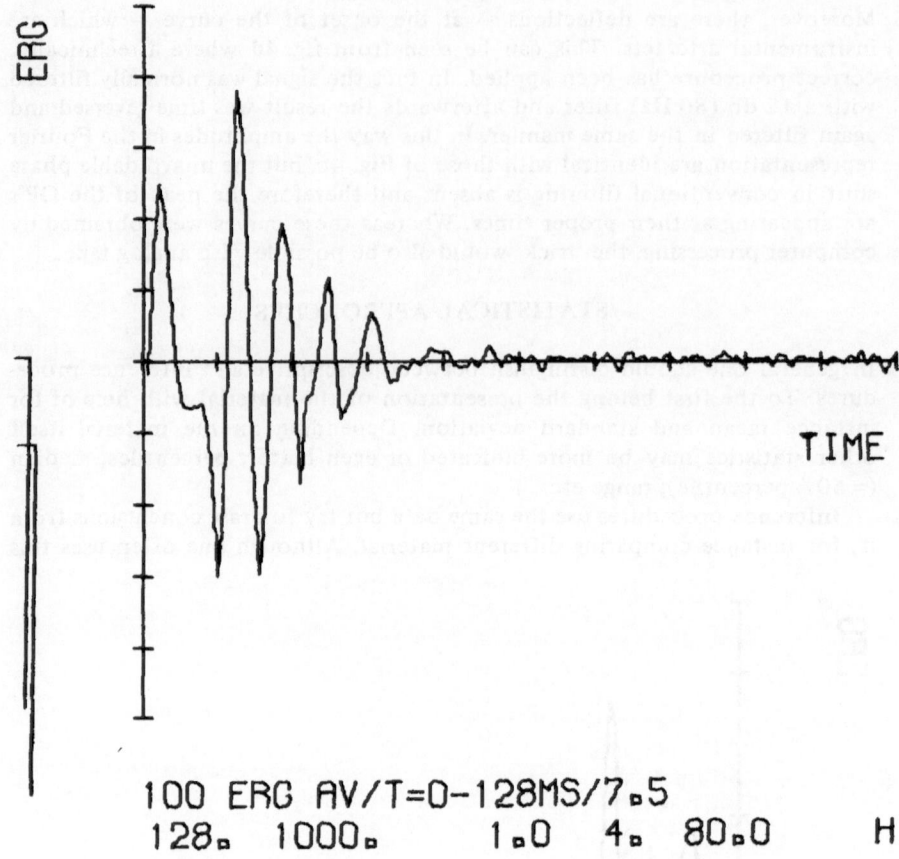

ERG

TIME

100 ERG AV/T=0-128MS/7.5
128. 1000.   1.0   4. 80.0   H

Fig. 4   Filtering of VP's. A. The original ERG with broad bandrecording; B. Filtering
with 10 Hz, 6 db; C. Filtering with conventional filter 80 Hz, 24 db. The VP's emerge
sharply. Note the time shift in the first sharp positive peak (arrow). D. Filtering with a
phase true procedure. The first sharp positive peak is now at its right place. The
excursions at the start in Fig. 4b due to the phase shift produced by the filter are now
absent.

the descriptive statistics, this is not necessary! The procedures are then
called parameter free.

For the present paper we will restrict ourselves to some problems, especially concerning electrophysiological signals. For the statistical principles
involved, we refer to standard literature.

For the type of signals we are treating at this moment normal distributions of the chosen features may be assumed. We first consider the problem
that one has acquired a homogeneous material. Two examples: a number of
responses in a supposedly identical situation of one subject or the responses
of supposedly identical subjects in also identical situations. This ideal situation is of course never reached, but it is conceived that the deviations are
purely due to chance.

32

Generally a value measured from a subject is considered to be indicative of abnormality if it belongs to a so called critical region. Such a region — or regions — consists of the extreme values of the distribution. For example in a normal distribution the probability of finding a value in the critical region indicated by the lower boundary $\mu+1.965$ is 2½%. It is selfevident that also a second critical region at the 2½% level exists ($\mu-1.965$).We will leave out the rather complicated problem how to assess the meaning of one or two sided critical regions and also the medical decision whether an improbable high value will be considered differently regarding its pathological aspects than a low one. We stress the fact that lying outside a boundary does not imply that the value is abnormal. For 5% regions, often used, every 20th normal will be on the average classified as 'abnormal'. For large deviations from the mean the assumption of normality of the distribution is seldom warranted. A blood pressure of zero will not occur in any normal subject!

We now consider the case that more than one feature is measured in each subject and we assume first that the features are statistically independent. Naïve statistics lead to the following reasoning. As each feature still has a probability of 5% to belong to its critical region the chance of indicating 1 feature out of N features as abnormal will be $1\text{-}(1\text{-}0.05)^N$. For 10 features this already means 40%! If one still wants to test the whole complex of features on a 5% level, each feature should then be checked against increased boundaries of $\mu \pm 2.85\sigma$. This is equivalent to a 0.5% level, if only that one feature should have been measured. One feels that here indeed rises a problem. Suppose we find an ERG feature of a certain subject beyond the chosen boundary, including the feature lenght could bring it into the range of normality. This looks must unwanted and even foolish. On the other hand if for instance the blood pressure was included it would be not so far sought to accept such contributi to our final dicision. A more sophisticated approach than that lead to the 2.85σ boundary, will be demonstrated for the case of two features. For instance one could think of the amplitudes of the a and b waves in the ERG of a normal population. Suppose the a-wave has a mean of $100\ \mu V$ and a standard deviation of $10\ \mu V$; for the b-wave the mean is thought to be $200\ \mu V$ with a standard deviation of $40\ \mu V$. The first thing that should be done is to normalize the measured values; subtraction of the mean, followed by division through the standard deviation. Every point in the plane of Fig. 5 now represents the outcome of one experiment. Point A means that the measurement had for the a-wave resulted in $100-0.8\times10 = 92\ \mu V$ and for the b-wave $200+1.2\times40 = 248\ \mu V$. The question is now whether a new measurement should be considered as belonging to this population. For one feature only the boundaries for two sided regions at the 5% level are indicated by arrows. The naïve statistics would produce the square in the figure.

A better approach using the two dimensional normal distribution would lead to the circle in case of complete independency of the feature.

The critical region is now the whole domain outside the circle. These remains a kind of ambiguity. The circle and the square cut the axis beyond the one dimensional boundary, and the circle lies outside the square on the axis. In terms of sensitivity the test is at this side less sensitive, which is reversal near the 45° positions.

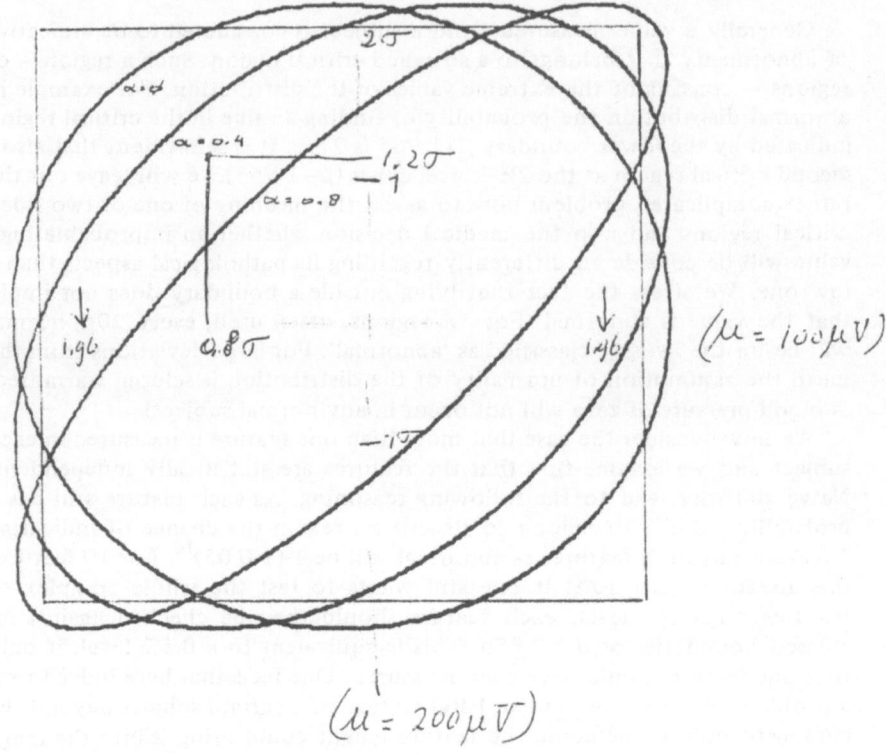

Fig. 5. Two dimensional statistics. The arrows point to 1,96σ the boundary for a 2½% one sided critical region. The square indicates the result of noise independent judgement. The circle is a better approach in case of independency. The ellipses are to be used if correlates between two features exist of resp. 0.8 and 0.6.

If now the two sets of data (the a- and b-waves) have a certain dependency, i.e. are correlated, the situation changes. Such dependency can be the result of rather trivial causes. A- and b-waves can be influenced identical by the size of the eyeball. This dependency is generally expressed by a correlation coefficient ranging from −1 to +1. A O-value means no dependency at all; +1 or −1 gives an absolute dependency; i.e. only one of the features would be sufficient to describe the material. In the case a correlation of +1 (or −1) the circle will shrink to a straight line! In our case a 45° line through the origin.

Such a strict relation between two physiological quantities are very rare and therefore the boundaries will be elipses as also shown in the figure. To show how complicated even with these simple assumptions, the practice of using multidimensional statistics is, we will consider the same point A as discussed before, with regard to an ellipse with a correlated coefficient of 0.6 between the two features. This point lies well within any test for normality for each feature independently. Only if we take the relation between the two variables into account one has te conclude to abnormality! If we take a simple example and suppose that the teo axis represent length and

34

weight which in reality show a correlation of 0.5 the conclusion will be that it deserves attention if a certain subject would be situated in point A. In this case that means he would be too heavy in relation to his length, which sounds like reasonable practice.

Actually electroretinographers have felt also this problem and therefore introduced measures like the a to b ratio or, as Karpe once proposed, physiological calibration. Especially for lange correlation coefficients ($\rho = 0.7$) we should evaluate the implication of the chosen statistical approach. As can be easily understood the rest domain approaches a straight line and very careful analysis of the whole experimental procedure should be performed. This necessity diminishes with decreasing correlation coefficient.

MACULAR ELECTRO-OCULOGRAPHY

J.C. HACHE, P. FRANCOIS & P. GOEMINNE

(Lille, France)

The EOG is a very interesting complementary method of the ERG but it has a too global viewing. As others did (namely HOCHGESAND et al.) we have tried to realize a more specific technique for a better study of the function of the macular area.

THEORETICAL CONSIDERATIONS

The variations of potential on the electrodes placed at lateral and medial canthus are related to the movement of electrical charges during ocular movements.

Our work is based on this hypothesis: the density of the electrical charges is proportional to the cellular density at the junction retina-pigmentary epithelium. We suppose that the distribution of the charges is realized as is shown on the first figure.

Thus, the density of the charges in the macular area is much greater than in the periphery. The density of the peripheral charges decreases slightly and progressively from the center to the ora serrata. Therefore, during large ocular movements, the potential variations depend on the displacement of the macular charges and above all on the displacement of the peripheric charges.

Moreover, at the occasion of the report of the latest Belgian Society, FRANCOIS, de ROUCK & GAMBIE have remarked on the correlation between the EOG alterations and the ERG scotopic alterations.

On the other hand during very small ocular movements, we notice that the electrical charges displacement in the orbita is above all due to macula. At one point of the orbita, the variation of the charge density due to peripheral retina is very small because the variation of the cellular density at this point is very small. On the back pole, with an ocular rotation of five degrees from the macula, the cellular density is divided by twenty, and a small eye rotation causes a very marked displacement of the charges.

METHOD OF EXAMINATION

Our method is based on this hypothesis:
We request from the patient eye movements of ten degrees (five degrees on each side). This can be achieved by means of two little red lights which are

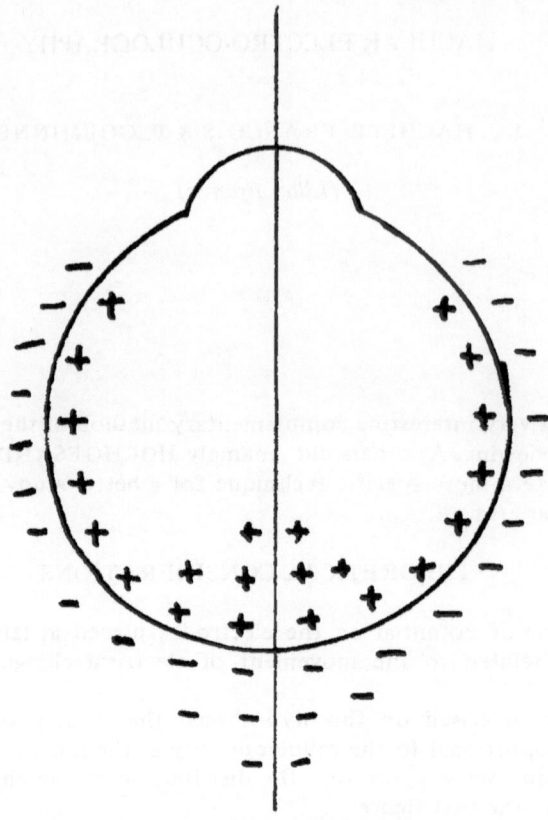

Fig. 1. Distribution of the charges.

switched on alternatively, as with the classical method, or in our automatic perimeter where the light spot is directed onto one point of the cupola under control of the computer. The examination protocole is the usual one: twelve minutes in darkness and twelve minutes in light. And we compute the ratio L/D of ARDEN. (figure 2)

However we have tried to improve the specification of the technic in making a red light background (λ six hundred and fifty nanometers). This will enable interesting correlations with the photopic components of the ERG obtained with a monochromatic red light (SOLE & ALFIERI).

The use of small eye movements has some disadvantages which reduce the signal/noise ratio.
1) The potentials are five or six times smaller than for the global EOG;
2) The errors of fixation of the lights are proportionately greater than for the usual EOG; 3) These errors are increased in case of wide central scotoma.

However we have verified that the responses are satisfactory if the angle of the movement is larger than the size of the scotoma.

We have to improve the signal/noise ratio. Thus we compute the average of ten successive movements and we do not take the first movements into consideration (as HENKES, VAN LITH et al. did).

This average is computed in real time by our computer PDP12 but the use of other methods to improve the S/N ratio is possible (for example GALLOWAY's method).

With normal patients we get the following results:

WHITE LIGHT BACKGROUND

	average	standard deviation
light	335 microvolts	43 microvolts
darkness	183 —	21 —
ratio	1.84	0.14

RED LIGHT BACKGROUND

light	305 microvolts	37 microvolts
darkness	183 —	21 —
ratio	1.56	0.11

We see that the photopic potentials obtained with a red illumination (1000 lux on the cornea) are somewhat smaller, and the ratio is also smaller, but now we use only this technic because it seems to be the best one for the pathologic applications.

PATHOLOGIC APPLICATIONS

We have studied 50 macular EOG's in pathologic cases. In these cases, we have compared macular EOG with standard EOG. When the standard EOG is altered by extensive damage of the retina and pigmentary epithelium, the macular EOG is also altered.

But the cases for which the standard EOG was inside normal limits and the macular EOG was altered are the most interesting.

We have studied four cases of fundus flavimaculatus or STARGARDT disease: the standard EOG is reduced: between 158 and 190; the macular EOG is altered.

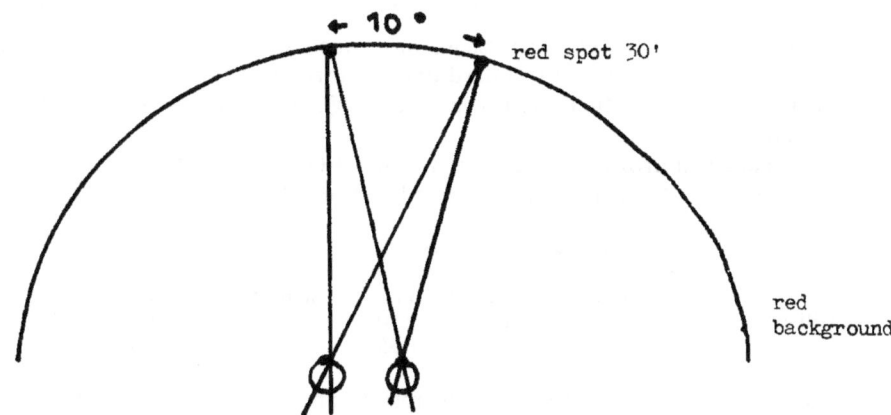

Fig. 2. Perimeter for the macular EOG.

	STANDARD EOG			MACULAR EOG		
	scotopic microvolts	*photopic* microv.	*ratio*	*scotopic* microvolts	*photopic* microv.	*ratio*
N° 1	635	1150	1.81	222	270	1.26
	710	1250	1.76	273	337	1.23
N° 2	640	1088	1.71	264	292	1.07
	590	975	1.65	244	271	1.08
N° 3	630	1150	1.83	154	201	1.30
	680	1290	1.90	216	270	1.39
N° 4	470	818	1.74	108	143	1.31
	420	665	1.58	112	108	0.97

In colloïd degeneration, the standard EOG is often normal. The macular EOG is altered (two cases), whereas the visual acuity is normal.

	STANDARD EOG			MACULAR EOG		
	scotopic	*photopic*	*ratio*	*scotopic*	*photopic*	*ratio*
N° 1 M. Suzanne	920	1650	1.79	140	178	1.27
	890	1570	1.76	158	194	1.24
N° 2 S. Marcel	877	1710	1.95	165	257	1.56
	867	1820	2.10	214	330	1.54

In vitelliform degenerations, the standard EOG is sometimes normal. We have one case with normal standard EOG, but macular EOG is abnormal (N° 1)

	STANDARD EOG			MACULAR EOG		
	scotopic	*photopic*	*ratio*	*scotopic*	*photopic*	*ratio*
N° 1 M. Anna	800	1600	2	130	170	1.31
	450	1000	2.2	140	190	1.36
N° 2 T. Maria	710	1320	1.86	145	166	1.14
	695	1270	1.83	131	138	1.06
N° 3 T. Fovianno	240	310	1.29	112	143	1.27
	230	290	1.26	110	132	1.20

In cases of unaffected carriers, we have one case (T. Maria, N° 2): it is a ten years old girl. Here the standard EOG is normal and the macular EOG is abnormal. For her father (T. Fovianno, N° 3), standard and macular EOG are altered.

In macular choroïditis, only the macular EOG can be altered, for example this case of a former unilateral macular choroïditis (left eye):

	STANDARD EOG			MACULAR EOG		
	scotopic	*photopic*	*ratio*	*scotopic*	*photopic*	*ratio*
G. Gilbert	870	1810	2.10	160	260	1.62
	846	1650	1.95	140	180	1.28

In cases of macular oedema the results are very interesting. We have found mainly low potentials and also low ratio in several cases. The best example is this case of traumatic retino-epitheliopathy (left eye):

	STANDARD EOG			MACULAR EOG		
	scotopic	*photopic*	*ratio*	*scotopic*	*photopic*	*ratio*
J. Claude	730	1365	1.87	233	415	1.79
	585	1170	2.00	208	313	1.49

We have also studied senile macular degeneration. Here the results are very variable.

In the same way we have no sufficient results in chloroquin retinopathy but it seems that it is perhaps a good method with ERG and static perimetry.

In conclusion, we think that with small movements, macular EOG is more specific than the standard EOG in macular alteration, but it is necessary to get many pathologic cases for a clinical evaluation of its utility.

Clinique Ophtalmologique et
Laboratoire de Biophysique
Unité d'Enseignement et de Recherche N° 3
Place de Verdun 59000 LILLE FRANCE

THE EXAMINATION OF THE FOVEOLAR AND PERIFOVEOLAR FUNCTION WITH THE AID OF FLICKER FUSION THRESHOLDS AND FLICKER ERG RESPONSES

J.J. MEYER*, S. KOROL**, G. OWENS**,
R. GRAMONI* & P. REY*
(Geneva Switzerland)

INTRODUCTION

The difficulty of evaluating small visual field losses is an important problem in ophthalmology BABEL et al. (1969) have proposed the use of flicker fusion thresholds, as plotted by DE LANGE, for detection and quantification of macular and perimacular visual field losses. The conclusion was that two thresholds only may express in central fixation the gravity and extension of a macular visual field loss. In every case examined, this method showed a greater sensitivity, than VA and kinetic perimetry. To evaluate the importance of a visual field loss, as well to determine its retinal or retrobulbar origin, the ophthalmologist has to compare perceptual responses with objective ones such as ERG and VER, each being obtained under different conditions of stimulation and apparently not suited to give information on the same retinal mechanisms.

In a previous paper (MEYER et al, 1974), we described different methods to facilitate the comparison of photopic averaged flicker ERG responses with subjective thresholds. The ERG were obtained with conventional clinical equipment after light preadaption and in the presence of different background illuminations. For the subjective thresholds we measured the minimum depth of modulation required to detect flicker at different frequencies of an intermittent light presented on a $1°$ test area surrounded by a steady light background (De Lange curves).

The results obtained from a set of normal subjects and pathological cases confirm the general validity of the De Lange model and suggest a good diagnostic device for clinical application. The study of cases with macular and perimacular chorioretinal degenerations shows that when the high and low frequency values of an attenuation curve are established, a comparison between subjective and objective responses becomes possible. We were unsure of the specificity of this method for chorioretinal lesions of less than $10°$.

The aim of this work was to test the method by considering both objective and subjective responses of subjects with foveolar and perifoveolar lesions. After a set of normal cases we have considered five other groups:
1. typical foveolar cases; 2. typical diffuse chorioretinal perifoveolar cases; 3. healed central serous chorioretinitis; 4. quinoline derivative retinal toxicity, 5. ethambutol retinal toxicity.

*   Institut de médecine sociale et préventive (Dir.: Prof. O. JEANNERET)
**   Clinique universitaire d'ophtalmologie (Dir.: Prof. J. BABEL)

Group 1. includes a case of acute foveolar sunburn of 1°;

Group 2. represents cases well known to have a pathological ERG;

Group 3. represents foveolar dysfunctions difficult to quantitate, but known to be present after partial or total recuperation;

Groups 4 and 5 contain cases known to have foveolar and perifoveolar dysfunctions, but difficult to quantitate with ERG.

MATERIAL AND METHODS

a. De Lange curves (psychophysical thresholds)

An intermittent test object of 1° visual angle on an illuminated background was the stimulus. The adaptation level of the undilated eye was kept constant by the background illumination at a distance of 50 cm. The light source was a modified TV tube which produced a sinusoïdal light, the modulation depth of which could be varied from 0 to 100% (DENIER VAN DER GON et al. 1958) and frequency from 1 to 100 Hz.

Fusion thresholds were determined by a successive approximation method (REY & REY, 1964), expressed as modulation percent and plotted versus frequency on a double log scale.

All the subjects were examined in a reference condition in which the brightness of the stimulus and background were equal to 170 cd/m^2 (= 100%).

b. Flicker ERG attenuation curves

The light source was a Van Gogh photostimulator presented on an indirectly illuminated wall 60 cm in front of the subject.

The pupil was dilated with Mydriaticum Roche (1%) and a scleral contact lens was used for electrical pick up. After light preadaptation (300 lux) for 3 min., the flicker ERG was recorded for five frequencies from 2 Hz to 64 Hz, with or without a background light (100 lux).

The ERG responses were amplified with an AC Tektronix preamplifier type FM 122, with low and high frequency cut-offs at 0,8 and 250 Hz and displayed on a dual beam Tektronix oscilloscope type A 502. A Biomac 1000 (Data laboratories) averaged 64 responses.

The ERGs were transformed into digital values for Fourier analysis. The different b-wave amplitudes and the Fourier components computed values were plotted as arbitrary values versus frequency on a double log scale, according to linear system analysis methods.

The examined eyes were:
- 11 normal eyes (persons aged 21 to 40),
- 5 eyes with foveolar (MA) diseases (persons aged 30 to 56),
- 8 eyes with diffuse chorioretinal degeneration (Re) (persons aged 14 to 54),
- 7 eyes with healed central serous chorioretinitis (CSC) (persons aged 34 to 62),
- 8 eyes in patients treated with ethambutol (My) (persons aged 30 to 59),

— 11 eyes in patients treated with quinoline derivatives (Qu) (persons aged 25 to 71).

The following examinations were made in one session:

1. Before eye dilatation and after 5 min light preadaptation, the CFF and the modulation % of seven frequencies of sinusoïdal modulated light were determined;

2. After eye dilatation the averaged ERG was recorded in the following conditions: a white light stimulus of 2 Hz, Van Gogh intensity 3 without background illumination ($WI_1 B_1$ condition).

A red light stimulus of 2 Hz, Van Gogh intensity 4 without background illumination ($RI_2 B_1$ condition).

A white light stimulus of 2, 12, 22, 44, 64 Hz, Van Gogh intensity 3 with background illumination ($WI_1 B_2$ condition).

RESULTS

A. Description of individual cases

1. *Objective responses in four different conditions* (Fig. 1)

— Most of pathological cases lie outside the reference zone which has a maximum of extension in condition 2 Hz, $WI_1 B_1$, and a minimum in the condition 44 Hz, $WI_1 B_2$.

— In the case of equal left and right eye impairment from medication toxicity, the corresponding ERGs are similar. In contrast, when one eye is more affected than the other eye (central serous chorioretinitis), the corresponding ERG is usually different.

— When the retinal intoxication continues, the ERGs are reduced ($m_1 a$, $m_1 b$, and $m_2 a$, $m_2 b$ curves corresponding to examinations made in an interval of one month).

— All different pathological ERGs seemed to be situated between two typical curves: one being a typical foveolar disease (Ma), foveolar sunburn lesion of $1°$, and the other a tapetoretinal degeneration (ta). In the former, we can observe at low frequency an enhanced b-wave amplitude. In the latter, at low and high frequencies there is reduced b-wave amplitude.

- Further, when one considers the relation between 2 Hz and 44 Hz responses, we can classify the ERG as follows:

Type	Low frequency	High frequency
1	Hypernormal response, a little delayed	Normal response
1'	Hypernormal response, a little delayed	Hypernormal response
2	Depressed response, much delayed	Depressed response
2'	Hypernormal response	Depressed response
3	Normal or depressed and much delayed response	Slightly diminished

45

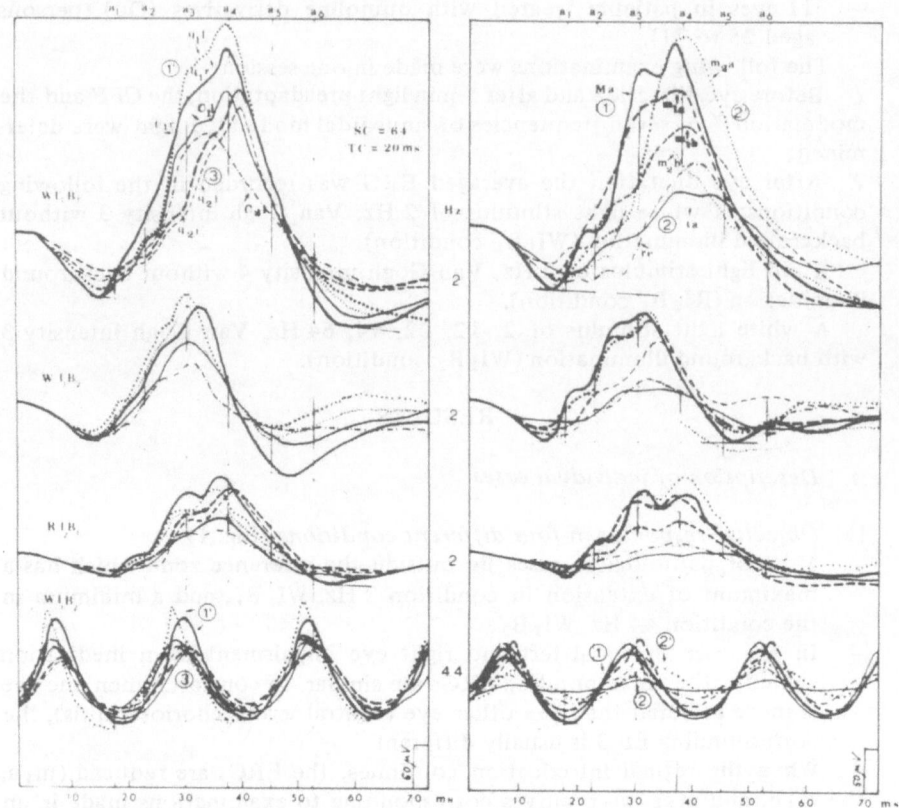

Fig. 1. Averaged flicker ERGs recorded in different stimulation conditions for some individual cases.
$WI_1 B_1$: white light, Van Gogh photostimulator intensity 3 without background light
$WI_1 B_2$: white light, photostimulator intensity 3 with background light (100 lux)
$RI_2 B_1$: red light, Wratten kodak no 26, photostimulator intensity 4 without background light
Shaded area: reference zone for normal values: left: q_1 and q_2: two different cases of quinoline derivatives intoxication l − left eye, r − right eye; c_1 and c_2: two different cases of healed central serous chorioretinitis l − left eye, r − right eye; right Ma: foveolar sunburn; m_1 and m_2: ethambutol intoxication a- and b- different examinations of the same subject (b- one month after a-); ta: tapetoretinal degeneration; re: central serous retinopathy; Numbers refer to different ERG types (see text); Abscissa: time in milliseconds (ms); Ordinate: frequencies in Hz.

— In the case of the pathologically enhanced response to low frequency, we observed, generally, an increase of the oscillatory potentials with the red stimulus condition.

2. *Corresponding De Lange curves of the same cases* (Fig. 2)
— the different ERGs also gave different curve types overrunning the reference zone.
— Fig. 2 shows five different curve types which can be grouped in three

types, when one considers only the relation between low and high frequency thresholds:

a. low frequency thresholds more depressed than high frequency ones (type 1, case Ma; type 1′, case C_1 r).

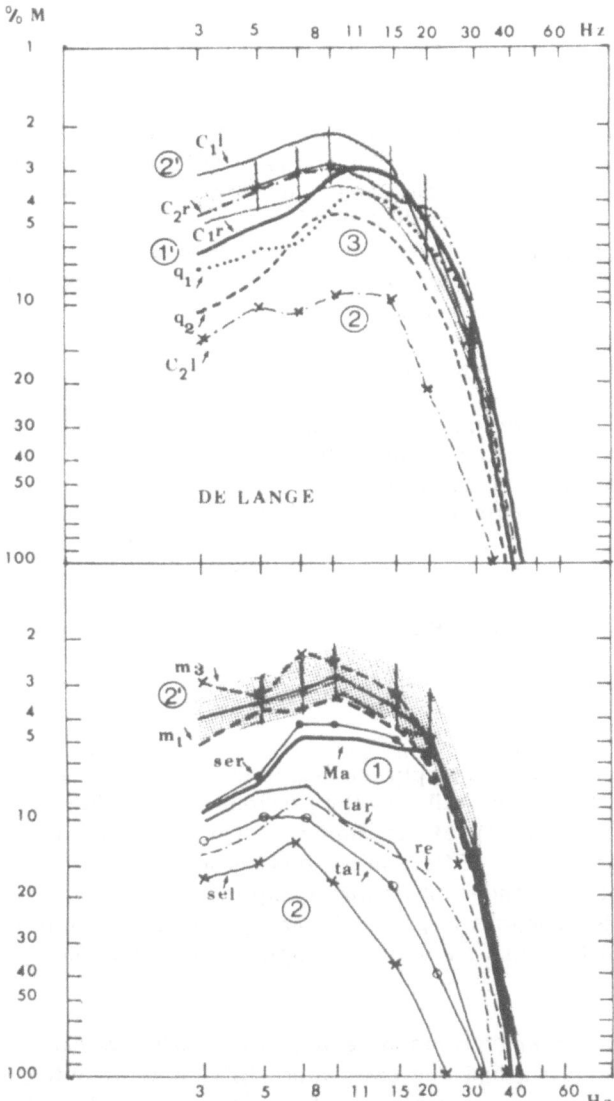

Fig. 2. De Lange curves established in normal and pathological cases. Individual curves correspond to the ERG represented in Fig. 1; se: chronic central serous chorioretinitis; re: retinoschisis; ta: tapetoretinal degeneration; (for other symbols, see Fig. 1); Shaded area: mean and standard deviation of 11 normal eyes; Abscissa: frequencies in Hz, log scale; Ordinate: modulation amplitude in %, log scale.

b. low frequency thresholds less depressed than high frequency ones (type 2, cases $C_2 1$, sel, tal, tar; type 2', case m_3).
c. Low frequency and high frequency thresholds depressed in the same proportion (type 3, case q_2).

COMMENT

These objective and subjective individual case results suggest a characteristic relation between ERG and De Lange curves.

In order to quantify the ERG morphological changes, we have applied our flicker ERG analysis method to the different groups. The method has been previously described (MEYER et al., 1974) and a summary of the main points is as follows: for De Lange data, one measures only thresholds; but in the case of the flicker ERG, one has to take in account both amplitude and latency changes as there is no simple phase-amplitude relation. One has to devise a system for quantifying the ERG morphological changes. This consists of two complementary methods:

a. *Amplitude measurement*: from a base line joining negative peaks one measures the maximum amplitude of the b-wave, as well as amplitudes for different latencies.

b. *Fourier analysis method*: for frequencies equal and higher to 12 Hz, one observes the attenuation of the computed first harmonic component, and changes in the behavior of other harmonics corresponding to different high frequency components of the 12 Hz ERG. The results are plotted on a double log scale to make a direct comparison with De Lange thresholds. We have shown that the maximum amplitude of the b-wave and the first harmonic of the ERG are similarly attenuated. One can obtain a more detailed analysis by considering other amplitudes and Fourier components.

B. *Quantitative results of the different groups*

1. *Analysis of objective responses*
With maximum b-wave amplitude measurement (Fig. 3), Ma is similar to Qu, My to Re, CSC is dissimilar to the previous groups. With the first harmonic measurement (Fig. 4), Ma is similar to Qu; the similarity is less evident between Re and My; CSC is similar to My group.

If other amplitudes or Fourier components are considered (Figs. 3, 4) group Qu is analogous to group Ma, and group My to group Re. The group CSC would look like Ma with the amplitude method, and like My with the Fourier method.

2. *Analysis of the corresponding subjective results (De Lange curves)*
For group Ma we had one case whose ERG is represented in Fig. 1. For group Qu we have represented the four cases examined. In the other groups the results are too heterogenous, and we have represented these cases as subgroups. Fig. 5 shows a similarity of group Qu with our typical foveolar case. Group My can be compared to group Re; both groups contain normal and subnormal curves characterised by the low and high frequency relation. Group CSC is composed of mixed types, somes curves are of foveolar type,

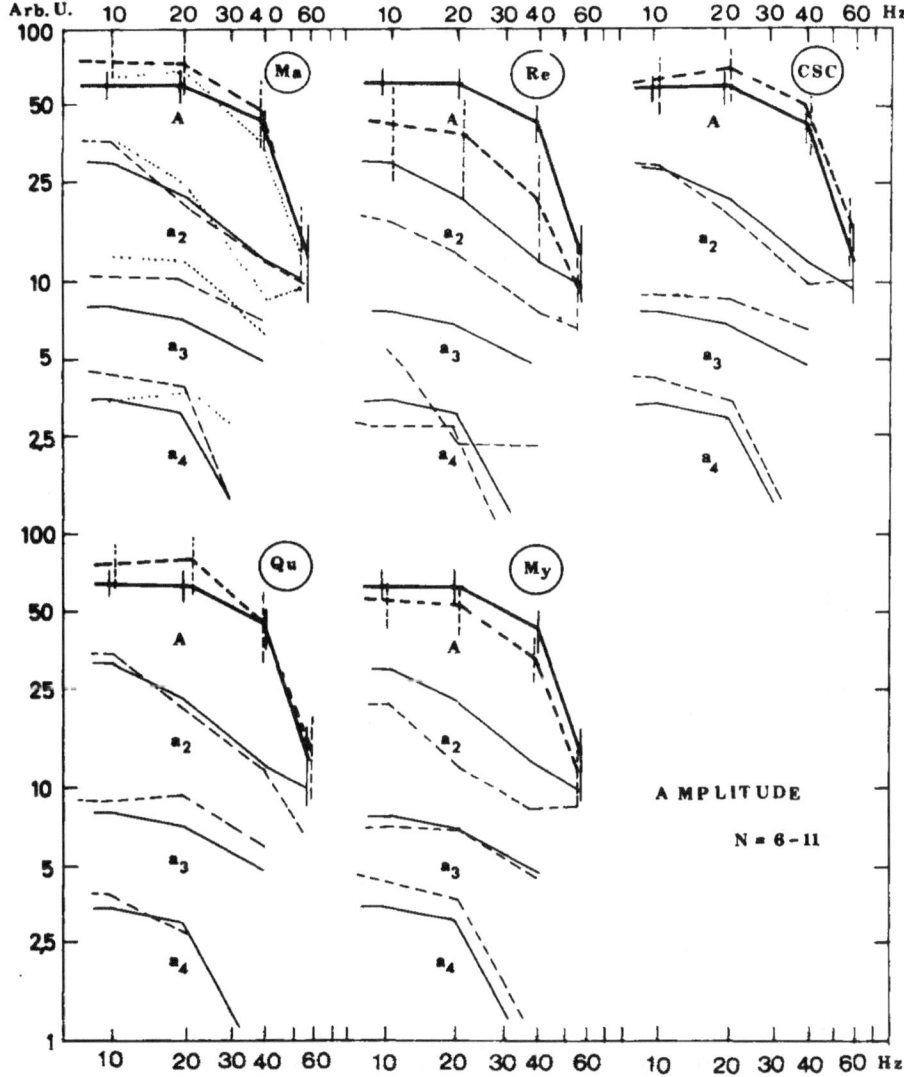

Fig. 3. Flicker ERG attenuation curves; b-wave amplitude method. A: maximum amplitude; a_2: amplitude at 22.5 ms; a_3: amplitude at 33.0 ms; a_4: amplitude at 37.5 ms; Ma: foveolar cases; Re: diffuse chorioretinal degeneration and other peri-foveal cases; CSC: healed central serous chorioretinitis; Qu: quinoline derivative treated patients; My: ethambutol treated patients; Continuous curves: normal values; broken curves: pathological cases; dotted curves: case with foveolar sunburn; vertical lines: standard deviation; N: number of examined eyes; Abscissa: frequencies in Hz; Ordinate: amplitudes in arbitrary units.

49

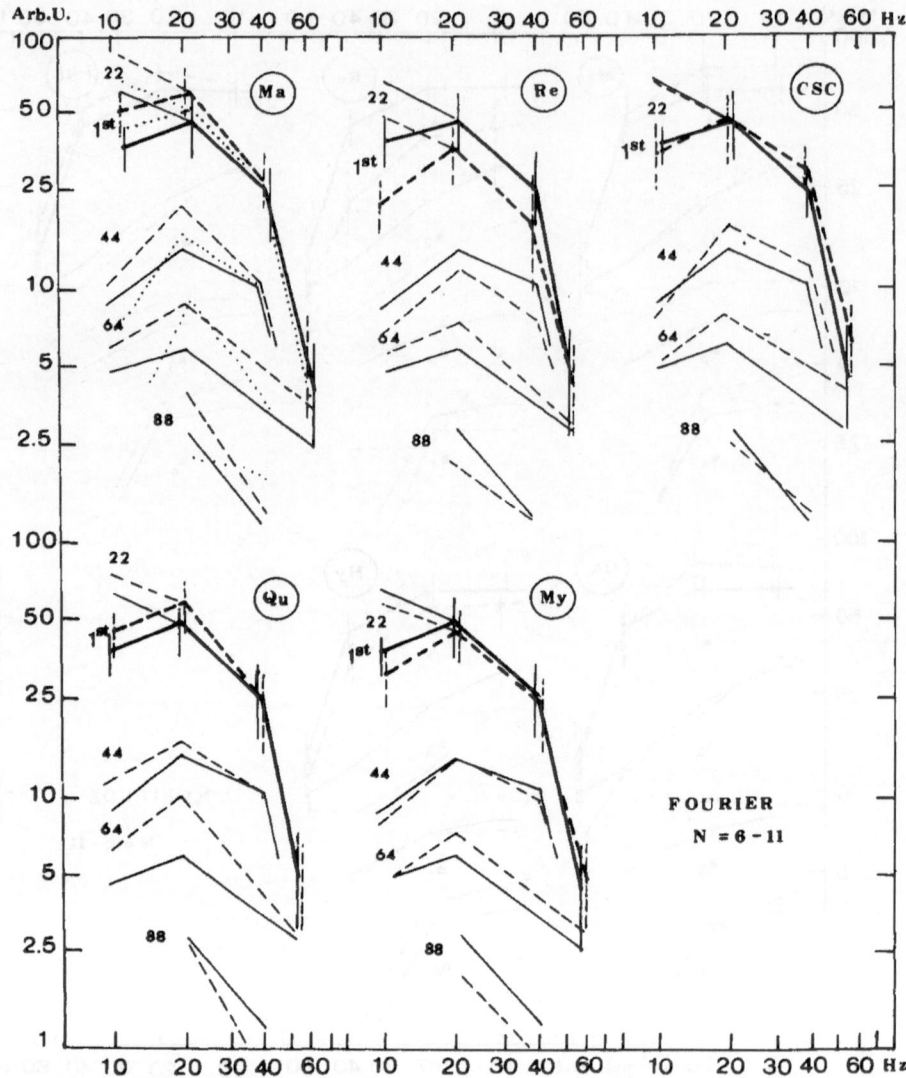

Fig. 4. Flicker ERG attenuation curves; Fourier component method. 1st: first harmonic amplitude of the flicker ERG responses for different stimulus frequencies; 22, 44, 64 and 88: frequencies of different other Fourier components of the 12 Hz response; Ma: foveolar cases; Re: diffuse chorioretinal degeneration and other perifoveal cases; CSC: healed central serous chorioretinitis; Qu: quinoline derivative treated patients; My: ethambutol treated patients; Continuous curves: normal values; broken curves: pathological cases; dotted curves: case with foveolar sunburn; vertical lines: standard deviation; N: number of examined eyes; Abscissa: frequencies in Hz; Ordinate: amplitudes in arbitrary units.

other of My or Re types.It is to be noted that n = 6 subgroup and LE represent seven eyes diagnosed as normal.

One can see a general pattern for each group in the objective responses and a similarity amongst some of them. At first sight, one cannot see this general pattern for each group in the subjective responses, except for groups Ma and Qu. However, when the high frequency low frequency thresholds relationships are considered for the subgroup or individual cases, one can see

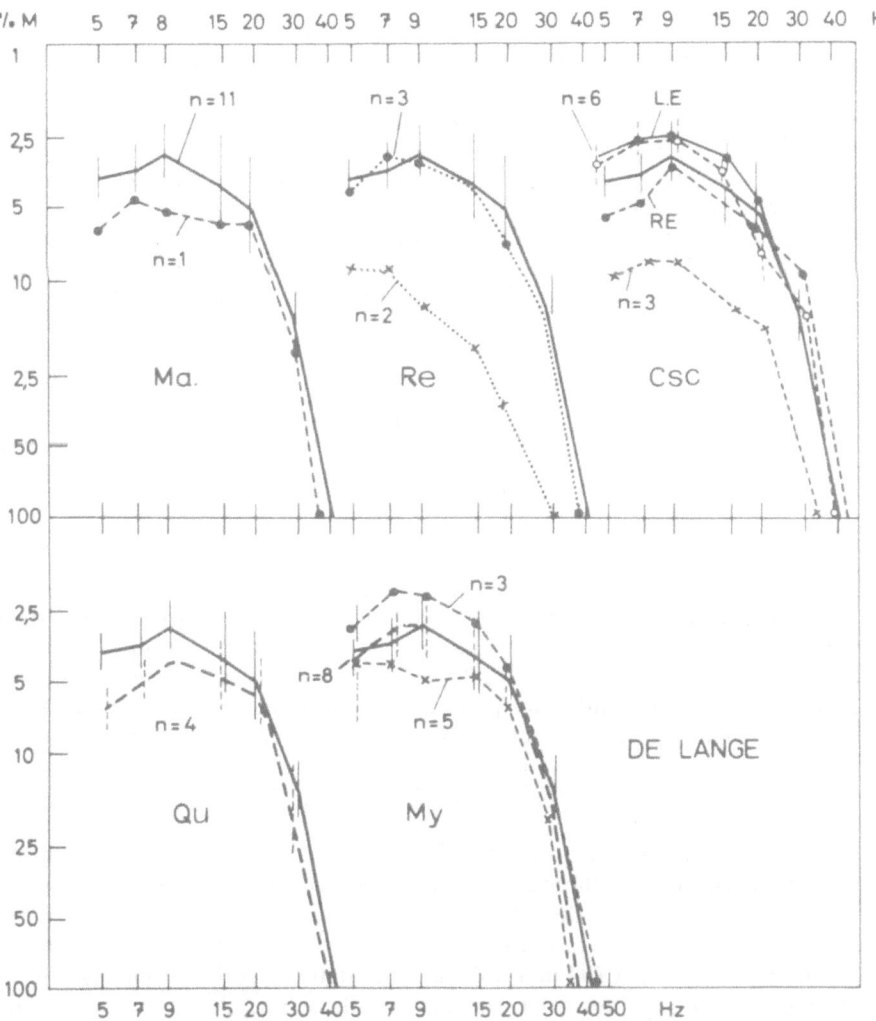

Fig. 5. De Lange curves for the different groups of Fig. 3 and Fig. 4. Continuous curves: normal values; Broken and dotted curves: pathological cases; Vertical lines: standard deviation; N: number of examined eyes; LE and RE: left and right eye of the same case; (for other symbols, see Fig. 3 or Fig. 4); Abscissa: frequencies in Hz; Ordinate: modulation amplitude in %.

a similarity also for ex. groups Re and My. The group CSC is again composed of mixed type curves.

To summarize these observations on individual, as well as grouped data: we can classify our curves in three main classes:

— two of them are characterised by an inbalance of high and low frequency response attenuation in comparison with a reference condition.

a. in the first class, low frequency responses are more attenuated than high frequency ones. We find two types:
- responses with normal high frequency (type 1)
- responses with enhanced high frequency (type 1')

b. in the second class, high frequency responses are more attenuated than low ones. We find two types:
- responses with enhanced low frequency (type 2')
- responses with depressed low frequency (type 2).

— The third class is characterised by a vertical displacement of the whole curve. We find one type:
- responses with all thresholds enhanced (type 3)
- responses with all thresholds depressed were not observed. If one considers pathological groups and types, one finds the following relationships:

Group	type
Ma	1
Qu	1,3
Re	2,2'
My	2,2'
CSC	1,1',3

As the group containing types 1 and 2 were known to correspond respectively to foveolar and perifoveolar cases, there are reasons to associate them with a localized (1) or a perifoveolar involvement (2) of a lesion. The groups containing essentially 1' type (CSC) and 2' type (My, CSC) were characterised by cases with a minimal pathology. One would associate these types with the beginning of a respectively foveolar and perifoveolar lesion.

DISCUSSION AND CONCLUSION

We have already seen in a previous work (MEYER et al., 1974) that the perceptive flicker thresholds assist in the detection of retinal dysfunction with a greater sensivity than the visual acuity and kinetic perimetry. In this study, the De Lange data confirmed this assertion. One can note that with our objective flicker ERG method we could detect significant changes in the cases known to give normal ERG results with normal clinical methods. This may be due, possibly, to a normal stable photopic stimulation condition and our method of analysis of averaged flicker responses. Ordinarily, one uses high intensity and low frequency stimulation in a dark room after bright light adaptation. One can also observe a general parallelism concerning the specificity of the tests: flicker attenuation curves, as well as De Lange curves, confirm the presence of two systems: a low frequency one and a high frequency one, whose relative disturbance depends on the extension and gravity of perifoveolar lesions.

That we can observe a general parallelism does not mean that both methods are equivalent. If foveolar fixation is possible, the De Lange method should be sensitive for detecting foveolar dysfunction. Diffuse perifoveolar dysfunction can be detected by flicker ERG more accurately. We found in both tests a paradoxical effect. We can observe that in case with foveolar involvement, the flicker ERG b-wave is enhanced, whereas it is depressed in the case of perifoveolar dysfunction. On the other hand, a perifoveolar dysfunction enhances the De Lange low frequency thresholds, which are usually depressed by a foveolar involvement.

We can logically conclude that there may exist from fovea to perifovea different mechanisms which may influence each other directly or indirectly by horizontal connection effects. In the case of glycine injection of rabbit eyes, KOROL et al. (1973, 1974) found that the b-wave form changed depending on frequency and stimulation intensity. Microscopy and autoradiography show a localisation of glycine around amacrine cells. These mechanisms may also be influenced by centrifugal effects. Ethambutol has previously been described as affecting only the optic nerve (MORTON GRANT, 1974). However, we could detect a pathological ERG of perifoveal type in the ethambutol group. This supports the hypothesis that the perifoveolar type may be caused indirectly by a change in the centrifugal action on the retina giving an enhanced b-wave, as seen in optic neuritis (FEINSOD & AUERBACH, 1969).

One can discuss the enhanced amplitudes and oscillatory potentials we observed in most cases of foveolar or perifoveolar retinopathy with a blue-yellow acquired color impairment. Again, this effect would be an indirect stimulation of perifoveolar red mechanisms. It is interesting to compare these results with those from cases with red-green defects where we could observe morphological changes for both objective and subjective examinations (MEYER, 1972).

These results show that it is possible to accentuate different photopic mechanisms, as well as enhance the photopic-scotopic duality of the visual system (ALFIERI & SOLE, 1965, 1968 ALFIERI et al., 1968). It is advantageous in studying foveolar dysfunctions to choose stimulation conditions that will reveal, at an earlier time, the inbalance of these mechanisms in pathological cases. Furthermore, with the combination of adaptation, frequency, stimulus intensity and color, the test specificity is enhanced.

SUMMARY

This study compares and verifies the efficiency of two functional tests based on intermittent light stimulation. One is the De Lange curve, the other the flicker ERG recorded in defined photopic conditions and analysed with two different methods. The cases studied belong to a reference group and other groups including foveolar lesions, perifoveolar and diffuse retinopathy, healed central serous chorioretinitis, ethambutol and quinoline derivative retinal intoxication. The results show that both objective and subjective methods are sensitive and show some parallelism: both methods aid in distinguishing foveolar and perifoveolar involvements; a possible comparison between the two tests is also possible.

Some hypotheses are made for explaining this paradox: a high sensitivity of the one degree De Lange test in the case of perifoveolar involvement as well as a high sensitivity of the flicker ERG test for foveolar involvement.

Some suggestions are made for further development of this dynamic photopic test.

REFERENCES

ALFIERI R. & SOLE P., Electroretinogramme chez l'homme, ondes e et vision des couleurs. *C.R. Soc. Biol.*, 159: *2362-2367* (1965).

ALFIERI R. & SOLE P., Adapto-electroretinogram (AERG) in monochromatic light in man; In: The clinical value of electroretinography, 5th Symp. ISCERG, Ghent 1966, p. *215-220*, Karger, Basel (1968).

ALFIERI R., SOLE P. & SCIOLDO-ZURCHER P., Harmonic analysis of the electro-retinogram; In Advances in electrophysiology and pathology of the visual system, 6th Symp. ISCERG, Erfurt 1967, p. *305-317*, Georg Thieme, Leipzig (1968).

BABEL J., REY P., STANGOS N., MEYER J.J. & GUGGENHEIM P., The functional examination of the macular and perimacular region with the aid of flicker fusion thresholds. *Doc. Ophthal.*, 26: *248-256* (1969).

DENIER VAN DER GON J.J., STRADKEE J. & VAN DER TWEEL L.H., A source for modulated light. *Phys. Med. Biol.*, 3: *164-173* (1958).

FEINSOD M. & AUERBACH E., Changes in the electroretinogram (ERG) in lesions of the optic nerve. Summary in: *Electroenceph. clin. Neurophysiol.*, 27: *216* (1969).

KOROL S., The effects of glycine on the rabbit retina: averaged ERG and averaged visual evoked responses. *Experientia*, 29: *984-985* (1973).

KOROL S., MEYER J.J. & LEUENBERGER P.M., The effects of glycine on the rabbit retina. Averaged ERG and microscopic anatomy. 13th Symp. ISCERG. Clermont-Ferrand (1974).

MEYER J.J.: Exploration de la fonction visuelle à l'aide de la lumière intermittente: courbe d'attenuation perceptive et électroretinogramme de papillotement. Thèse no 1574, 125 p., Université de Genève, (1972).

MEYER J.J., KOROL S., OWENS G., GRAMONI R. & REY P., The functional exami-nation of the human photopic visual system with the aid of psychophysical flicker thresholds and ERG flicker responses, *Doc. Ophthal.*, in press.

MORTON GRANT W., Toxicology of the eye. Drugs, chemicals, plants, venoms. Charles C. Thomas, Springfield, Ill., pp. *1201*, 2nd ed., (1974).

REY P. & REY J.P., Fréquence de fusion optique. Comparaison de trois méthodes de mesure avant et après le travail. *Le Travail Humain*, 26, *135-145*, (1964).

ERG AND EOG IN DIAGNOSIS AND
PROGNOSIS OF BULL'S EYE MACULOPATHY

H.E. HENKES, M. VAN MIERLOBENSTEYN &
G.H.M. VAN LITH*

(Rotterdam, The Netherlands)

The so-called bull's eye of the macular region can only be diagnosed using an ophthalmoscope. The diagnosis does not imply a definite aetiology; it merely refers to an annular depigmentation around the central foveal area, due to local atrophy of the pigment epithelium. Fluorescein angiography accentuates the loss of pigment epithelium cells.

The condition may be symptomless, but can be accompanied by serious functional defects of the central retinal area and, more often than not, of the whole of the retina.

Thusfar, two major causes were held responsible for this condition:

1stly: an iatrogenic disorder, almost exclusively restricted to chloroquine ingestion; and

2ndly: a hereditary disorder, more particularly the dystrophy of the cone system.

Apart from these causes, we have seen some other cases, of as yet unclassified nature.

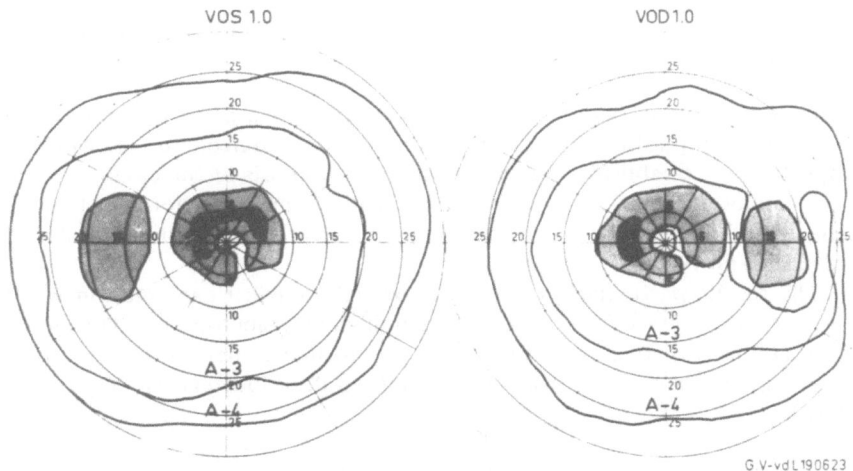

Fig. 1. *Case 1:* Annular perifoveal scotoma in bull's eye maculopathy due to chloroquine overmedication.

*   Eye Clinic, Erasmus University Rotterdam

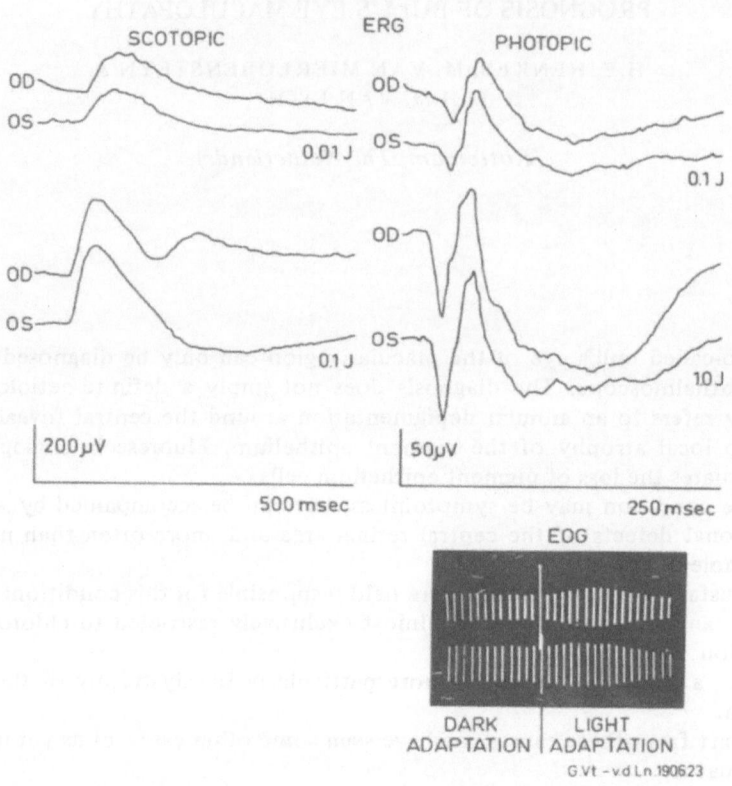

Fig. 2a. *Case 1:* Normal ERG following global stimulation. The EOG light-rise is sub-normal.

It goes without saying that the case history (use of certain drugs, existence of photophobia, time of onset, familiar occurrence, etc.) is of primary importance in establishing the diagnosis and prognosis of the case.

In many a case the diagnosis of the underlying condition can be ascertained, and the prognosis corroborated by electro-ophthalmological tests, viz. ERG and EOG.

The results particularly of electro-ophthalmological examination will be discussed in view of five categories of bull's eye maculopathy. The electro-ophthalmological technique used, and the normal values for the set-up employed in the present investigation, have been described earlier (VAN LITH, 1973).

I. CHLOROQUINE RETINOPATHY

Though in the advanced stage of chloroquine retinopathy with a full-blown bull's eye macula, retinal functions frequently show severely abnormal ERG's and EOG's, the early case of chloroquine bull's eye retinopathy may show still normal electric activity. However, if a disturbance is encountered, such a disturbance may be found either in the EOG, or in the ERG (usually in the rod system), or in both. According to FRANÇOIS & DE ROUCK (1972), the electro-ophthalmological disturbances preceed the changes found with fluorescein-angiography.

Case 1: A 53-year old woman was first seen in 1972 because of visual complaints. Though the visual acuity was still 1.0, an annular perifoveal scotoma was detected (Figure 1), without, however, any funduscopic alterations. In July of 1973 a faint bull's eye maculopathy was noticed. It then came out that the patient took Resochine tablets since 1968 for unclear reasons.

Colour vision and dark adaptation were normal. Electroretinography revealed a normal response on global stimulation (Figure 2a). The EOG however showed a subnormal light-rise. The LP/DT-ratio was 1.50 and 1.20 for the right and left eye respectively. A 10 degree's macular stimulus produced nearly normal photopic ERG responses (90 percent R.E.; 80 percent L.E.). The VECP's were rather low, but otherwise normal (Figure 2b).

Conclusion: a case of chloroquine bull's eye maculopathy is described with beginning loss of retinal function and a severely changed EOG response.

II. CONE DYSTROPHY AND CONE–ROD DYSTROPHY

In cone dystrophy the cone system response becomes progressively affected while the rod system is functioning normally (KRILL & DEUTMAN, 1972; KRILL et al., 1973). In the early stages, the macular photopic response may be affected selectively while the global photopic response may be still intact.

In the later stages, the scotopic mechanism may show additional signs of deterioration. This, then, becomes a cone-rod dystrophy.

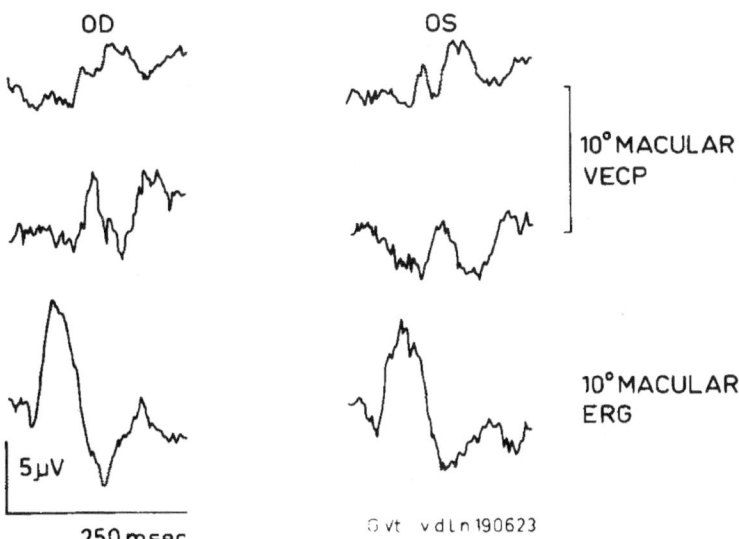

Fig. 2b. *Case 1:* The photopic ERG following macular stimulation is slightly reduced in amplitude. The VECP's are rather low, but otherwise normal.

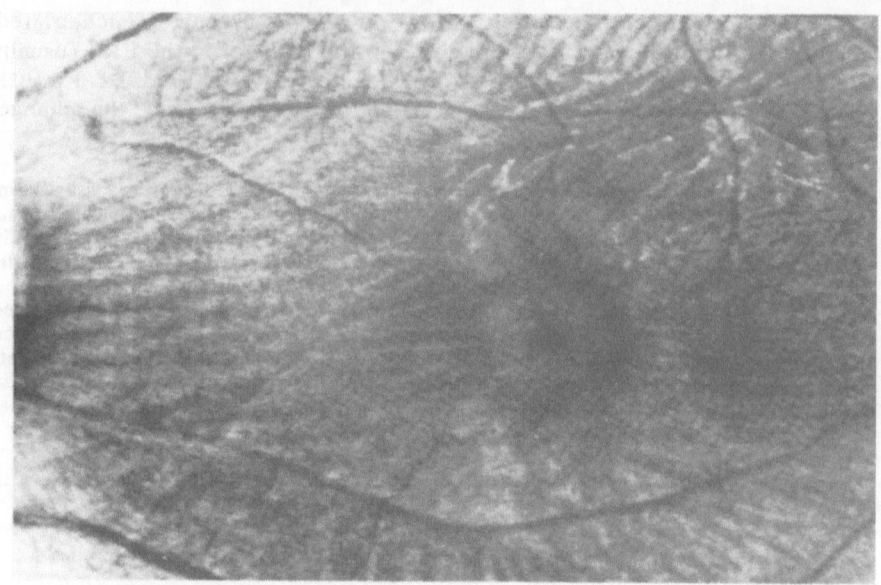

Fig. 3a. *Case 2:* Advanced cone-rod dystrophy showing faint, still incomplete bull's eye maculopathy.

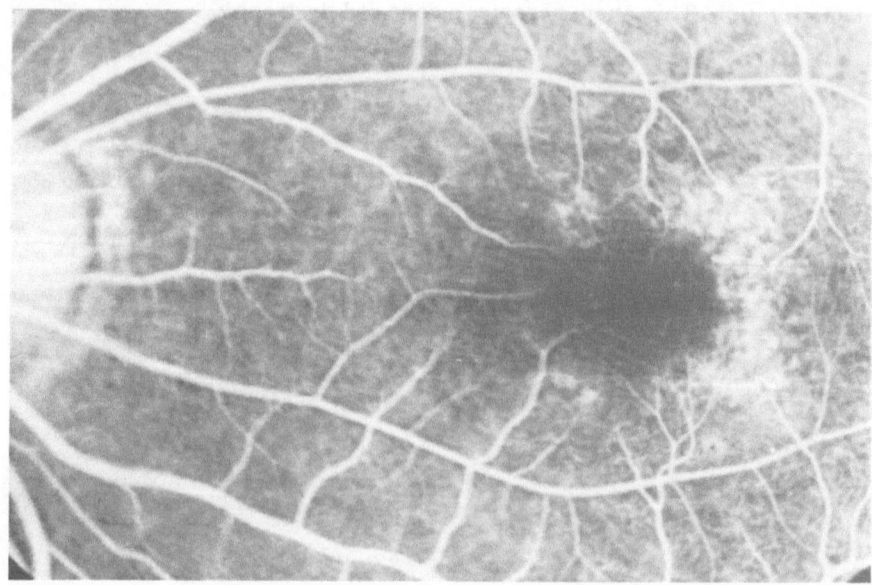

Fig. 3b. *Cas 2:* Fluorescein angiography accentuates the loss of pigmentepithelium cells.

If progression goes on, the electrical response of both retinal systems may even become extinguished. This condition necessitates a differential diagnosis with retinitis pigmentosa sine pigmento.

Case 2: A 19-year old man complained of a slight reduction of vision and colour deficiency. No family history of visual defects could be elucidated. The maculae showed symmetrically a faint depigmented area, partially surrounding an intact fovea. Fluorescein angiography enhanced the, as yet incomplete, bull's eye aspect (Figures 3a and 3b). The fundus vessels showed some narrowing. A patchy appearance in the periphery, due to peripheral pigment epithelial defects was observed.

Visual acuity was 1.0 in both eyes. Both eyes still showed full visual fields for the largest object and of highest intensity (Figure 4). For the other stimuli a decreased retinal sensitivity was observed. A paracentral scotoma was the most important finding.

Normal colour vision on Farnsworth's D-15 test was found. The dark adaptation curve revealed a rather strong photopic and a mild scotopic defect in the cone and rod segments of the curve.

The EOG light-rise was absent (Figure 5). Both retinal systems showed an activity level far below the normal (approx. 10% of normal for both eyes).

Conclusion: Notwithstanding the almost normal fundus picture − apart from the macular area − an advanced cone-rod dystrophy had to be diagnosed. Retinitis pigmentosa sine pigmento was considered, but rejected on account of the (para)central scotomas and the absence of marked alterations of retinal vessels and optic disks.

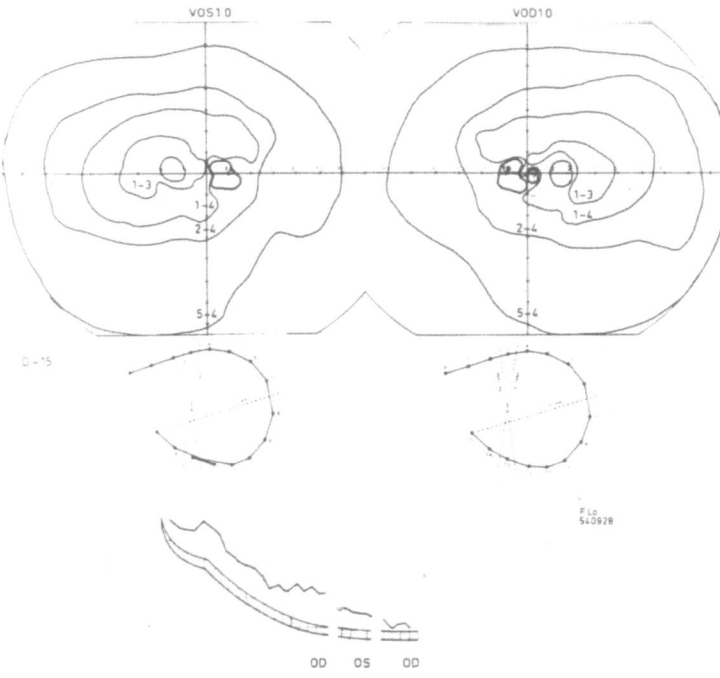

Fig. 4. *Case 2:* Visual fields show paracentral scotomas. Normal colour vision. Dark adaptation shows considerably increased photopic threshold but almost normal scotopic threshold.

III. STARGARDT'S DISEASE

In Stargardt's disease – with or without fundus flavimaculatus – the photopic ERG on global stimulation of the retina is, generally speaking, intact. If affected, the photopic response is less disturbed than the scotopic response. However, if the disease is limited to the posterior pole, the differential diagnosis may be difficult with regard to foveal cone dystrophy. Other data may then be of help to corroborate the diagnosis, e.g., the existence of photophobia, and of nystagmus.

> *Case 3:* A 19-year old man complained of deteriorating vision since 3 years. His visual acuity was 0.8 in 1970 and had diminished to 0.2 when we saw him in 1973.
>
> No complaints of photophobia.
>
> No member of the family had visual complaints; consanguinity of parents could not be established. The macular region showed a beaten-bronze centre surrounded by a bull's eye (Figure 6a, b). Both eyes showed central scotomas (Figure 7). The Farnsworth D-15 panel was normal.

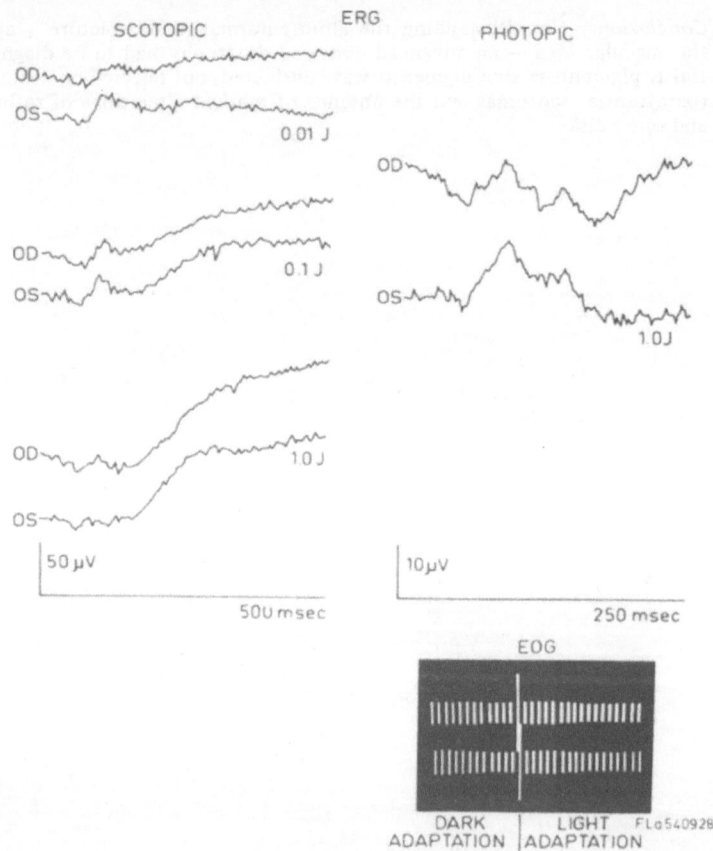

Fig. 5. *Case 2:* Both retinal systems are highly affected and produce only rudimentary responses. In the EOG, the light peak/dark trough ratio is 1.00 for R. and L. eye.

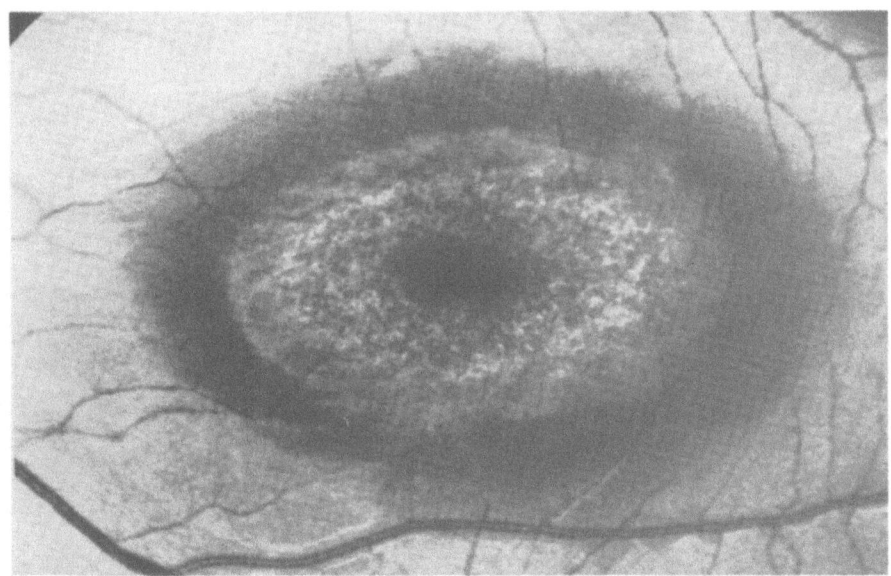

Fig. 6a. *Case 3:* Stargardt's disease showing a bull's eye maculopathy.

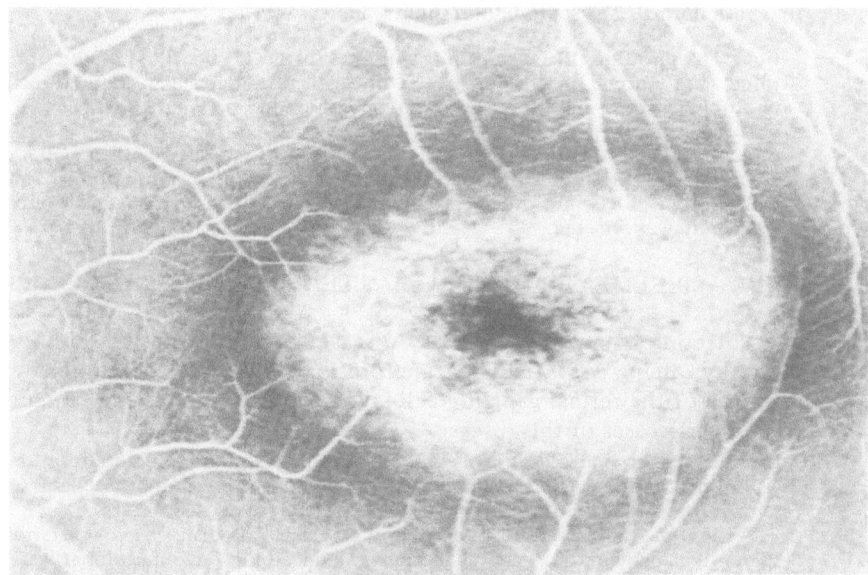

Fig. 6b. *Case 3:* Fluorescein angiogram.

Dark adaptation showed a slightly elevated cone branch. Final rod threshold was 1 log unit too high. The EOG showed normal values of 2.35 in the right eye and 2.60 in the left eye (Figure 8a).

The scotopic ERG was completely normal in both eyes after global stimula-

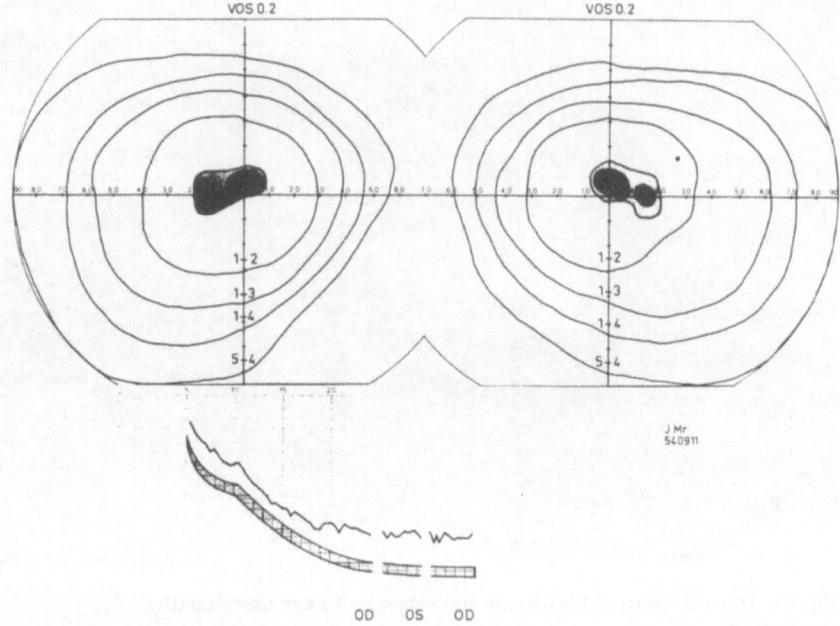

Fig. 7. *Case 3:* Visual fields demonstrate central scotomas. Cone system adaptation is slightly above normal. The scotopic threshold is increased.

tion. The photopic ERG was almost normal in the R. eye (90% of the normal value) and normal in the left eye. Only after local, macular stimulation the photopic response and the VECP's were greatly reduced (Figure 8b).

Conclusion: This patient suffered from Stargardt's disease with a bull's eye aspect lacking the fundus flavimaculatus-aspect. As neither photophobia, abnormal photopic ERG, nor defective colour vision were found, a diagnosis of cone dystrophy was rejected.

IV. SPIELMEYER-VOGT – (BATTEN-MAYOU) DISEASE

I ṭ̃ents suffering from this hereditary disease sometimes show a bull's eye maculopathy. Being essentially a tapetoretinal dystrophy combined with degeneration of the retinal ganglion cell layer, the ERG is mostly extinguished, even in early cases of this disease.

Case 4: An 11-year old girl was referred to us because of rapid deterioration of vision. She suffered from a slow but progressive deterioration of intellect. Consanguinity of the parents existed and there were affected relatives.

Vision was approx. 0.1. Funduscopy revealed pale disks, narrow arterioles, spider-like pigmentations in the periphery and a bull's eye maculopathy (Figure 9). Visual fields were difficult to assess, but were still relatively intact (Figure 10).

Colour vision was probably defective, but neither the HRR-plates, nor the Farnsworth D-15 panel could be executed due to lack of understanding.

EOG recording was not possible.

The ERG was severely changed: photopic responses were very much reduced (approx. 10% of the normal values), and the scotopic ERG was extinguished (Figure 11).

62

In conclusion: A child suffering from Spielmeyer-Vogt-(Batten-Mayou) disease showing a bull's eye appearance in the macula.

V. BULL'S EYE MACULOPATHY OF UNKNOWN ORIGIN ('ESSENTIAL' BULL'S EYE MAEULOPATHY)

Several sporadic cases of bull's eye maculopathy have been encountered, showing, apart from progressive loss of visual acuity, practically normal retinal functions.

In none of the cases a history of chloroquine medication or signs of cone dystrophy could be elucidated.

Case 5: A 51-year old man, complaining of loss of central vision, was first seen in April 1973. His vision was fingers counting at 5 meters in the right eye and 0.3 in the left eye.

Funduscopy revealed a bull's eye almost restricted to the fovea (Figure 12a), accentuated by fluorescence angiography (Figure 12b).

Visual fields showed central scotomas (Figure 13). Colour vision tested with the HRR-plates and Farnsworth D-15 panel was unaffected, as was the D.A. curve, the EOG and global ERG (Figure 14).

An internal medicine examination gave normal findings.

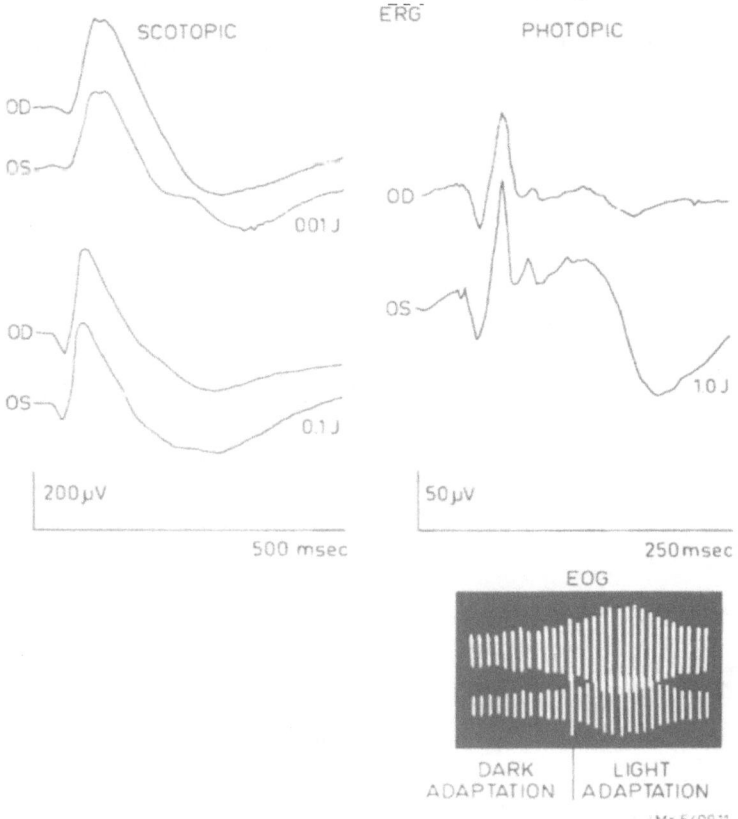

Fig. 8a. *Case 3:* The global ERG shows normal values for the scotopic system. The photopic system gives a slightly reduced activity in the R.E. but normal activity in the L.E. The EOG is normal.

63

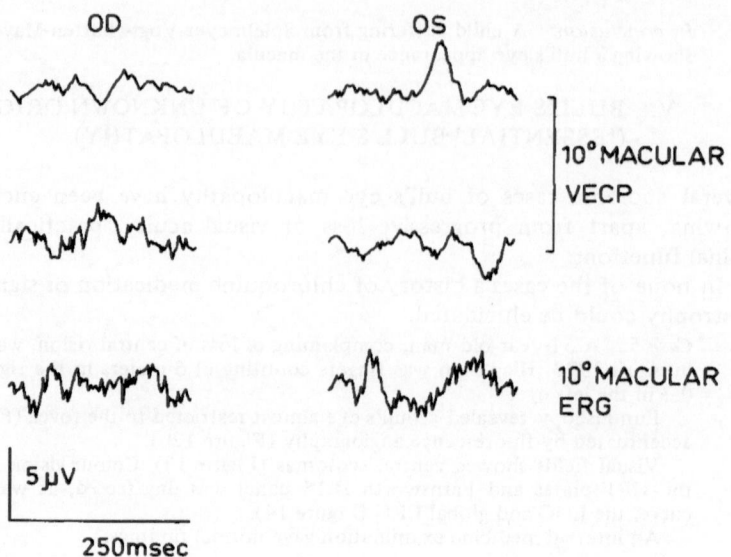

OD OS

10° MACULAR
VECP

10° MACULAR
ERG

5 µV

250msec

ig. 8b. *Case 3:* Local macular stimulation (10 degrees) gives markedly reduced hotopic responses in the R.E., both in the ERG and in the VECP.

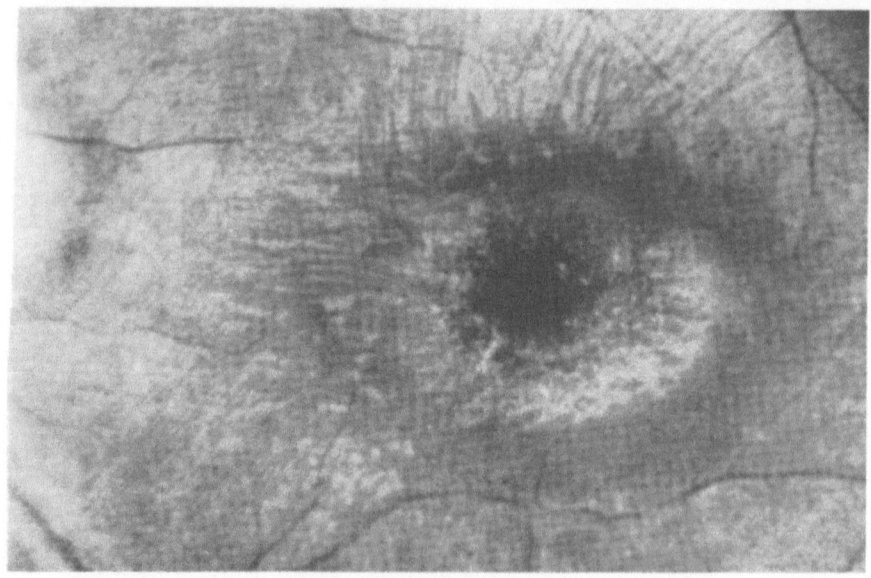

Fig. 9. *Case 4:* Bull's eye in Spielmeyer-Vogt-(Batten-Mayou) disease.

Conclusion: This patient was suffering from a progressive 'essential' bull's eye macular lesion.

Due to the age of onset of visual complaints and the lack of relevant symptoms, the diagnosis: cone dystrophy was rejected.

DISCUSSION

From the case histories discussed, it emerges that electro-ophthalmological examinations can be of great help in establishing the diagnosis in bull's eye maculopathy. In some categories ERG and EOG are indispensable (cone-dystrophy; cone-rod dystrophy); in others they will be of great help in establishing an early diagnosis (chloroquine retinopathy).

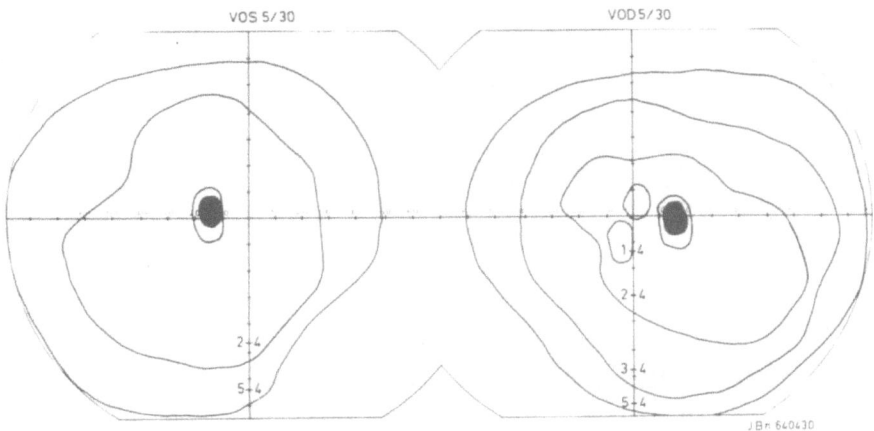

Fig. 10. *Case 4:* Visual fields seem to be intact. Colour vision is probably defective, but tests can not be executed correctly.

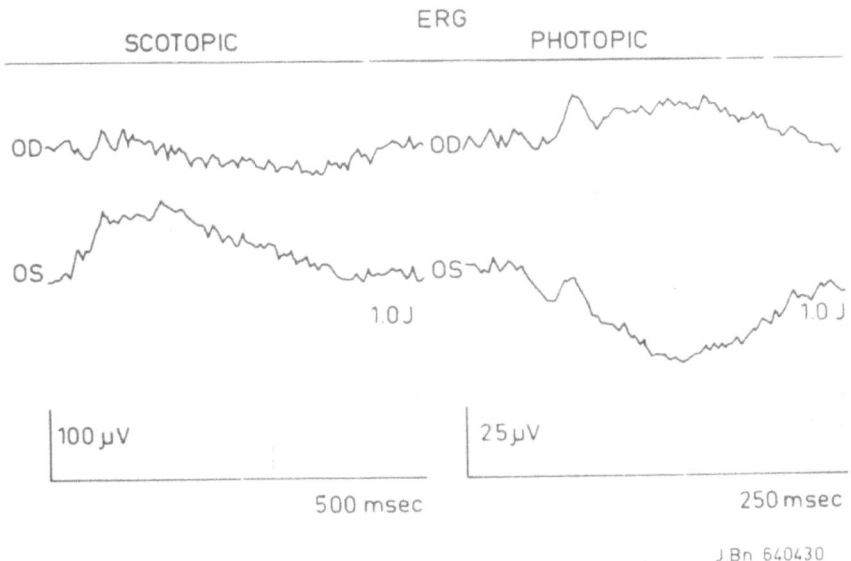

Fig. 11. *Case 4:* Even the highest stimulus luminance available, provokes only minimal scotopic activity. Photopic activity is present, but highly reduced. EOG recording is not possible.

65

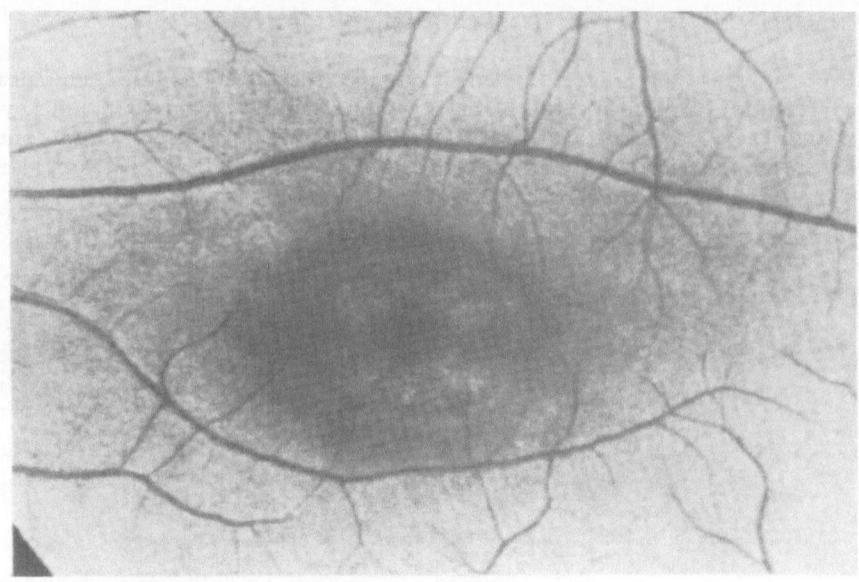

Fig. 12a. *Case 5:* 'Essential' bull's eye maculopathy.

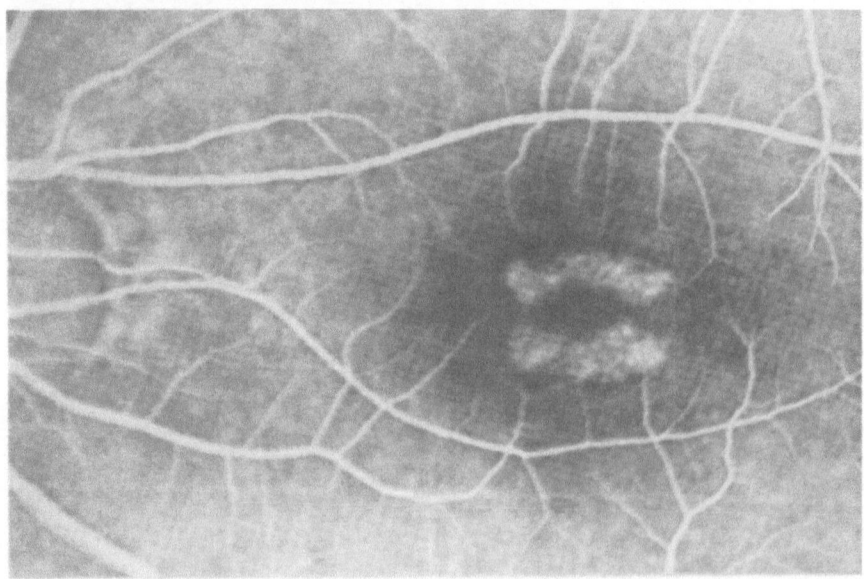

Fig. 12b. *Case 5:* Fluorescein angiogram.

There is no correlation between the electro-ophthalmological response pattern and the extensiveness (or intensity) of the bull's eye.

This is conceivable from the fact that global ERG and EOG do not correlate with local retinal pathology. Abnormalities in the global ERG and

EOG are indications for widespread retinal pathology, existing far beyond the limits of the bull's eye proper.

A relation between local, i.e. macular ERG-responses and bull's eye maculopathy may exist, based upon the existence of local macular pathology, but *not* upon the existence of a bull's eye.

Apart from the 5 categories of bull's eye maculopathy discussed above, a 6th group of bull's eye maculopathy was reported only recently (DEUTMAN; 1974). DEUTMAN described a hereditary bull's eye dystrophy (the so-called benign concentric annular macular dystrophy) in which ERG's and EOG's give variable results in the different affected family members, ranging from normal to definite abnormal values. Both retinal systems are affected, whereby the bipolar cell layer seems to suffer more than the photoreceptors.

SUMMARY

With the help of 5 representative case histories, 5 categories of bull's eye maculopathy are discussed from the viewpoint of electro-ophthalmological characteristics:

viz. chloroquine retinopathy; cone- and cone-rod dystrophy; Stargardt's disease; Spielmeyer-Vogt-(Batten-Mayou) disease and 'essential' bull's eye maculopathy.

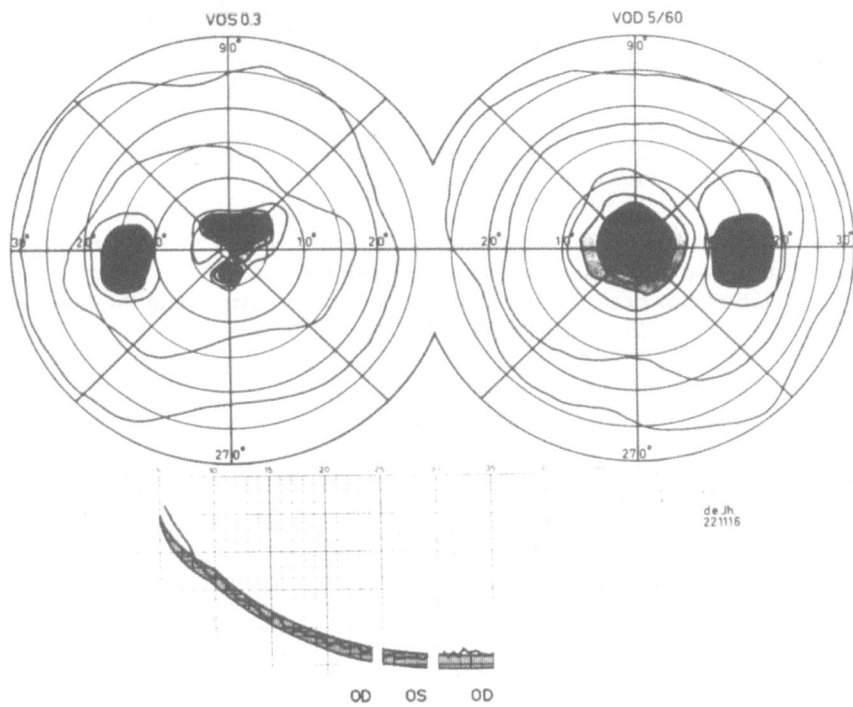

Fig. 13. *Case 5:* Central scotomas and normal dark adaptation are recorded.

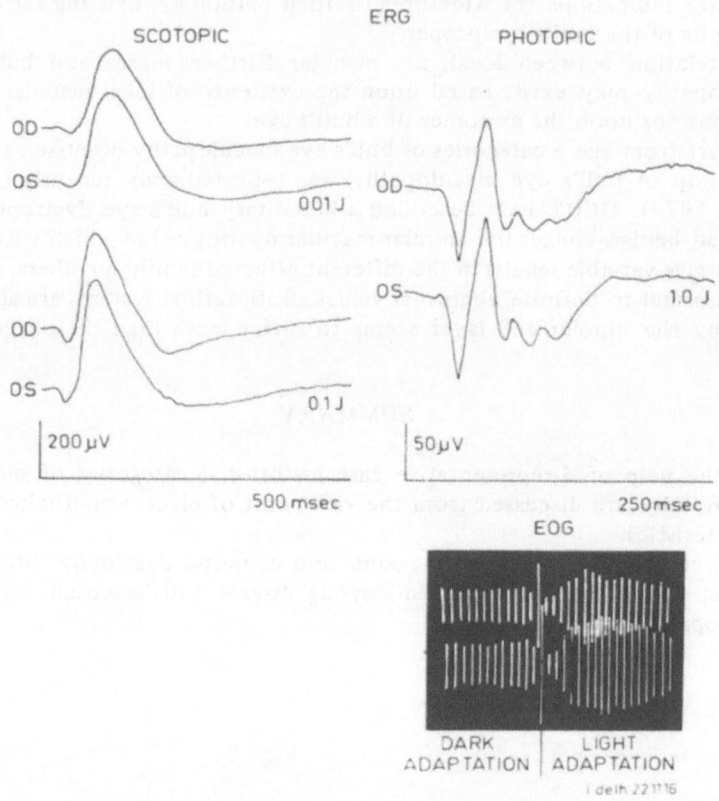

Fig. 14. *Case 5:* Normal values of photopic and scotopic activity are found after global stimulation of the retina.

It is shown that electro-ophthalmological procedures are indispensable in establishing the diagnosis of the underlying condition.

A relationship between the electrical response pattern and the bull's eye maculopathy could not be established.

REFERENCES

KRILL,,A.E. & DEUTMAN, A.F.: Dominant macular degenerations: the cone dystrophies. *Amer. J. Ophthal.* 73: *352-369* (1972).

KRILL A.E., DEUTMAN, A.F. & FISHMAN, M.: The cone degenerations. *Docum. Ophthal.*, 35: *1-80* (1973).

DEUTMAN, A.F.: Benign concentric annular macular dystrophy. *Amer. J. Ophthal.*, 78: *384-396* (1974).

FRANÇOIS, J. & DE ROUCK, A.: Rétinopathie chloroquinique. *Bull. Soc. Belge d'Ophtal.* 160: *581-590* (1972); id. *Ophthalmologica* 165: *81-99* (1972).

VAN LITH, G.H.M.: Electro-ophthalmology II. Indications and Interpretation. in: Photography, Electro-ophtalmology and Echo-ophthalmology in Ophthalmic Practice. Documenta Ophthalmologica Proceedings Series vol. 3: *257-270.* Junk, the Hague (1973).

CLINICAL AND ELECTROPHYSIOLOGICAL FINDINGS OF A CASE OF FUNDUS FLAVIMACULATUS

K. IMAIZUMI, R. TAKAHASHI, K. MITA & H. HOSHI

(Morioka, Japan)

INTRODUCTION

The retinal abnormality of fundus flavimaculatus can easily be diagnosed erroneously as tapetoretinal degeneration when one depends merely on ophthalmoscopic findings, not performing psychophysical and electrophysiological testings (CARR, 1965). KLIEN & KRILL (1967) emphasized the usefulness of fluorescein fundus angiography for the differential diagnosis of fundus flavimaculatus. Several reports of this disease have been made in foreign countries, but very few in Japan (YURI, et al., 1969, OGINO, et al., 1970, WATANABE, et al., 1971).

The purpose of the present paper is to describe our clinical findings and the characteristic view of fluorescence patterns in fundus angiography obtained from a typical case.

CASE REPORT

The patient was a Taiwanese, 25-year-old male, in military service, who visited our clinic in June, 1973, with a complaint of visual disturbance in both eyes.

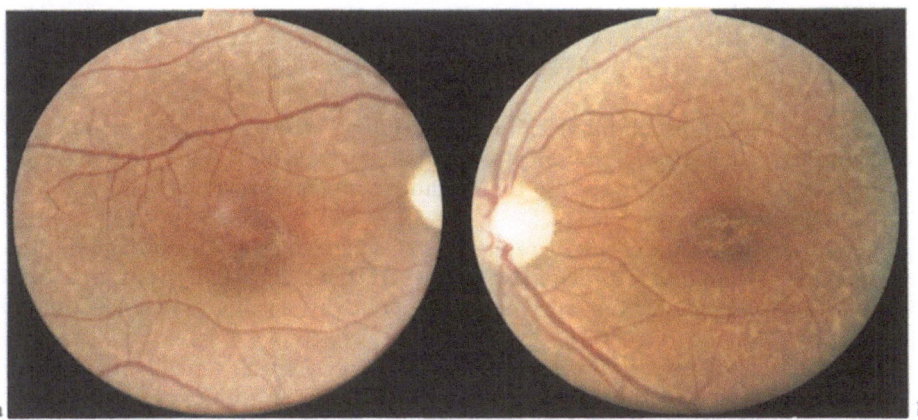

Fig. 1. a. Right eye: b. Left eye. Note isolated, deep-seated, opaque, pisciform flecks in the paramacular and midperiphery region, and atrophic degenerated area (3/4 size of the disc) in the foveal region.

Present history: In November, 1969, he joined the military force and in December a cloudiness in vision was noticed in both eyes. In January, 1970, he noted a blur around the sight when aiming a rifle, and in April, he had difficulties when reading books at night. In 1971, his vision of both side had dropped to 0.1. In December, 1972, he was diagnosed as bilateral retinitis centralis by an ophthalmologist in Taiwan. At that time, according to his father, who was also an ophthalmologist, no flecks were observed in the fundi but an oedematous opacity was found in the macular region.
Family history: There is no history of consanguinity. No one complaints of poor vision or night blindness in the family.
Past history: Nothing significant, but tonsillitis with a high fever of 40 °C in January 1965, and in summer of 1971.
Systematic examination: Other than the ophthalmological problems, no abnormality was found in the systemic examination.
Present condition: The visual acuity of the right eye is 0.06 (n.c.) and 0.06 (0.1 x −1.OD) of the left. The anterior segment, ocular media and intra-ocular tension were all normal in both eyes. Ophthalmoscopically, the macular region was seen to be pathologically altered, having an inconspicuous reddish color to the extent of about 3/4 of the optic disc diameter. (Figure 1, a and b). A peculiar glistering sheen was also observed in this area, with an overlying pigmentation. A minor haemorrhage was found in the macula of the right eye at our first examination. Deepseated yellowish flecks were disseminated in the paramacular and midperipheral retinal regions, but not in the degenerated portion of the macula or at the margin of the optic disc.

The retinal flecks were either yellowish or yellow-white. Their shape, size, opaqueness and density varied to some extent. In most cases the shapes of the flecks were round, linear or in pisciform, and some were confluent. Some flecks, located at midperiphery of the fundi, had fine powdery pigment deposits at their borders, giving a dirty appearance. With slit lamp examination, the surface of these flecks appeared to be relatively flat. The condition was similar in both eyes. The optic nerve and the retinal vessels were normal.

FUNCTIONAL EVALUATION

Methods: The psychophysical examinations of the visual field, color sense and dark-adaptation, and electrophysiological examinations such as ERG and EOG were performed by the methods reported previously (IMAIZUMI, 1969).

Fluorescein fundus angiography was also carried out in accordance to the procedure employed previously (IMAIZUMI, et al., 1972), but this time photographs were taken at every 1/3 second by a super sequence fundus camera (Topcon, TRC-F3).
Results: As shown in Table 1, determination of visual field by a Goldman perimeter revealed that it was in the normal range in both eyes for the outer isopter with the highest intensity. However, there were depressions in all directions at 15° in the right eye and 10° in the left. Approximately a 4° absolute scotoma was detected in each eye by a Bjerrum perimeter. Both

eyes showed an abnormality of yellowblue color vision. In dark-adaptation tests, similar results were obtained in both eyes, with a high threshold of the cone process and a delayed rod-cone break. The threshold of the rod process showed a delay but the final threshold level was within the normal range.

Electrophysiologically, both the photopic and scotopic ERGs were observed as almost normal in each eye, while EOG in the right eye was subnormal and in the left distinctly abnormal (Figure 2).

With fluorescein fundus angiography, at five seconds after the injection of fluorescein, dots of leakage of the dye corresponding to the flecks appeared earlier than choroidal flush (Figure 3). However, even when a photograph was taken without fluorescein injected, as shown in Figure 4, a very similar fluorescent patterns was observed. This phenomenon demonstrates that the flecks possibly yield pseudo-fluorescence and this is one of very characteristic findings in this case. The fluorescent spots, which correspond

Table 1. Clinical and Electrophysiological Findings.

function \ side	visual fields (Goldmann)	scotometry (Bjerrum)	color sense	dark adaptation (Goldmann-Weeker)		ERG		EOG
				primary process	secondary process	photopic	scotopic	
right	4/v isopter normal central depression 15° all direction	absolute scotoma approxim. 4°	yellow-blue defect	slightly increased threshold. delayed	delayed, final rod threshold normal	almost normal	almost normal	flat type d=100μV Q=1.33
left	4/v isopter normal central depression 10° all direction	absolute scotoma approxim. 4°	yellow-blue defect	slightly increased threshold. delayed	delayed, final rod threshold normal	almost normal	almost normal	flat type d=63μV Q=1.21

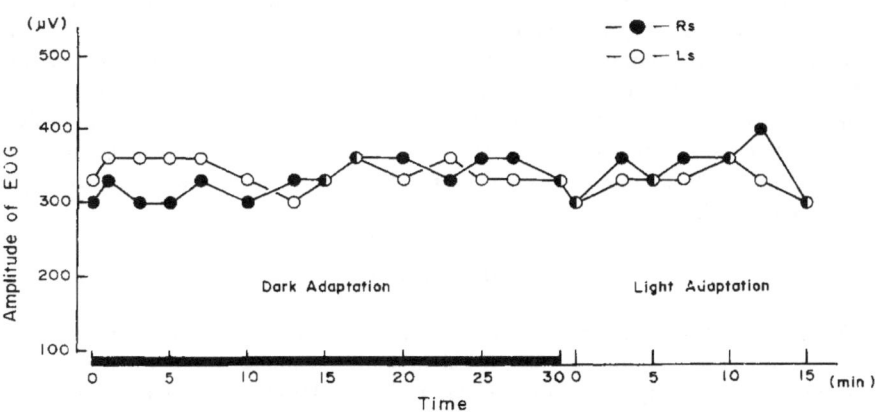

Fig. 2. EOG recorded from this case.

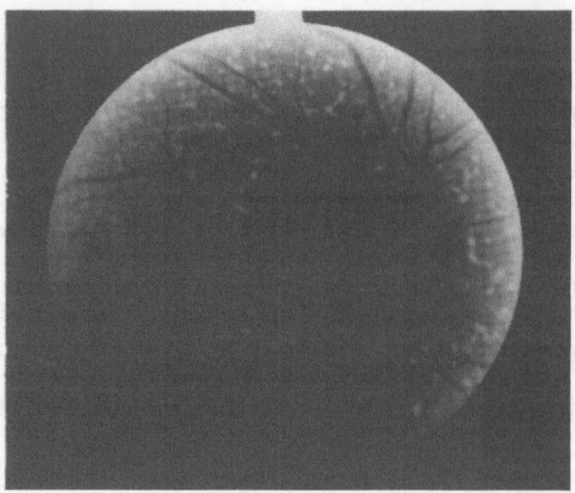

Fig. 3. Right eye. Aspect of 5.1 sec after intravenous fluorescein injection. Flavimaculatus lesions showing pseudo-fluorescence.

to the flecks and appeared from the early arterial phase, became most distinct in the venous phase. Some of those spots increased in size in the venous phase with time. (compare Figure 5, a and b and Figure 6, a and b). The number of the fluorescent spots seemed to exceed that of the flecks. Furthermore, fluorescent spots were observed even around the macula where the flecks were scarecely seen by ophthalmoscopy. It was peculiar that the distinctly visible flecks at midperiphery did not show marked fluorescence in the early arterial phase, whereas clear fluorescent spots appeared at the paramacular and peri-papillar regions, where the flecks were not distinct by the ophthalmoscopic observation. When the dye completely disappeared from retinal vessels, the fluorescence in the flecks also faded out to a considerably extent, but, as shown in Figure 7, remained subsequently for a period of time. The outline of each of the remaining fluorescent spots was relatively sharp. Since the patterns of remaining fluorescence at the late venous phase closely resembles that obtained without injection of the dye (Figure 4), it is assumed that the fluorescence-staining is at least for a major part of the spots, due to the phenomenon of pseudo-fluorescence. In the macular region, fluorescence appeared at the early arterial phase, increased in brightness faster than that of the flecks. An extravasation or delayed retinal circulation-time could not be recognized through the entire course of the angiography.

DISCUSSION

The results of experiments of visual functions on the present typical case of the fundus flavimaculatus resembled in many respects those on other cases reported previously by others (HOLLWICH, 1963, FRANCESCHETTI & FRANCOIS, 1965, CARR, 1965, KRILL & KLIEN, 1965, KRILL, 1966, ERNEST & KRILL, 1966, KLIEN & KRILL, 1967, AMALRIC, et al.,

1967). Considering from the results of the examinations of visual acuity, visual fields, color sense, dark-adaptation threshold and ERG, the disorder of visual function in the present case seems to be attributable mostly to the lesion of the macula; therefore, the present case might belong to group II of this disease, a type with atrophic macular lesion, as classified by KLIEN & KRILL (1967).

The ERG of fundus flavimaculatus has been reported to show a minor abnormality or to be mostly normal. KRILL (1966) realized, however, by an analysis of b-wave amplitudes during dark-adaptation process, that in

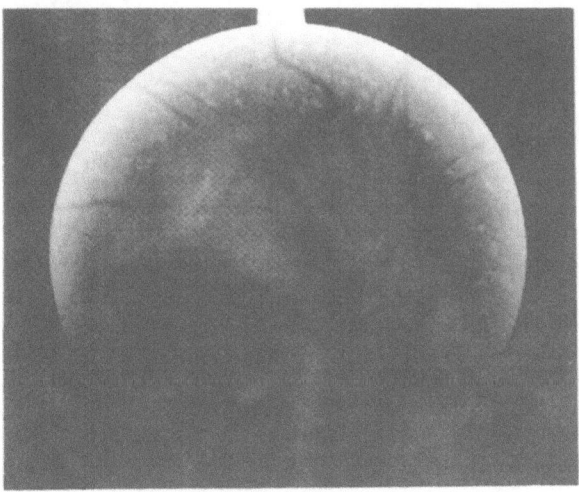

Fig. 4. Right eye. This was taken under the same condition as Fig. 3 without injection of the dye. Note similarity in appearance to Fig. 3.

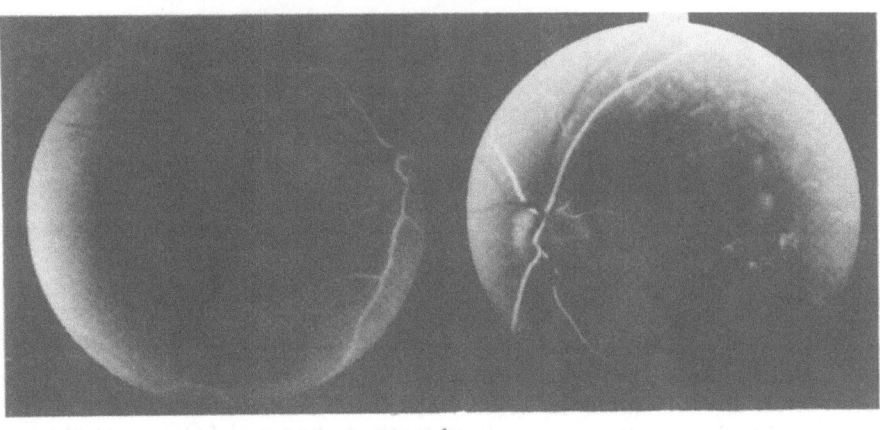

a   b

Fig. 5. The early arterial phase at 12.5 sec in a, and 12.8 sec in b after the dye injection. The border of the flecks is indistinct.

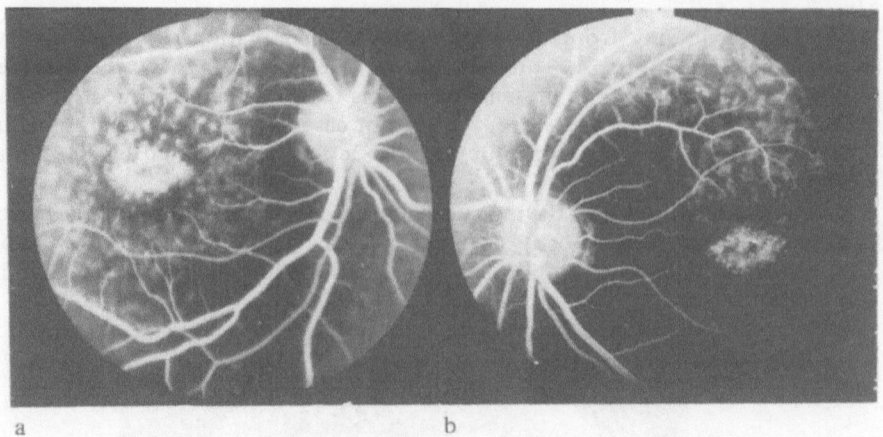

a   b

Fig. 6. The venous phase at 22.6 sec in a, and 24.3 sec in b after the dye injection. There are more fluorescent spots than ophthalmoscopically observed lesions in the paramacular region.

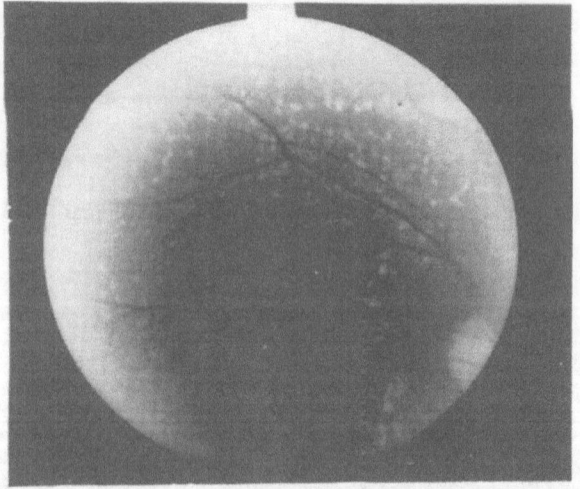

Fig. 7. Right eye. Approaximately 52 minutes after the dye injection. Flavimaculatus lesions show fluorescence-staining with a relatively clear border, closely resembling Fig. 4. Note the dye has completely disappeared from the retinal vessels.

14 cases out of 15, there was a delay in growth of b-wave amplitude with increasing dark-adaptation.

There are very few reports concerning EOGs recorded from fundus flavimaculatus, but in the present study marked abnormal EOGs were obtained from both eyes. KLIEN & KRILL (1967) reported that EOGs from 14 cases (25 eyes) out of 18 cases (33 eyes) were subnormal, and suggested that the abnormality of EOG was responsible to a widely spread disorder of the

74

pigment epithelial cells. No comments were made, however, referring to the normal EOG obtained from 4 cases (8 eyes).

KLIEN & KRILL (1967) felt, on the basis of an enucleated globe with this disease, that a principal histopathological change was a deposit of acid mucopolysaccharide in pigment epithelial cells, which possibly represented the characteristic flecks, seen by ophtalmoscopic examination. In fact, the flecks seen in the present case were located deep in the retina and the surface was revealed to be smooth by slit lamp examination.

KRILL (1965, 1966) emphasized the importance of fluorescein fundus angiography in the differential diagnosis of flecked retina syndrome. There have been some reports concerning the findings of the angiography of this disease (ERNEST & KRILL, 1966, KLIEN & KRILL, 1967, AMALRIC, et al., 1967, OGINO, et al., 1970, WATANABE, et al., 1971), and most of them pointed out a characteristic that fluorescent dots appeared from the early arterial phase coincidently with the flecks, then increased in brightness during the venous phase, and persisted until the dye had disappeared from the retinal vessels.

However, as described above, we recognized the flecks were fluorescent, perhaps due to a pseudo-fluorescence, even prior to the early arterial phase. Furthermore, fluorescence of the flecks persisted even after the injected dye completely disappeared from the retinal vessels. Such a pattern of angiography is evidently different from that seen in retinitis pigmentosa, where shows a delayed retinal circulation time (IMAIZUMI, 1972) Therefore, the statement in other articles, that fluorescence remains long in the flecks of fundus flavimaculatus, should be reconsidered.

SUMMARY

A typical case of 25-year-old male with fundus flavimaculatus has been reported. The peripheral visual fields were normal, but a central scotoma and a slight disturbance of dark-adaptation threshold were found. Normal ERG and heavily depressed EOG were obtained. In the fluorescein fundus angiography, pseudo-fluorescence was recognized within the flecks before the early arterial phase. Fluorescence-staining of the flecks persisted even after the injected fluorescent dye completely disappeared from the retinal vessels.

REFERENCES

AMALRIC, P., KMENT, H. & RENKY, H.: *Klin. Mbl. Augenhk.*, 150: *625-636* (1967).
CARR, R.E.: *Arch. Ophthal.*, 74: *163-168*: (1965).
ERNEST, J.T. & KRILL, A.E.: *Amer. J. Ophthal.*, 62: *1-6*: (1966).
FRANCESCHETTI, A. & FRANCOIS, J.: *Arch. Ophthal. (Paris)*, 6: *505-531* (1965).
FRANCESCHETTI, A.: *Trans. Amer. Acard. Ophth. Otolaryn.*, 69: *1048-1054* (1965).
HOLLWICH, F.: *Klin. Mbl. Augenkl.*, 143: *817-829* (1963).
IMAIZUMI, K.: *Acta. Soc. Ophthalm. Jap.*, 73: *2347-2496* (1969).
IMAIZUMI, K., TAZAWA, Y., IMAIZUMI, S. & MITA, K.: Fluorescein Angiography (ISFA), Igakushoin LTD, Tokyo, *212-218* (1972).
KLIEN, B.A. & KRILL, A.E.: *Amer. J. Ophthal.*, 64: *3-23* (1967).
KRILL, A.E. & KLIEN, B.A.: *Arch. Ophthal.*, 74: *496-508* (1965).

KRILL, A.E.: *Jap. J. Ophthal.*, 10 (Suppl),: *293-300* (1966).
OGINO, T., HASEBE, N., UCHINO, M. & YOSHIDA, M.: *Jap. Review Clin. Ophthal.*, 64: *319-322* (1970).
WATANABE, T., TAMAI, A. & MATSUURA, H.: *Folia. Ophthal. Jap.*, 22: *88-91* (1971).
YURI, H., AKABANE, N. & TAZIMA, Y.: *Jap. J. Clin. Ophth.*, 23: *604-608* (1969).

A PATTERN STIMULUS FOR OPTIMAL
RESPONSE FROM THE RETINA[1]

C. BARBER & N.R. GALLOWAY

(Nottingham, England)

INTRODUCTION

The importance of edges and sharp intensity contours in visual stimuli has led to great popularity for the checkerboard pattern stimulus since SPEHL-MAN (1965) reported a bigger response from a flashed checkerboard pattern than from a plain flash. Other patterns have been compared with it but is generally acknowledged to be the most effective type of stimulus for producing a large evoked response (WHITE, 1969; VAN DER TWEEL & SPEK-REIJSE 1973). In clinical applications, and particularly where threshold detection may be involved, this is clearly an advantage.

The amplitude of the evoked response depends upon the size of checks in the pattern (SPEHLMAN, 1965; RIETVELD, TORDOIR, HAGENOUW, LUBBERS & SPOOR, 1967; HARTER & SUITT, 1970; HARTER & WHITE, 1970) and it has been shown that there is an optimum check size, subtending a visual angle of 10'-30' of arc, for maximal response (RIET-VELD et al 1967; HARTER & WHITE, 1970). Using checks of 20.5' RIET-VELD et al (1967) showed that for both photopic and scopotic response the contribution from the retina outside a subtense of 4° was minimal. However, MICHAEL & HALLIDAY (1971) have shown that with 50' checks the contribution from the peripheral retina (4°-16° subtense) is roughly equal in magnitude to that from the central 4°. HARTER (1970) demonstrated the dependence of optimum check size on retinal eccentricity.

Hence, it appears that a checkerboard can be optimised for central or peripheral stimulation, but not for both simultaneously. To do this the check size must increase progressively with eccentricity of retinal stimulation. We describe here a preliminary attempt to design such a stimulus. This should, if successful, produce a larger response than a checkerboard of any check size.

METHOD

Design of Stimulus Pattern

HARTER (1970) has produced data relating the optimum check size (for the production of maximum amplitude of one component of the VER) with

1. This study was supported by a clinical research grant from the Sheffield Regional Hospital Board. We would like to thank Mrs. C. Sills for valuable technical assistance.

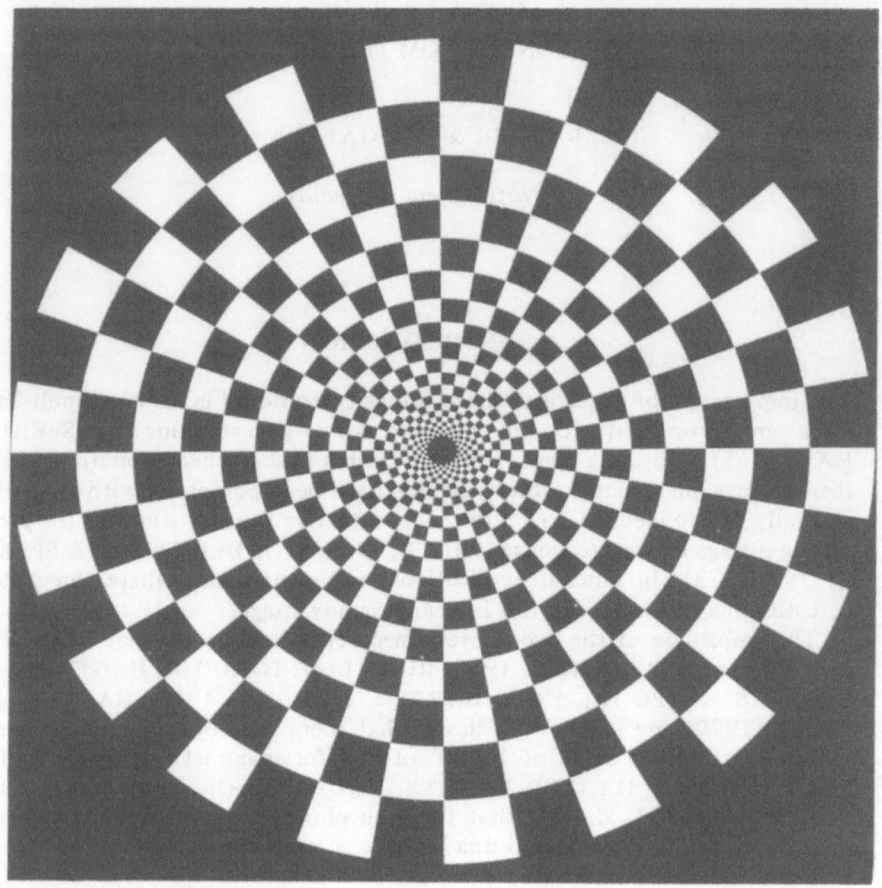

Fig. 1. The dartboard pattern used as stimulus.

retinal eccentricity which can, within certain limits, be approximated to a linear relationship. This relationship and the fact that, for a given check size, a square elicits a larger response than a diamond shape (RIETVELD et al, 1967) is used to derive the angle between successive radial divisions ($\theta = 10°$) and the ratio of successive circular divisions ($r_{n+1}/r_n = 1.173$) in the stimulus pattern. (Fig. 1) We have called this a 'dartboard' stimulus. It was produced photographically on a 35 mm slide.

One immediately obvious difference between this pattern and a checkerboard is that this contains checks of various orientations. However, this should have no effect on the response. RIETVELD et al (1967) found the responses to a checkerboard to be unchanged as it was rotated through 360° and CIGANEK (1971) has produced similar responses from checkerboards orientated normally and rotated through 45°.

Such a pattern clearly lends itself to pattern reversal techniques although in this study it was used solely as a flashed pattern.

Stimulation and Recording System

The stimulus patterns were flashed onto a back-projection screen by equipment derived from a slide projector. The light beam was chopped by means of a semicircular shutter driven by an electronically controlled stepper motor. This gives wide and independent variation of flash duration and repetition rate.

The subjects viewed the screen from a distance of 0.94 m so the pattern subtended a total visual angle of 30°. The checks in the dartboard subtended 5' at an eccentricity of 0.5° (inner limit) and increased to 140' at the periphery. A further seven slides of checkerboards with checks subtending 10', 15', 20', 30', 45', 60' and 120' respectively, were used, and one of these (10') was also defocussed to provide a 'blank' slide. An opaque dot, which coincided with the central blank area of the dartboard pattern, was sited in the centre of the screen and this, dimly illuminated so as to be visible at all times, was used as the fixation point.

The stimulus was flashed onto the screen for a period of 100 ms at a frequency of 1.1 Hz. The rise-time was 10 ms. The intensity was set at approximately 3.5 log units above threshold for the conditions of the experiment. A constant noise source masked auditory stimuli from the rotating shutter.

Normal silver/silver chloride EEG electrodes were used; the active electrode placed 2.5 cm above the inion on the midline and the indifferent electrode on the right ear lobe. A vertex position was used for guard. The bandwidth of the amplifying system was 0.1-100 Hz (3 dB points) and the responses were averaged (using a Datalab 102A) before being read out on an XY plotter (Bryans 26000) and recorded on magnetic tape.

Subjects

Two male and two female subjects were used with ages ranging from 21 to 44. All had visual acuities of 6/5, and normal visual fields.

Experimental Design

The nine stimulus patterns (blank, seven checkerboards and dartboard) were presented in random order to each subject on four separate occasions. Subjects were seated comfortably in a dental chair with adequate neck support, but no chin rest or bite bar, and told to fixate on the central spot and concentrate on the stimulus. Each run of 128 flashes was preceded by one minute of dark adaptation and two flashes to gain the subject's attention.

RESULTS

Visual comparison of the responses evoked by the dartboard stimulus shows them to be qualitatively similar to those from checkerboards. The superimposed traces show good intra-subject consistency (Fig. 2).

Components which are visible in nearly all responses are a positive peak

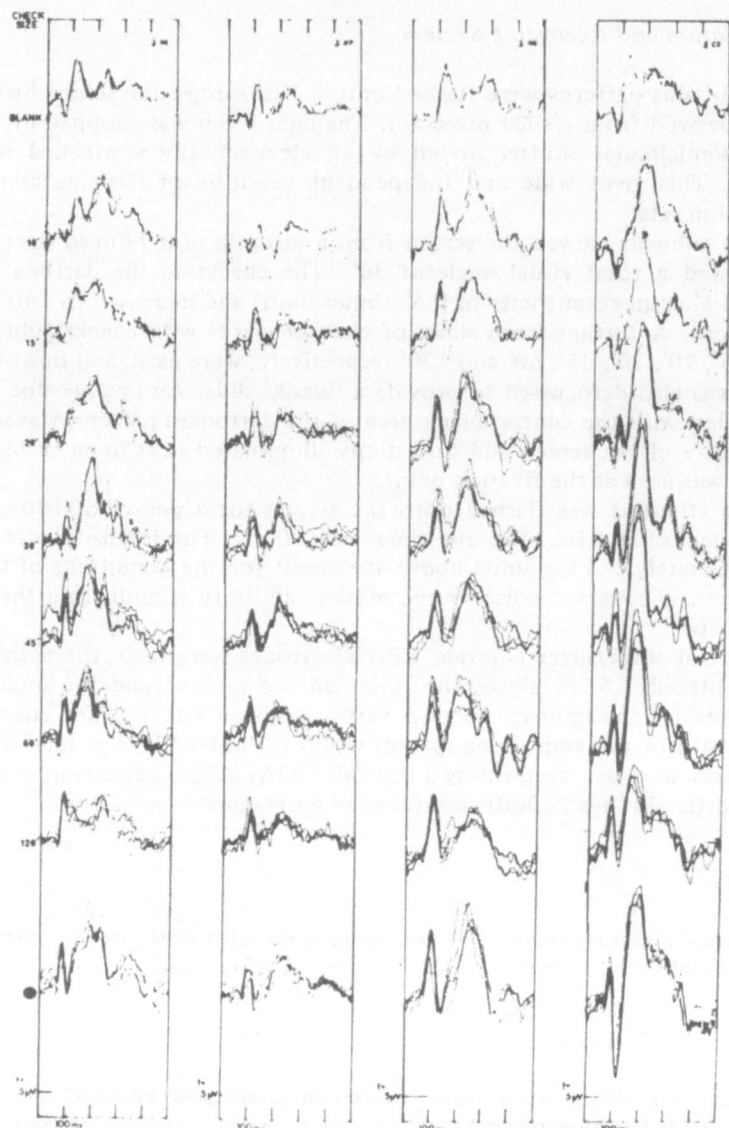

Fig. 2. The VER's produced. Superposition shows consistancy of each subject's responses and large inter-subject differences. Each superimposed trace is the average of 128 responses.

at 90-100 ms latency, a negative peak at 105-130 ms latency and a positive peak at 180-250 ms latency. (Fig. 3) The second and third of these are identified as the 'surface-negative' and 'surface-positive' components used by HARTER (1970) and mentioned by SPEHLMAN (1965) and RIET-VELD et al (1967). All three components are similar, but of greater latency, to those reported by SPEKREIJSE, VAN DER TWEEL & ZUIDEMA (1973)

80

for pattern appearance and designated I, II and III respectively. This notation will be used hereon. The responses do, in fact, seem to be almost entirely 'on' responses (Fig. 4).

The shape of the curves relating amplitudes of components II and III to check size (Fig. 5) is similar to that reported for central stimuli by RIETVELD et al (1967) and HARTER & WHITE (1970), but the peak occurs at 35' of arc instead of the 10'-30' reported by these authors. The amplitude of component I increases with check size, the rate of increase falling off for the larger checks.

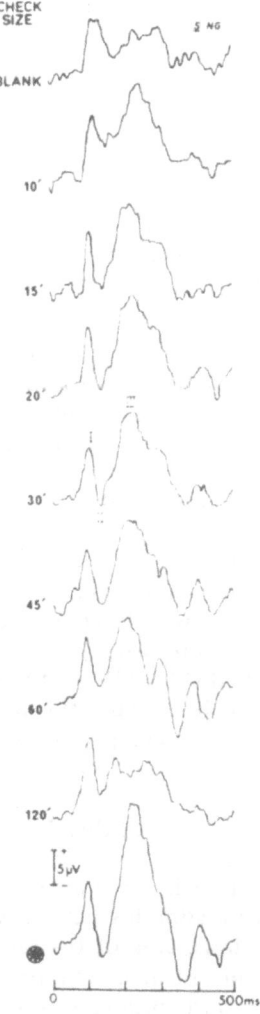

Fig. 3. One set of VER's showing the variation in checkerboard response with check size, and the similarity of form but larger amplitude of the dartboard response (denoted by ●). Note components I, II and III. Stimulus duration 100 ms, total field 30°. Each trace is the average of 128 responses.

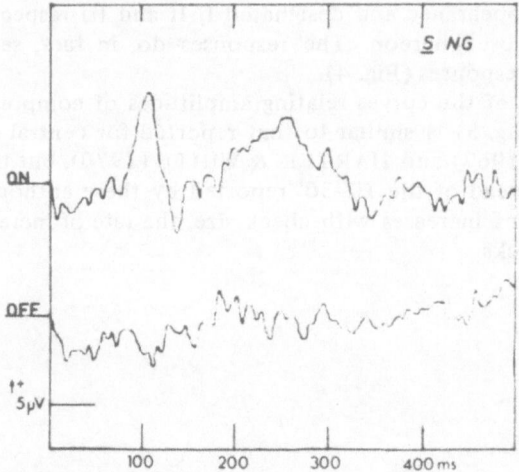

Fig. 4. Responses to pattern-appearance and pattern-disappearance with dartboard stimulus (average of 128 responses). The 'on' response is very similar to the flash response and there is little 'off' response. This may be due to the fairly slow (10 ms) rise-time and fall-time of the flash.

The most prominent feature of both checkerboard and dartboard responses is the triphasic wave I-II-III. To provide a quantitative criterion for the comparison of responses the peak amplitude of II relative to the mean peak amplitude of I and III was determined. The variation in this criterion with check size shows the expected peaking, although there is considerable inter-subject variation in optimum check size (Fig. 6).

The response size evoked by the dartboard stimulus is shown, for each subject, on the same graph. In all cases it is considerably larger than the best checkerboard response; there is an average increase of some 30%. It is interesting to note that the subjective effect of the darboard seemed greater. Some subjects reported an impression of a 'jumping-about' of the checks similar to that described by REGAN (1972) for pattern reversal stimulation.

In some cases it was possible, using the dartboard stimulus to obtain quite reasonable records by averaging only a small number of responses (Fig. 7).

DISCUSSION

The main result is to show that it is possible, using even grossly simplifying approximations, to produce a stimulus pattern which evoked a more nearly optimum response from a large area of the retina. This pattern, which we have called a 'dartboard' produced qualitatively similar, but significantly larger, evoked responses than the best checkerboard for each of the subjects tested.

The form of the checkerboard responses is very similar to those described by SPEKREIJSE et al. (1973). The latencies are greater for each component but this may be due to the slower rise-time of our stimulus and

82

the correspondingly slow fall-time may explain the virtual absence of an 'off' response (VAN DER TWEEL, SPEKREIJSE & REGAN, 1969). The similarities are suprising, however, in view of the fact that SPEKREIJSE et al. used a constant luminance pattern appearance system whereas these responses were produced by a simple flashed pattern and must contain a large luminance component. The gradual increase in amplitude of com-

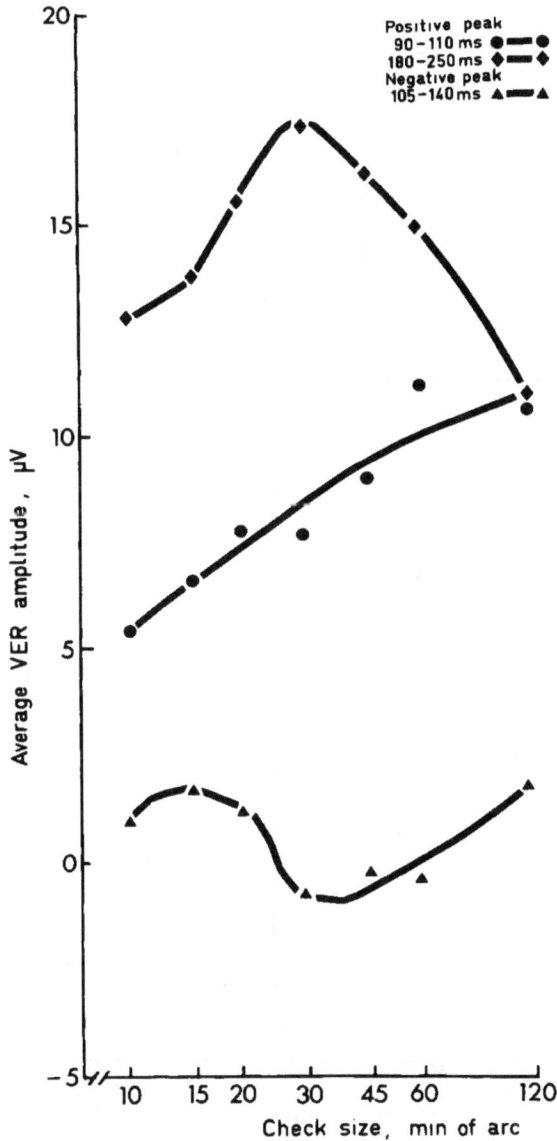

Fig. 5. Amplitudes of the components I, II and III in the checkerboard response as a function of check size. Data have been combined across subjects and replications; each point represents the average of 16 VER's.

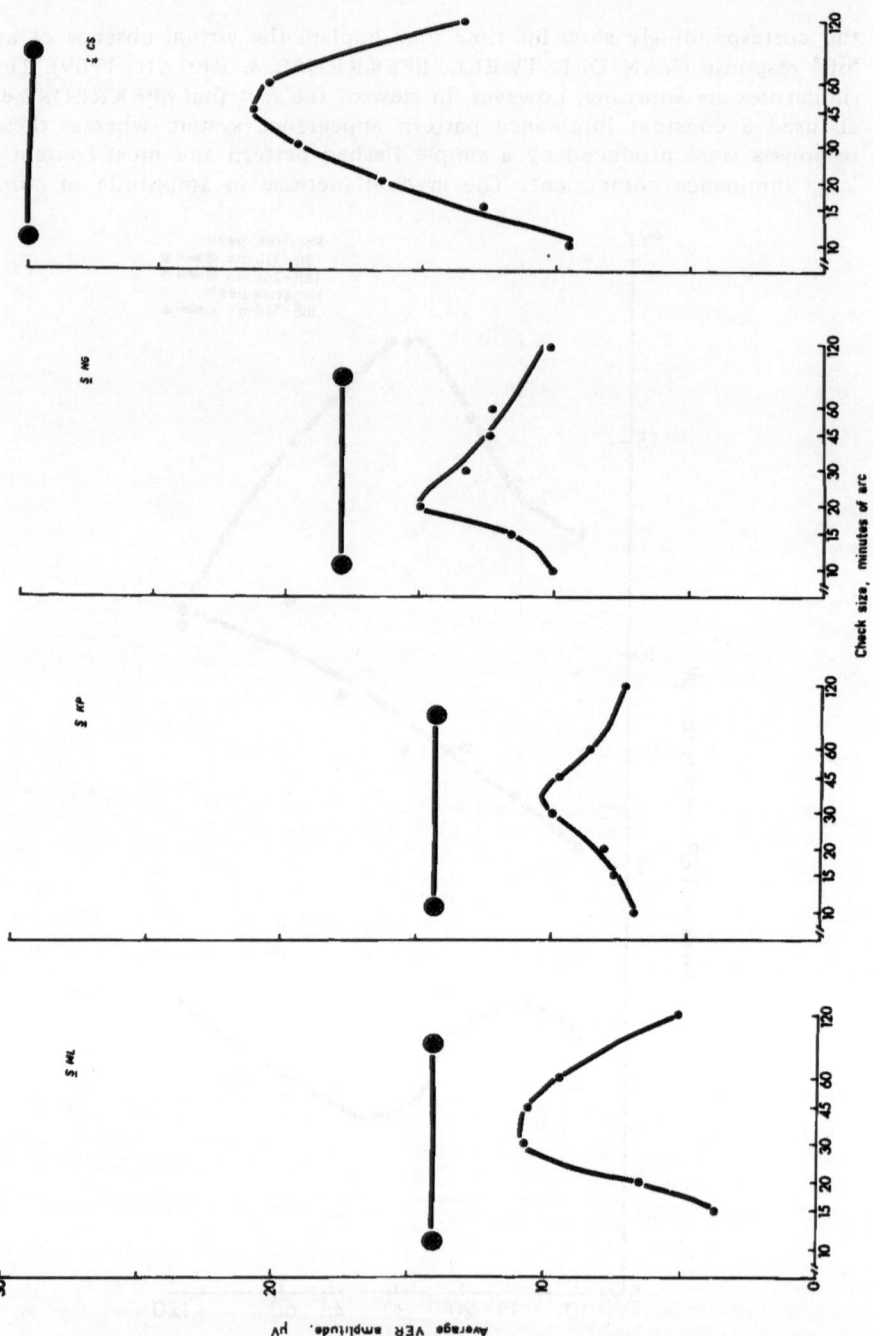

Fig. 6. VER amplitude (mean of peak-to-peak amplitudes I-II and II-III), for checkerboard responses as a function of check size. The value obtained for the dartboard response is shown thus: ⬤ — ⬤. Data have been combined across replications; each point represents the average of 4 VER's.

ponent I with check size is in accordance with the view of JEFFREYS (1971) that this component originates in the peripheral area. For a large field of small checks the response is essentially a pattern plus luminance response from the fovea plus a luminance response (unresolved pattern) from the peripheral area. Increasing the check size must increase the proportion of pattern response from the peripheral area, suggesting that this component is pattern-specific. The optimum sheck size for maximising components II and III was found to be 35' compared with 10'-30' reported previously (RIETVELD et al, 1967; HARTER & WHITE, 1970). The total stimulus field was larger in this study and presumably the shift reflects a greater peripheral contribution for the larger check size. The relatively large fixation spot used would also tend to diminish the central contribution and thus shift the peak away from the smaller check sizes.

Although the dartboard stimulus described does evoke considerably larger responses than an optimum checkerboard there are a number of modifications which suggest themselves. The most obvious concerns the central 1°. This is really too large to use as a fixation spot and may well reduce the response amplitude by some 10%; an obvious disadvantage in a stimulus intended to evoke a large response. The centre could simply be filled by a (say) 20' checkerboard, but this would give a discontinuity at the junction. A better way would be to double each side of the checks at a convenient radius. If this were done at 3° the relation between check size and eccentricity would be a better fit to the data produced by HARTER (1970). It has been shown by EASON, WHITE & BARLETT (1970) that, for approximately 9° fields, the optimum check size in a checkerboard pattern is dif-

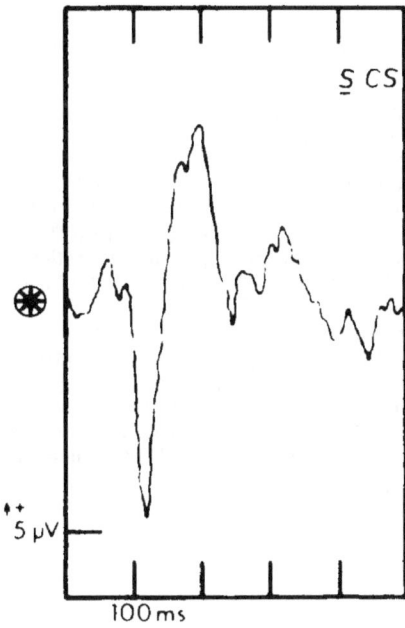

Fig. 7. VER to dartboard stimulus; average of only 8 responses.

ferent for upper and lower field stimulation. A more sophisticated improvement would be to take account of this variation.

SUMMARY

When using a checkerboard pattern for the stimulation of visually evoked cortical potentials the check size required for a maximal response is dependent upon the eccentricity of the check from the optic axis. A stimulus is described with a check size which increases progressively with eccentricity; this has been designed to elicit a maximal response from the peripheral as well as central retina. Responses obtained when using this stimulus pattern are compared with those obtained using various sized checks in uniform checkerboard patterns.

REFERENCES

CIGÁNEK, L. Binoculor addition of the visual response evoked by dichoptic patterned stimuli. *Vision Res.* 11, *1289-1297* (1971).

EASON, R.G., WHITE, C.T. & BARTLETT, N. Effects of checkerboard pattern stimulations on evoked cortical responses in relation to check size and visual field. *Psychon. Sci.*, 21, *113-115* (1970).

HARTER, M.R. Evoked cortical responses to checkerboard patterns: effect of check size as a function of retinal eccentricity. *Vision Res.*, 10, *1365-1376* (1970).

HARTER, M.R. & SUITT, C.D. Visually evoked cortical responses and pattern vision in the infant: a longitudinal study. *Psychon. Sci.*, 18, *235-237* (1970).

HARTER, M.R. & WHITE, C.T. Evoked cortical responses to checkerboard patterns: effect of check size as a function of visual acuity. *Electroenceph. Clin. Neurophysiol*, 28, *48-54* (1970).

JEFFREYS, D.A. Cortical source locations of pattern-related visual evoked potentials recorded from the human scalp. *Nature*, 229, *502-504* (1971).

MICHAEL, W.F. & HALLIDAY, A.M. Differences between the occipital distribution of upper and lower field pattern-evoked responses in man. *Brain Res.*, 32, *311-324* (1971).

REGAN, D. In: Evoked potentials in psychology, sensory physiology and clinical medicine. Chapman and Hall, London. (1972).

RIETVELD, W.J., TORDOIR, W.E.M., HAGENOUW, J.R.B., LUBBERS, J.A. & SPOOR, Th. A.C. Visual evoked responses to blank and to checkerboard patterned flashes. *Acta Physiol. Pharmacol. Neerl.*, 14, *259-285* (1967).

SPEHLMAN, R. The averaged electrical responses to diffuse and to patterned light in the human. *Electroenceph. clin. Neurophysiol* 19, *560-569* (1965).

SPEKREIJSE, H., VAN DER TWEEL, L.H. & ZUIDEMA, Th. Contrast evoked responses in man. *Vision Res.*, 13, *1577-1501*.

VAN DER TWEEL, L.H. & SPEKREIJSE, H. Psychophysics and electro-physiology of a evoked by changes in spatial brightness contrast. Proc. 7th. Int. Symp. ISCERG, Instanbul *1-12* (1969).

VAN DER TWEEL, L.H. & SPEKREIJSE, H. Psychophysics and electro-physiology of a rod-achromat. Proc 10th Int. Symp. ISCERG, Los Angeles, *163-174* (1972).

WHITE, C.T. Evoked cortical responses and patterned stimuli. *Am. Psychol.*, 24, *212-214* (1969).

TOPOGRAPHICAL ANALYSIS OF THE PATTERN EVOKED RESPONSE (PER): ITS APPLICATION TO THE STUDY OF MACULAR AND PERIPHERAL VISION IN NORMAL PEOPLE AND IN SOME PATHOLOGICAL CASES

NICOLE LESEVRE[1]

(Paris, France)

For some years, we have been studying the human Pattern Evoked Response (PER) recorded on the scalp and processed by computer, in order to analyse its spatio-temporal organization (LESEVRE REMOND, 1970, 1972, LESEVRE 1973).

It has been said that this PER is almost entirely due to the central foveal area with very little contribution from the peripheral retina (RIETVELD et al. 1967, COBB et al. 1967, REGAN 1972 etc...). Some other authors — after having developed a topographical analysis of the PER over large areas of the scalp and using asymmetrical stimulation (such as half field, quadrants or octants) — have recently suggested that some components of this complex response might reflect the effect of extra-macular stimulation (MICHAEL HALLIDAY 1971, JEFFREYS 1971, 1972, LESEVRE REMOND 1970, LESEVRE 1973, LESEVRE et al. 1973).

The following work has been undertaken in order to estimate and measure — in the case of symmetrical stimulation — the relative contribution of the central and peripheral retina to the various components of the Pattern Response.

This has been done in people with normal vision, as well as in patients with impaired peripheral vision.

METHODOLOGY

1. *Stimulation*

The Pattern Evoked Responses of 10 normal people (young adults with normal binocular vision) and 3 patients with vision limited to the central $2°$ or $4°$ area have been obtained and studied under the following conditions: The stimulus used was a $20°$ square checkerboard made of $40'$ checks. Because the check size is an important stimulus parameter when central and peripheral stimulation of the retina are compared (HARTER 1970), we have also made controls with $20'$ checks, as it seems that this check size gives the best pattern response in the case of central stimulation (RIETVELD 1967, HARTER 1970, LESEVRE REMOND 1972).

(1) Maître de Recherche INSERM. From L.E.N.A. (Dr. A. Remond) Hôpital La Salpétrière, 75634 Paris Cedex XIII.

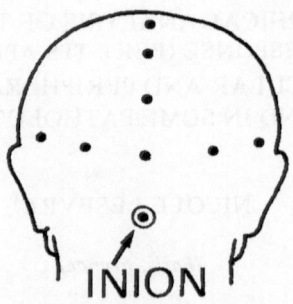

INION

INTER-ELECTRODE
DISTANCE 4 cm

Fig. 1.

Two types of responses have been studied: (a) the response to the appearance of the checkerboard on a luminous background ('on' response). (b) the Pattern Reversal Response obtained with a technique similar to that described for the first time by COBB et al. 1967 (a displacement of the checkerboard is made in order to replace a white square by a black one and *vice versa*, with no change of the overall luminance).

For both types of responses the frequency rate was random around 1 and a half per second (the checkerboard is 'on' for 650 ms and 'off' for about the same time).

The relative contribution of the central and peripheral area to each component of both types of responses have been studied in the following way: (a) presentation of checkerboards of increasing area: $2°$, $5°$, $10°$, $20°$; (b) presentation of patterns consisting of a 20° checkerboard on which a grey uniform central disk was placed, which did not change luminance and did not move during the pattern stimulation; the central uniform disks were of increasing area: $2°$, $5°$, $10°$.

In the 7 experimental situations, the subject was asked to fixate on a point placed at the center of the checkerboard or the uniform disk.

Stimulation was always given for both eyes simultaneously. Two runs, of 70 successive stimulations each, were always made for each of the 7 experimental situations.

2. *Electrophysiological recordings*

The evoked response was recorded with 10 electrodes in line forming a cross montage as seen on Fig. 1, the interelectrode distance being 4 cm. The longitudinal part of the cross is on the midline and goes from a point situated on the Inion (or a little below the Inion) to a point placed 16 cm anterior to the Inion. The transverse part crosses the midline 4 cm above the Inion and extends 8 cm on the right and 8 cm on the left, oriented towards the external border of both eyes (Fig. 1).

In order to have a better image of the potential field over the scalp, bipolar and monopolar derivations were simultaneously recorded. In the case of mono-

20° CHECKERBOARD. (ON)

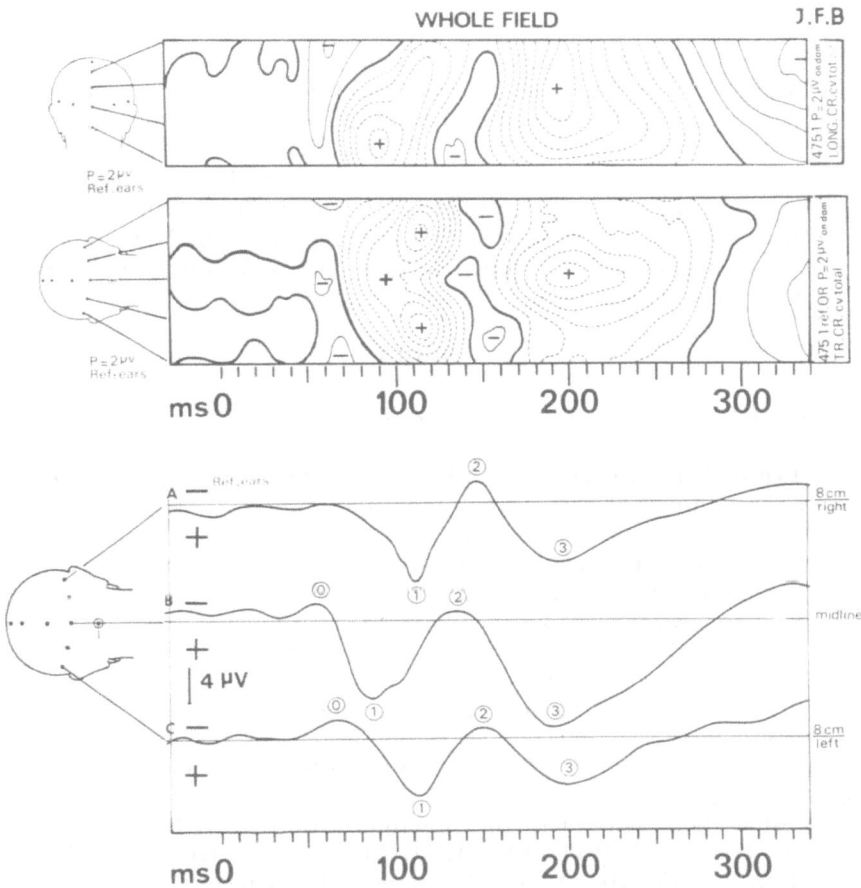

Fig. 2. Typical PER ('on' response) obtained from a normal subject by stimulating with a 20° checkerboard.

Upper part: Spatio-temporal maps of potentials referential to the ear lobes, recorded simultaneously on both arms of the cross montage.

The checkerboard appears at time 0. Only the first 340 ms of the 'on' response are represented here.

As regards polarity, the positive potentials are represented by broken lines, the negative potentials by plain thin lines. Each extrema of potential are marked at the exact place of the scalp where it occurs by the sign + (positive potentials) or − (negative potentials).

Amplitudes are given in the form of isopotential lines. There is a difference in amplitude of 2 μV between two successive isopotential lines.

Lower part: part of the same data seen above but represented in the form of chronograms of potential:

B obtained from the electrode located at the center of the cross, A and C obtained from the most lateral electrode, situated 8 cm away from the midline on the right (A) and on the left (C).

polar derivations, the reference electrode was usually from the two ear lobes (or, in some cases, from a frontal region). The horizontal and vertical eye movements (EOG) were always recorded simultaneously from two other channels in order to control fixation.

3. Data processing

The EEG data was digitized 'on line' (sampling period of 2 ms during the whole epoch of stimulation, that is approximately 1.300 ms). The digital data was then processed by computer (B.G.E. Gamma M 40), which calculated each average response and presented it in the form of a chronogramm and a spatiotemporal map (Fig. 2). Each isolated response occurring during or just after an eye movement was eliminated from the average.

The following results (chronograms and maps) all correspond to *potentials* (monopolar recordings).

RESULTS

I. Study Performed on People with Normal Vision

A. Typical Pattern Response to whole field stimulation (Fig. 2)

Let us first review what the nature is of a typical pattern 'on' response to whole field stimulation (20°), when recorded by an active electrode placed on the midline, 3 to 4 cm above the Inion, and a reference electrode taken from the two ear lobes: The PER appears as being made up of 3 principal components: wave 1, positive, culminating approximately 70-90 ms after the onset of the stimulus; wave 2, negative, peaking between 100 and 130 ms; and wave 3, a long-lasting positive component, beginning 150 to 170 ms after the stimulus and peaking around 200-250 ms. (Fig. 2: Lower part). We have also observed an earlier negative wave of low amplitude which we have called wave 0, as it is not clearly seen in all subjects (Fig. 2.: Lower part).

Most authors agree with this description (SPEHLMANN 1965, RIETVELD et al. 1967, JEFFREYS 1971, LESEVRE REMOND 1970, 1972, BARBER & GALLOWAY in this volume). The latencies vary, of course, according to the physical parameters of the stimulus (X-luminance, contrast, check size, frequency), but remain unchanged when the experimental situation does not change; whereas the amplitude of each component does vary in the same subject from one time to another, even when experimental conditions do not change.

The Pattern Reversal Response is also characterized by 3 successive components but usually of opposite polarity compared to that of the appearance response (COBB & MORTON 1967, REMOND & LESEVRE 1971, HALLIDAY 1972, SPEKREIJSE et al. 1973).

Our own contribution to this description has been a topographical analysis of the PER ('on' response or pattern reversal) achieved with the spatiotemporal mapping method of REMOND (1965). This analysis has shown the following facts (Fig. 2: Maps):

— as far as *transversal* organization is concerned, the response is very symmetrical: each midline peak is followed some 10 to 20 ms later by two

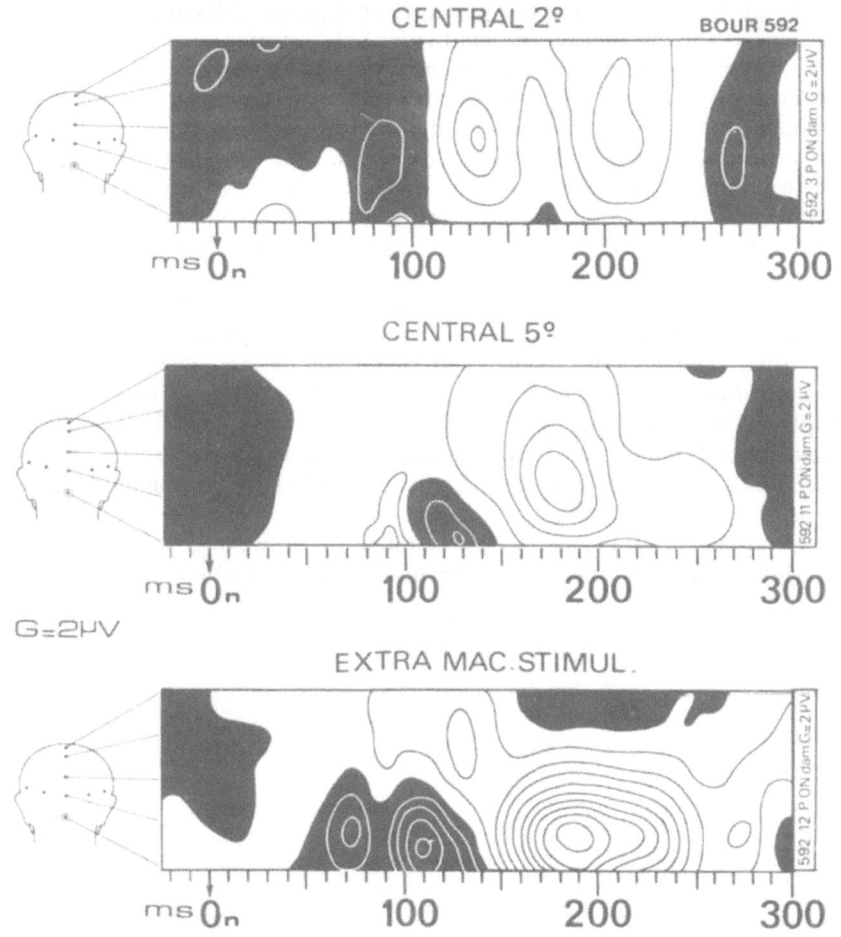

Fig. 3. Topographical study of the PER ('on' response) obtained from a normal subject (different from that of Fig. 1), on the longitudinal part of the cross montage, in 3 different experimental situations:
— upper map: 2° checkerboard
— middle map: 5° checkerboard
— lower map: central 5° uniform disk, covering the center of a 20° checkerboard.
The reference electrode is frontal.
In these maps – and those of the following figures – regions of positivity are in white (with isopotential lines in black) and regions of negativity in black (with isopotential lines in white).
The difference of amplitudes between 2 successive isopotential lines is 2 μV.
Only the first 300 ms of the 'on' response are shown here.
This figure illustrates:
1) The very posterior situation of wave 1 (white) and 2 (black) in the two upper maps (culmination lower than the Inion) compared to that of the lower map (culmination around 4 cm above the Inion); in the lower map wave 1 is only marked by a relative positivity between 2 negative peaks (Waves 0 and 2).
2) The decrease in amplitude of wave 3 (peaking a little before 200 ms) from the lower map to the upper map (peripheral stim. = 18 μV; central 5° = 8 μV, central 2° = 4 μV).

lateral peaks culminating in symmetrical regions, 6-8 cm away from the midline, on the left and on the right (Fig. 2: lower map).

— as far as antero-posterior organization is concerned (the only type of organization we shall be concerned with in this paper), the maxima of potential of the two early waves culminate in posterior regions, (1 to 4 cm above the Inion according to the subject), whereas wave 3 — the long-lasting positive wave — culminates on the midline in more anterior regions (6 to 10 cm above the Inion according to subjects). (Fig. 2: upper map).

This topographical organization of the PER — that is, the absolute place of the maxima of potentials on the scalp and the direction of isopotential lines seen on the maps — does not change, for one and the same normal subject, if the placement of the electrodes and the place of the stimulus in the visual field do not change. This topographical organization constitutes an individual print, somewhat like a finger print, which can be found over months and even years. On the other hand, one does find some topographical differences from one normal subject to the other; but inspite of these absolute inter-individual differences, the relative topographical differences between components remain the same for all the normal subjects we have tested. In other words, the tendency for wave 3 to peak in more anterior regions than the early waves has always been observed.

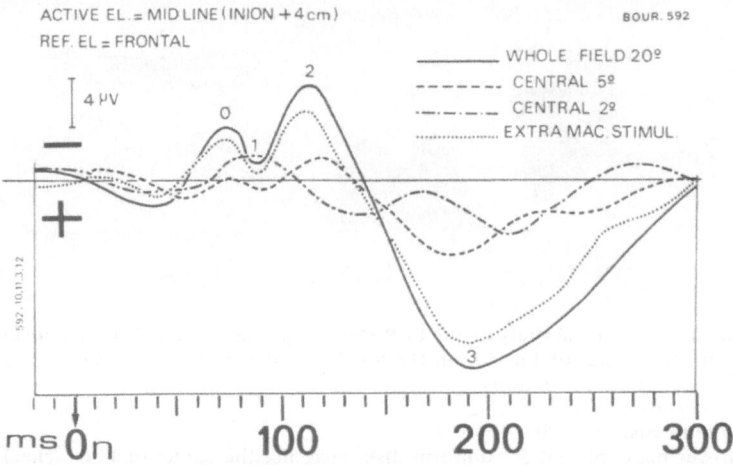

Fig. 4. Comparison of amplitudes of the PER obtained from only one derivation (center of the cross linked to a frontal electrode) from one same subject (same as in Fig. 3) in 4 different experimental situations.
The curves corresponding to 3 of these situations are part of the data shown in the maps of Fig. 3; the response to a fourth situation — whole field — has been added.
Only the first 300 ms of the 'on' response are represented here.
When observed from this only derivation the amplitudes of the 3 components increase when one stimulates only (dotted line) or also (full line) the peripheral retina.
Only a topographical analysis — like that seen in Fig. 3 — can explain why these amplitude comparisons are not correct for the early waves (because they change topography according to the retinal area stimulated) whereas they are correct for wave 3 (which does not change topography).

B. Comparison between whole field stimulation and selective central or peripheral stimulation (Figs. 3, 4 and 5).

A systematic study was achieved by comparing amplitudes, latencies and topographies for the 3 principal components of the PER ('on' response or pattern reversal) obtained in the 7 different experimental conditions utilized. The following results have been obtained:

1. *Early waves*

When observed on the midline of our montage, the two early components change topography as a function of the retinal area stimulated (Fig. 3):

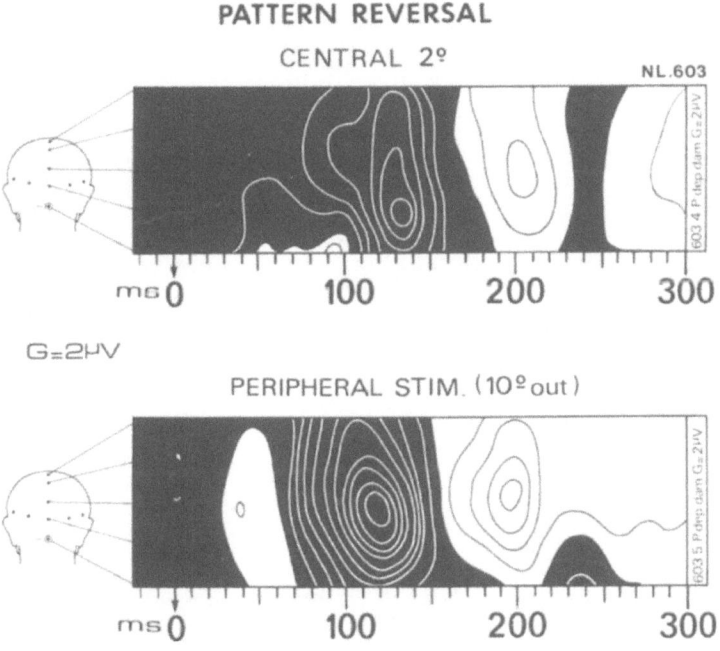

PATTERN REVERSAL

CENTRAL 2°

NL.603

ms 0   100   200   300

G=2µV

PERIPHERAL STIM. (10° out)

ms 0   100   200   300

Fig. 5. Pattern reversal response obtained from a normal vision subject (different from that of other figures), on the longitudinal part of the cross montage, in two different experimental situations:
– 2° checkerboard (upper map)
– 10° uniform disk hiding the center of a 20° checkerboard. (Lower map)
There is an amplitude difference of 2 µV between two successive isopotential lines.
Reference electrode = ear lobes.
Wave 1 (white), beginning around 50 ms in both situations, peaks lower than the Inion on the upper map and 8 cm above the Inion on the lower map.
wave 2 (black) begins around 100 ms and peaks 4 cm above the Inion in the upper map, whereas it begins earlier and peaks 8 cm above the Inion in the lower map.
wave 3 (white), which culminates around 200 ms, does not change topographically but increases in amplitude from 4 µV (upper map) to 8 µV in the case of selective peripheral stimulation.

93

a),– When compared to that obtained with whole field stimulation, the topography seen in the *selective macular stimulation situation* is characterized by a displacement towards more posterior regions of the scalp, such that the maximum of potential culminates lower than the Inion. The maximum of potential being out of our 'montage', no exact measure of amplitude can be taken, so that comparing amplitudes makes no sense in such a case (Fig. 4).

The more the stimulation is limited to the central 2° area, the more

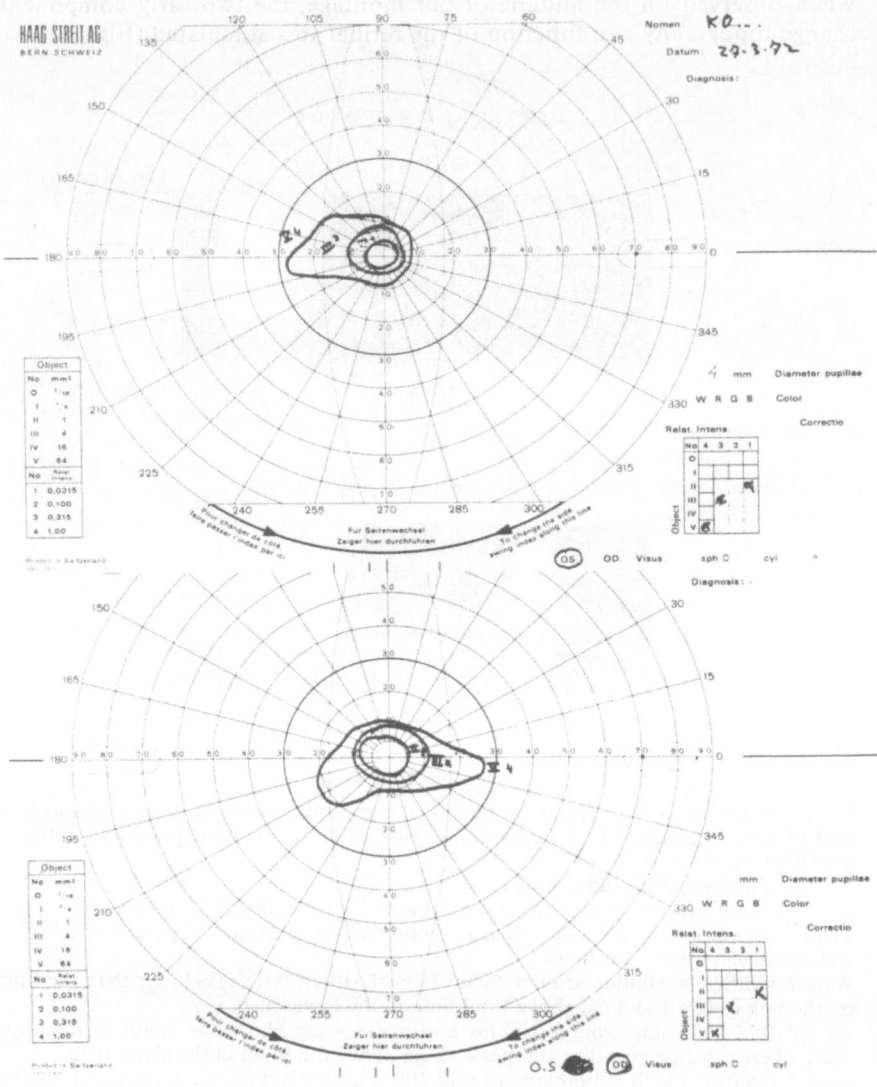

Fig. 6. Visual field of patient whose PER is shown Fig. 8 (Refsum disease).

posterior is the topography of these two components (Fig. 3: two upper maps).

b), – when compared to that observed with whole field stimulation, in the case of *selective peripheral stimulation*, the topography of the early components becomes more anterior, culminating 6 to 10 cm above the Inion, in the same region where wave 3 culminates in the case of whole field stimulation (Fig. 3: lower map).

– The same topographical differences – culmination in regions lower than the Inion for selective foveal stimulation and in much more anterior regions for selective peripheral retina stimulation – have also been observed in the case of *Pattern reversal response* (Fig. 5).

2. *Later wave*

The topography of wave 3 does not change according to the retinal area stimulated, whereas its amplitude does (Figs. 3, 4 and 5):

– In the case of *selective peripheral stimulation*, the amplitude of wave 3 increases or at least remains about the same, compared to that obtained for whole field stimulation.

– In the case of *selective macular stimulation*, the amplitude of wave 3 decreases to such an extent that, in most people, it is barely seen when only the central 2° is stimulated.

These results suggest the following conclusions: (1) When comparing responses from central and peripheral areas, amplitude measurements must take into account the topography of the maximum potential, as far as the two early waves are concerned. Thus, if only one derivation is used (fig. 4), it is not possible to compare these components from amplitude measurements; whereas amplitude may be utilized in the case of wave 3 since its topography does not change according to the retinal area stimulated.

– 2) Wave 3 seems to be essentially related to stimulation of the peripheral area of the retina.

– 3) When one wants to study essentially the macular part of the response under the best conditions, one needs to place some electrodes lower than the Inion.

II *Responses obtained from patients with impaired peripheral vision* *

Only 3 patients with 'tubular vision' (vision limited to the central 2° to 4°) have been systematically studied up to now (unfortunately, it has not yet been possible to study patients with a limited central scotoma).

We shall describe the results obtained from two of them, keeping in mind that this type of experiment-which is long and tiring even for normal subjects – is usually difficult to perform in patients often having fixation problems.

Concerning the etiology of these two cases of 'tubular vision', one is retinal, the other is cortical; but both have approximately the same restricted visual field:

* *Acknowledgments:* we wish to thank Dr. F. CHAIN & M. LEBLANC who performed the neurological and part of the ophthalmological examinations of the patients whose PER have been analysed in this work.

The first case is a man of 43 years for whom the diagnosis of 'REFSUM's disease' has been made. The first signs of a tapeto-retinal degeneration occurred in childhood. He actually has a restricted visual field as seen in Fig. 6, with a visual acuity of 6/10 for both eyes. He has practically no night vision (adaptometry curve: Fig. 7).

His pattern 'on' responses to whole field and to selective macular stimulation are shown in Fig. 8, and compared to those of a normal subject. The following results should be emphasized:

— In the case of *whole field response*, the differences with normal responses are striking: there is no wave 3; the early positive wave 1 culminates lower than the Inion, whereas no wave 2 (negative) can be seen. (Indeed, the negative and positive waves which culminate on the first electrode of the montage, 16 cm above the Inion, are probably a rest of alpha activity which, for this patient, was unusually important with eyes open, and extended towards anterior regions of the scalp).

— In the case of *selective macular stimulation*, the patient's response is much more like the normal response, though its onset is delayed: wave 1 peaks at 90 ms in the normal subject, whereas it peaks at 120 ms for the patient.

The second patient is a man of 50 years, in whom a episode of cerebral anoxia occurred after he had tried to hang himself. This led to cortical blindness. Actually, his vision seems to be limited to the central 2° of 3° area, as far as one can tell. His visual field was very difficult to measure. because of his difficulty in controlling his eye movements in the visual field. (This occurred to such an extent that the diagnosis of 'Balint Syndrome' had been first suggested.)

His pattern 'on' responses, obtained by stimulating with a 10° (upper map) or a 5° (middle map) checkerboard; and with a 20° checkerboard, the center of which was hidden by a 10° uniform disk, (lower map) are characterized by:

— a total absence of wave 3 in all three situations;

— the similarity of the response obtained with a 10° and a 5° checkerboard, these responses being made up of only the two early components which culminate, at normal latencies, much lower than the Inion, in a way resembling the central 2° response of normal people.

— a total absence of response in the case of extra-macular stimulation (no significant difference from noise level).

DISCUSSION AND CONCLUSIONS

a) *Early components*

We have seen that in people with normal vision, as well as in patients with only central vision, waves 1 and 2 show a maximum potential lower than the Inion. Moreover, in the normal vision group, selectiva extra — macular stimulation still produce these early waves. In such a case, their topography is extended much more towards anterior regions. These results are in agreement with what is known about the cortical retinal mapping of the striate area, and probably also the extra striate areas (at least area 18). Indeed,

96

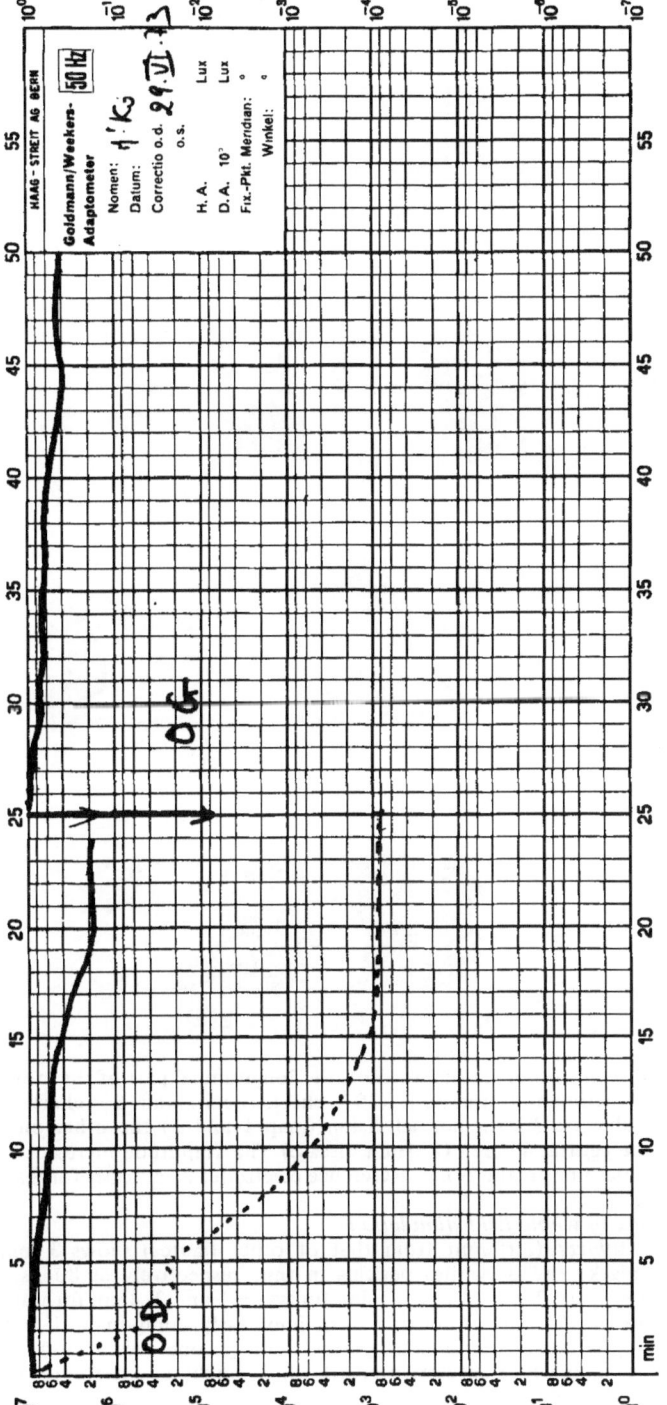

Fig. 7. Adaptometry curve of same patient as that of Fig. 6 and 8.

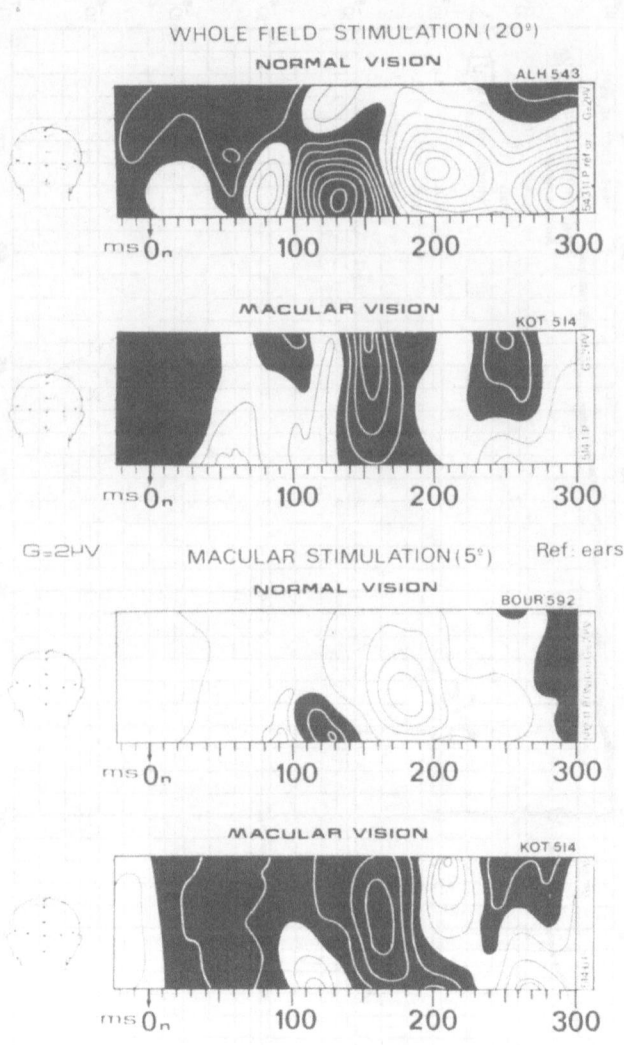

Fig. 8. PER ('on' response) obtained on the longitudinal part of the cross montage in 2 different experimental situations (20° checkerboard and 5° checkerboard from 3 different subjects: 2 with normal vision (map 1 and 3) the other one with vision limited to the central 4° area (Refsum disease) The amplitude increases of 2 μV from one isopotential line to the other. Reference electrode: 2 ear lobes for map 1- 2 and 4; frontal for map 3.

1) *In the case of whole field stimulation*
The normal subject (different from that of other figures) shows 3 components: 1 (white), 2 (black) and 3 (white) peaking in time respectively at 80 ms, 130 ms and 200 ms, and in space 2 cm above the Inion for waves 1 and 2, 4 cm for wave 3.
The response of the patient shows a very poor early component 1 and no wave 3 whatever. In the most anterior part of the montage one sees a kind of rhythmical activity (black and white successive areas) which might be interpretated as a rest of alpha activity (see text).
2) *For selective macular stimulation*, the patient has a better wave 1 peaking below the Inion, and still no wave 3.

98

electrophysiological data obtained in monkeys, and to a lesser extent in man, suggest that the two foveal dipoles are near the occipital pole and that peripheral dipoles are more anterior. Various, – and often contradictory – hypothesis have been suggested with respect to the underlying cortical generators of these two components (HALLIDAY 1972, JEFFREYS 1971, 1972, VAUGHAN 1968, LESEVRE et al. 1973). In any case, our data suggest that both components come from areas with a retinotopic organization.

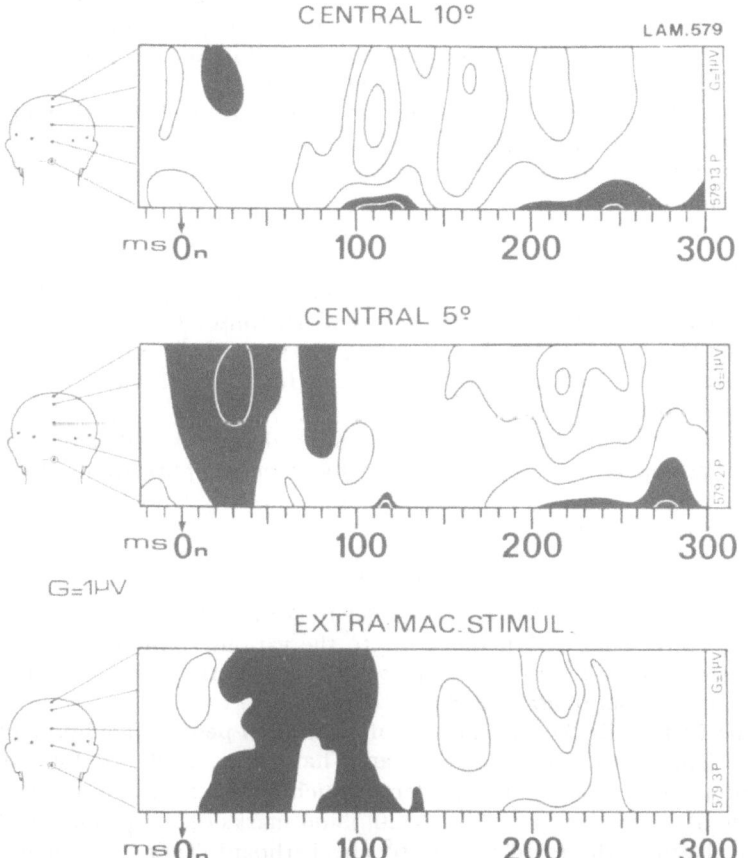

Fig. 9.   PER ('on' response) obtained on the longitudinal part of the cross montage, in three different experimental situations, from a patient with vision limited to the central 3 or 4° area (cortical origin: see text)
Reference electrode: right ear lobe.
There is an amplitude difference of 1 μV between two successive isopotential lines.
the responses to a 10° or a 5° checkerboard are very similar: made up of 2 early components (white and black) peaking lower than the Inion at normal latencies (70 ms and 120 ms); no wave 3 can be seen.
no response whatever can be seen for extra-macular stimulation (the anterior, irregular waves peaking 12 to 16 cm above the Inion might be interpreted as related to the EOG (eye movements 'artefacts')

99

b) *Late component*

We have seen that in people with normal vision wave 3 increases when selective peripheral stimulations are given and decreases with selective macular stimulation; furthermore, that in both patients with exclusive central vision, wave 3 is totally absent.

These results strongly suggest the importance of a peripheral retinal contribution to this late wave. Besides, the relatively anterior topography on the scalp of this wave confirms this hypothesis. Nevertheless, with regard to the visual cortical areas involved in this late wave, many unsolved problems do remain. Unlike that of the early components, the topography of the late wave on the scalp does not change depending on the part of the visual field stimulated (LESEVRE 1972). Would this last result, contrary to the foregoing data, suggest that this late wave 3 does not have its origin in an area having a retinocortical organization?

With respect to the results obtained from the patients we are also faced with many unsolved problems. For instance, why are the early waves delayed when the deterioration of the peripheral vision is of retinal origin and why are not they delayed when it is of cortical origin?

Why is the full-field response in the case of the 'tapeto retinal degeneration' smaller than the selective central 2° response? May it be caused by an inhibitory or overlapping mechanism? If this is the case, how can it be explained that a peripheral retina without function inhibits or overlaps the central retinal area?

Despite it seems to us that a topographical analysis is already very useful insofar as it guards the clinician against an 'over simplification' of the VER, considering it as a 'all or nothing' response based mainly on amplitude and latency values.

SUMMARY

This work has been undertaken in order to evaluate the relative contribution of the central and peripheral retina to the various components of the Pattern Evoked Response (P.E.R.) in people with normal vision as in patients with impaired peripheral vision.

The Pattern Evoked Responses of 10 normal people and 3 patients with vision limited to the central 2° area have been analyzed by computer (spatio-temporal maps). The patterns which served as stimuli were checkerboards of increasing size (2° to 20°) and masks of increasing size (2° to 10°) placed in the middle of a 20° checkerboard. Two types of responses were studied: a) the 'on' response (response to the appearance of a pattern on a luminous background) and b) the pattern reversal response (white square replaced by a black one and vice versa without any change of the overall luminance). The responses were recorded with 10 electrodes (simultaneously bipolar and monopolar leads) forming a cross montage the center of which was situated on the midline 4 cm above the inion.

A — The results obtained from *normal people* showed that:

— The maxima of potential of the two early waves (80 and 120 ms) culminate in more posterior regions than that of the late positive wave (200 ms).

— compared to that of whole field stimulation, the response to selective macular or foveal stimulation is characterized by a displacement of the two early waves towards more posterior regions (below the inion) whereas in the response to selective peripheral stimulation these two waves are displaced towards more anterior regions (6 to 8 cm above the inion).

— The late positive wave decreases in amplitude and tends to disappear in the case of selective macular or foveal stimulation.

B — In all situations the responses obtained from *patients* with impaired peripheral vision were characterized by a very posterior topography of the two early waves (which culminated lower than the inion) and by a complete absence of the late positive wave.

These results suggest the importance of peripheral retina contribution to the late part of the pattern evoked response. The change in topography of the two early waves according to the part of the retina stimulated (central or peripheral) shows the necessity of achieving a topographical analysis of the evoked potential in clinical applications and the danger of only taking into account values of amplitude measured on only one or two derivations.

REFERENCES

COBB W.A., MORTON H.B. & ETTLINGER E., Cerebral potentials evoked by pattern reversal and their suppression in visual rivalry. *Nature* (Lond.), 216: *1123-1125* (1967).

HALLIDAY A.M. Discussion on component Analysis and Topology. TRACE (Paris) 6, 1, *39—46* (1972).

HARTER M.R. Evoked cortical responses to checkerboard patterns: effects of check size as a function of retinal eccentricity. *Vision Res.*, 10: 1365-1376 (1970).

JEFFREYS D.A. Striate and extrastriate origins of pattern-related visual evoked potential (VEP) components. *J. Physiol. (London)*, 211: *29-30* (1971)

JEFFREYS D.A. Component Analysis of the spatial contrast EP. TRACE (Paris), 6: 1-30-38 (1972).

LESEVRE N., Potentiels évoqués par des patterns chez l'homme: influence des variables caractérisant le stimulus et sa position dans la champ visuel. In: 'Activités évoquées et leur conditionnement chez l'homme normal et en pathologie mentale' — Ed. INSERM, Paris, *1-22* (1973).

LESEVRE N., & REMOND A., — Influence des contrastes sur les réponses évoquées visuelles. *Rev. Neurol.*, 122: *505-616* (1970).

LESEVRE N., & REMOND A, — Potentiels évoqués par l'apparition de patterns: effets de la dimension du pattern et de la densité des contrastes. *Electroenceph. clin. neurophysiol.* 32: *593-604* (1972)

LESEVRE N., JOSEPH J.P., RENAULT B. & FINDJI F. A neurophysiological 'model' of the human pattern evoked potential based on charges observed according to the part of the visual field stimulated. *Electroenceph. clin. Neurophysiol*, 34, 7, 722 (1973).

MICHAEL W.F. & HALLIDAY A.M. 1971 — Differences between the occipital distribution of upper and lower field pattern evoked responses in man. *Brain Research*, 32, *311—324* (1971).

REGAN D. — Evoked potentials in Psychology, Sensory Physiology and Clinical Medicine, Chapman and Hall L.T.D., London, *328* (1972).

REMOND A., Topological aspects of the organization processing and presentation of data. In PROCTOR, L.D. & ADEY W.R. (Eds.) The Analysis of Central Nervous System and Cardiovascular Data Using Computer Methods', NASA, Washington, *73-93* (1965).

REMOND A. & LESEVRE N – Etude de la fonction du regard par l'analyse des potentiels évoqués visuels (lumière diffuse, patterns et mouvements des yeux) In: La fonction du Regard, ed. INSERM, Paris, *127-175* (1971).

SPEKREIJSE, H., VAN DER TWEEL, L.H. & ZUIDEMA, Th. Contrast evoked responses in man. *Vision Res.* 13, *1577-1601* (1973).

VAUGHAN H.G. – The relationship of brain activity to scalp recordings of event-related potentials, in E. DONCHIN & D.B. LINDSLEY (Eds), Average Evoked Potentials Methods, Results and Evaluations, NASA, Washington, D.C. *45-94* (1968).

ELECTRO-OPHTHALMOLOGY IN SENILE
MACULAR DEGENERATIONS

Y. OGUCHI, S.F. KOORNSTRA-LUNT, G.H.M. VAN LITH &
A. WITZIER

(Rotterdam, The Netherlands)

INTRODUCTION

Electro-ophthalmological studies of patients affected with a senile macular degeneration have already been described in many previous reports (HENKES 1954, JACOBSON et al. 1956, FRANCOIS et al. 1956, 1957, 1967, JAYLE et al. 1959, RUEDEMANN et al. 1961, NAGATA et al. 1962, DIETERLE 1962, ZETTERSTRÖM 1964, PERDRIEL et al. 1964, KRILL 1966, ROUHER et al. 1966, ARDEN & BANKES 1966, BANKES 1967, PERDRIEL 1969, BIERSDORF & DILLER 1969, NIEMEYER 1969, RUEDEMANN 1969, MERIN & AUERBACH 1970, STANGOS et al. 1970, 1972, GLIEM 1971, SOKOL 1972 and GASS 1973). More often than not, they limit their dealings to the global ERG and EOG. Some authors find a decrease of the scotopic b-wave (HENKES, 1954, JACOBSON et al. 1956, FRANCOIS et al. 1956, DIETERLE 1962, KRILL 1966, NIEMEYER 1969 and GASS 1973), others a decrease of the photopic b-wave (JAYLE et al. 1959, RUEDEMANN et al. 1961, NAGATA et al. 1962, KRILL 1966, PERDRIEL 1969, NIEMEYER 1969 and STANGOS et al. 1972) or a decrease of the critical fusion frequency in the ERG (JAYLE et al. 1959, RUEDEMANN et al. 1961, NAGATA et al. 1962, ZETTERSTRÖM 1964 and KRILL 1966) and/or an abnormal EOG (FRANCOIS et al. 1957, STANGOS et al. 1972 and GASS 1973). When abnormal results are obtained, they are not consistently present. Therefore one can also find little or no changes in the ERG (NAGATA 1962, MERIN & AUERBACH 1970) and in the EOG (KRILL 1966, FRANCOIS et al. 1967). This so-called normal group is intelligible, as it is rather difficult to visualize a local retinal disturbance like a macular degeneration, with an ERG elicited from the whole retina. According to FRANCOIS & DE ROUCK (1964), only a disturbance in the macular area of more than three disc diameters will produce a significant alteration in the global ERG. This is generally not the case in macular degenerations.

Recently, new electro-ophthalmological examination methods, which may be of some help in diagnosing a macular degeneration, have been developed for clinical use. The visually evoked cortical potentials (VECPs) elicited under photopic conditions, represent mainly the function of the central 12° part of the retina (VAN LITH & HENKES 1970). If a pattern reversal stimulus is used instead of a flash stimulus, the representation of the VECPs is even limited to the central 2°-4° area (BEHRMAN, NISSIM & ARDEN 1972). Therefore, the pattern reversal evoked potentials can be expected to be a more exact method in evaluating the foveal function. The local electro-retinogram may also be a useful method in probing the macular function; the smallest recordable response can be obtained with a stimulus of 2° to 3° (ARMINGTON et al. 1961, VAN LITH & HENKES 1968). ARDEN & BANKES (1966) and BANKES (1967) described extinguished foveal ERGs in patients affected with a unilateral macular degeneration. BIERSDORF & DILLER (1969) also studied only macular degenerations by use of the local ERG. They came to the conclusion that macular degenerative patients could be differentiated from normal subjects when the visual acuity dropped to a range of 20/40 to 20/80. SOKOL (1972) studied a 40-year-old patient with a macular degeneration by means of a checkerboard stimulus. The VECPs showed an absence of any measurable signal.

In the present study, patients with senile macular degenerations were examined by means of the ERG and the VECPs, elicited both with local macular (M-ERG and M-VECP) and total retinal (G-ERG and G-VECP) flash stimuli. Furthermore, VECPs were determined with a checkerboard reversal pattern stimulus (P-VECP). The records have been compared with the ophthalmoscopic appearance of the fundus, visual acuity and visual field.

METHOD

The apparatus used for the total and local stimulation has been described in detail previously (VAN LITH et al. 1972). For the macular stimulation, only the 10° stimulus was used. The light source of the stimulus was a xenon flash of 1 joule. A density filter of 1 log unit was used both for the local and global stimulation. All flash responses in the ERG and the VECPs were obtained in the light adapted state, which was achieved with two halogen lamps with a blue filter (Schott BG 25) in front of them. Adaptive illumination of the globe was 3 logasb without the blue filter. After amplification (band width 0.15-500 Hz 6 dB/octave) the responses were averaged, the analysis time being 250 msec. For the local 10° ERG (M-ERG) and VECPs (G-VECP and M-VECP), 300 responses were averaged, while 30 responses were averaged for the global ERG (G-ERG). The VECPs were led off from a 5%-25% positioning of the electrodes in the midline, when the distance between the nasion and the inion was 100%. The ERG's were recorded with a Henkes contact lens. The pupil was dilated by means of Mydriaticum.

The pattern reversal VECPs were obtained by using checkerboard stimuli. The stimulus field subtended a visual angle of 30°. The size of each block was 1°. The stimulus frequency, which was acquired with a constantly moving mirror in front of the projector, was 4 cycles per second. 250 responses were averaged on a CAT computer. The analysis time amounted to 500 msec, thus 2 cycles were recorded. The VECPs were conducted from 15% positioning to the ear. The pupil was not in a state of dilation. Before this examination, the spectacle correction was examined very carefully in order that the subject view the checkerboard as sharply as possible.

The patients studied were from the eye hospital of the Erasmus University of Rotterdam. Visual acuity, refraction and the fixation of the patients were checked. Visual field was examined with a Goldmann perimeter. The macular alterations were observed ophthalmoscopically and fundus photographs were taken.

RESULTS

32 eyes of 17 patients were examined with flash stimulation and 28 eyes of 15 patients by pattern reversal stimulation. The affected eyes were classified into three groups; colloidal (9), disciform (10) and atrophic (13) macular degeneration. In Fig. 1 results of two patients are presented. The first patient has a non-corrigible visual acuity of 0.8 in his right eye. Funduscopically, depigmentation and increased granularity were observed in the macular area and hard white spots in the temporal area, 1 disc diameter away from the macular area. There was no foveal reflex. The visual field obtained with the Goldmann perimetry, was normal (Fig. 2). Electro-ophthalmological examination showed well-developed responses in the G-ERG (145 μV), M-ERG (9 μV), G-VECPs (12 μV), M-VECPs (9.5 μV) and P-VECPs (17 μV).

The second patient had a low vision of only 1/300 of his right eye. The funduscopic findings demonstrated a disciform macular degeneration. In the visual field, a 40° central scotoma was observed (Fig. 2). The amplitude of the photopic b-wave in the G-ERG (50 μV) and the b-wave in the M-ERG (3.5 μV) were low, viz. about 50% of the normal values. The G-VECPs (4 μV), M-VECPs (1.5 μV) and P-VECPs (1.0 μV) were also seriously deteriorated.

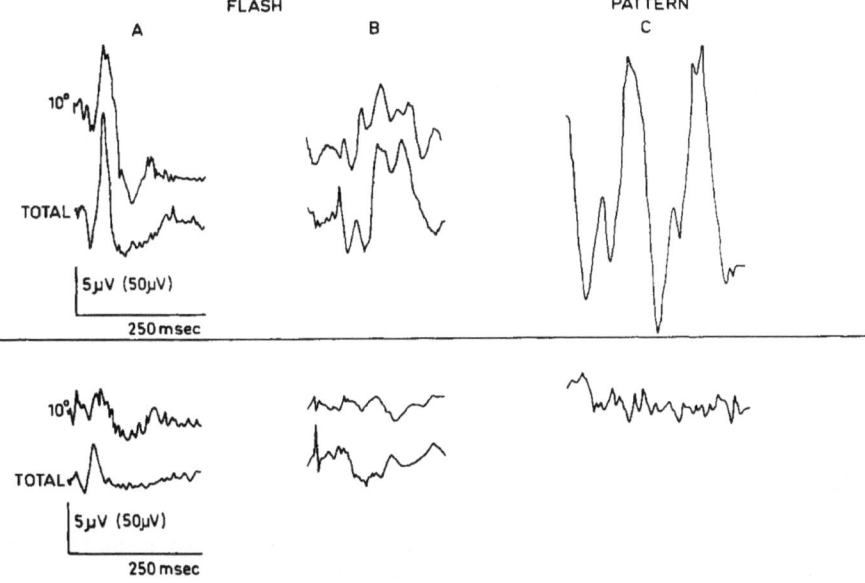

Fig. 1. Electro-ophthalmological results of slightly affected (upper recordings) and severely affected senile macular degeneration (lower recordings). Left 2 recordings: M-ERG and G-ERG; Middle 2 recordings: M-VECP and G-VECP; Right recording: P-VECP. Calibration is 5 μV, except for G-ERG which is 50 μV.

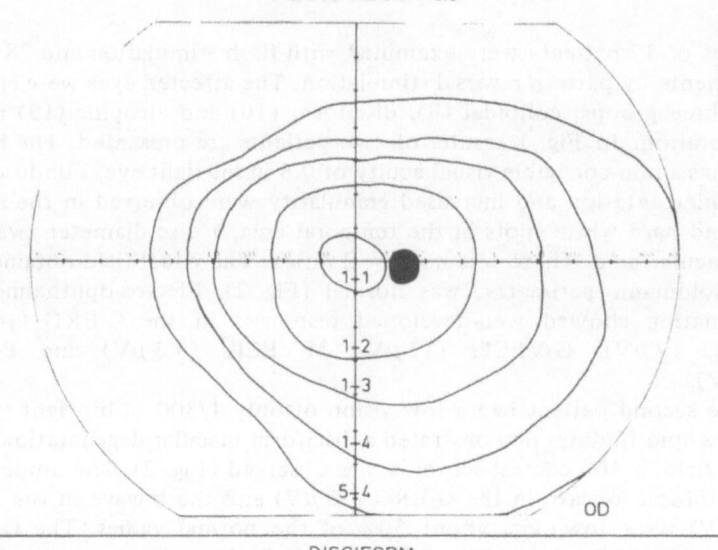

MACULAR DEGENERATION

ATROPHIC

VISUAL ACUITY 0.8

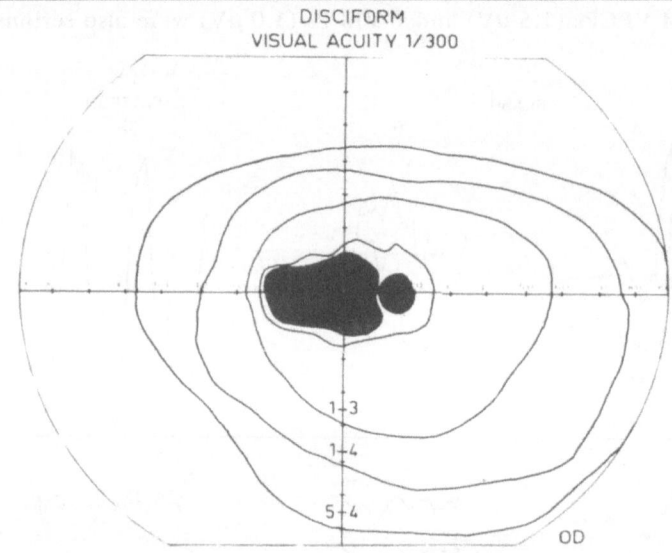

DISCIFORM

VISUAL ACUITY 1/300

Fig. 2. Visual field of slightly affected (upper) and severely affected (lower) patient.

In the entire group of patients, a wide range of responses in the ERG and VECPs were found, from extinguished to well-developed. We first compared the results of our patients with a normal group of the same age. The age of the patient group varied from 53 to 82 years old (70 on the average), that of the normal group from 53 to 71 (60 on the average). The number of eyes in the normal group examined by G-ERG, G-VECP, M-ERG, M-VECP and

P-VECP were 18, 22, 20, 20, and 13 respectively. The combined two groups examined up till now, were not large enough to be evaluated statistically. Some tendencies could be observed between the patients affected with a macular degeneration and the normal subjects.

As for the G-ERG, the height of the photopic b-wave varied from 90 μV to 200 μV in the normal subjects, in the affected group from 30 μV to 150 μV. Approximately 70% of the patients had a photopic b-wave lower than 90 μV (Fig. 3). In the G-VECPs, the difference between both groups seemed to be even less. In the M-ERG the results were better than in the G-ERG, but not as good as those in the M-VECPs. In the normal group, the responses of the M-ERG varied from 8 to 22 μV, in the pathological group from 3 to 24 μV. In the M-VECPs, the differences were more pronounced. The affected group had amplitudes ranging from 0 to 10 μV, the normal group from 6 to 15 μV. Only 8 eyes in the affected group had responses within the range of the normal group. Of these 8 eyes, 6 had a visual acuity of better than 0.6, one of 0.38 and one 1/60.

In the P-VECPs, too, there was much variation in amplitude viz. from 0 to 17 μV in the patients and from 10 to 18 μV in the normals. In 6 pathological eyes, the height of the amplitude was above 10 μV, of which 5 had a visual acuity of over 0.7 and one of 3/30.

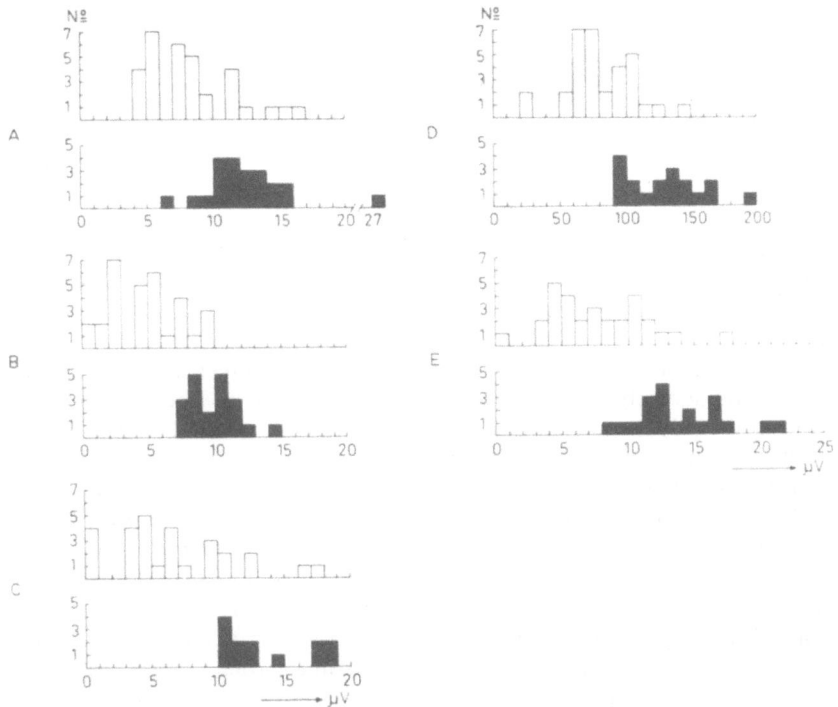

Fig. 3. Electro-ophthalmological results of a senile macular degeneration group (open columns) and a normal group (black columns). From A to E: Data of G-VECP, M-VECP, P-VECP, G-ERG and M-ERG. Abscissa: amplitude of responses. Ordinates: number of patients.

107

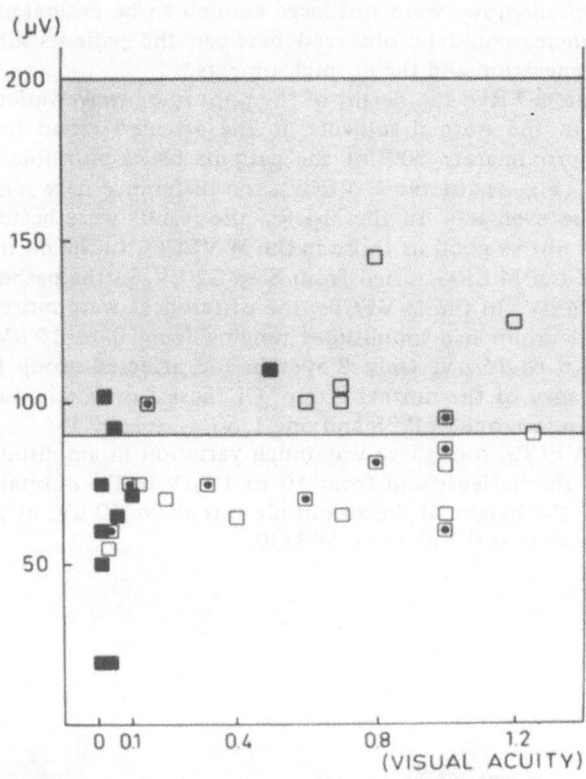

Fig. 4. G-ERG and visual acuity; ■: disciform senile macular degeneration; □: atrophic senile macular degeneration; ▣: colloidal senile macular degeneration. Shadow indicates normal range.

In the affected group, the funduscopic appearances varied from slight changes to severely affected lesions. The severity of the fundus changes could not easily be classified, however. Therefore, visual acuity was compared with the ERG and VECPs. In Figure 4, the amplitude of the photopic b-wave in the G-ERG is plotted versus the visual acuities. There is a tendency that low responses are obtained in the cases with a low acuity, but there is no clear correlation. For the G-ERG we expected such a bad result, but not for the G-VECPs, since the latter is mainly dependent on the central retinal area. The results of the G-VECPs, however, were even worse in comparison to those of the G-ERGs. No correlation at all occurred between the amplitude and visual acuity. Even in some patients with a poor visual acuity in combination with a large central scotoma, high potentials were obtained. In Figure 6 the height of the M-ERG and in Figure 7 that of the M-VECPs are presented. There are still no clear relations, although in the disciform type, the magnitude of potentials are always low when there is a lowered visual acuity and a loss of sensitivity in the central visual field.

Comparative results are obtained in the P-VECPs (Fig. 8). High cortical potentials are observed in patients with a good visual acuity and low potentials in those with a poor vision, yet there are a few patients who combine a good visual acuity with a low pattern response or a low vision with high potentials.

When we compare the electro-ophthalmological finding of patients with a normal visual field with those of patients who have a visual field displaying a central scotoma, some additional conclusions may be drawn. In the intermediate group, no clear relations were seen between the electro-ophthalmological results and the visual field. In the group of 7 cases with a normal visual field, there was a wide variation in the VECPs obtained by flash and pattern stimuli. In the G-ERG and M-ERG, however, one tendency was observed. In the G-ERG, 6 cases showed more than 80 μV in b-wave amplitude and one 60 μV. In the M-ERG, 6 cases had a b-wave of more than 9 μV, while one had a b-wave of 5 μV. In the group of eight subjects with a central scotoma, the G-ERG, M-ERG, M-VECP and P-VECP always presented lower amplitudes than those in the former group. In the G-VECP, there were no clear differences.

The differentiation among three types of macular degenerations should certainly be taken into account, too. There were, however, no definite distinctions among the colloidal, disciform and atrophic types. The only apparent exception lies in the extremely low M-VECPs and P-VECPs in

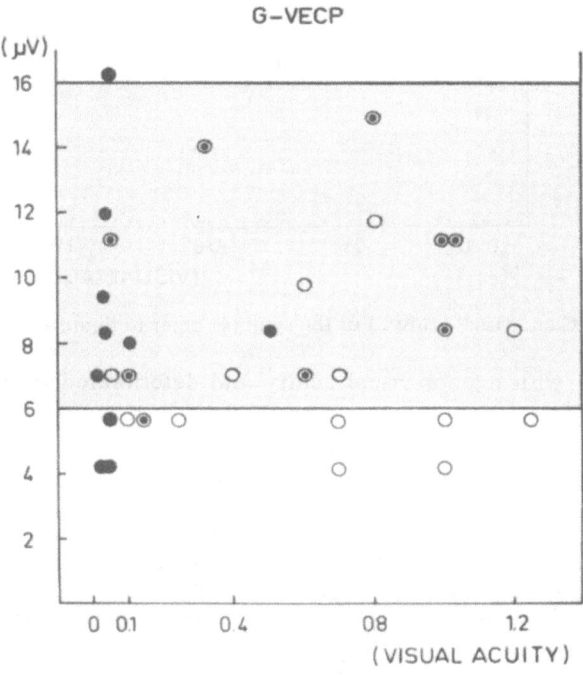

Fig. 5. G-VECP and visual acuity; •: disciform senile macular degeneration; o: atrophic senile macular degeneration; ⊙: colloidal senile macular degeneration. Shadow indicates normal range.

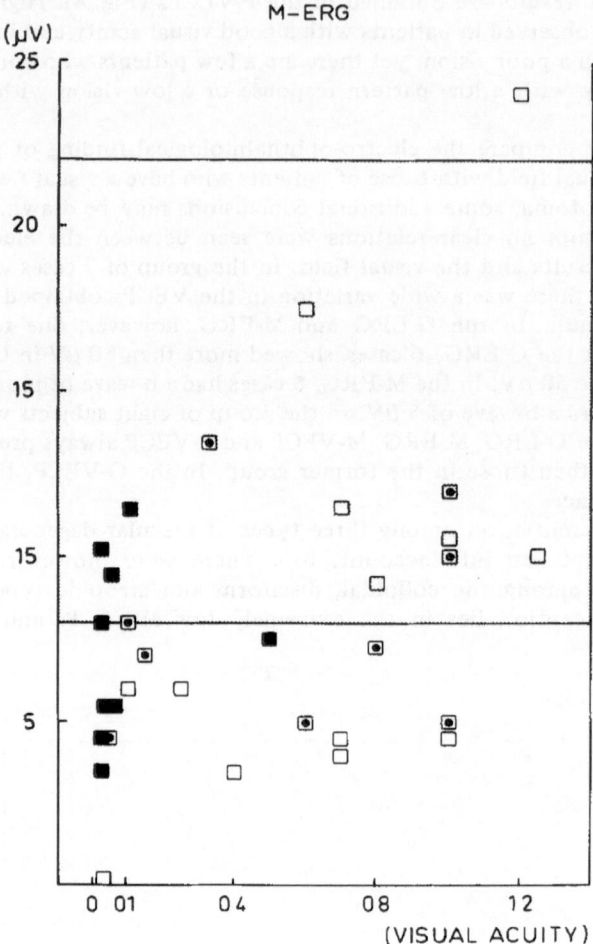

Fig. 6.   M-ERG and visual acuity. For the symbols, refer to figure 4.

combination with a poor visual acuity and deteriorated visual field in the disciform type.

DISCUSSION

It is natural that in senile macular degenerations much variation exists in the electro-ophthalmological results, since visual acuity, visual field and funduscopic appearance also vary very much. This large variation induces the first and very important question of whether there are any differences in the electro-ophthalmological results between an affected and a normal group. The second question is whether or not any correlations are to be found in patients with senile macular degeneration upon comparing the electro-ophthalmological results with other findings, such as visual acuity, visual field and ophthalmoscopic appearance.

As for the first question, it is hard to differ clearly the affected group from a normal one by use of the G-ERG. In this study, the G-ERG is lowered in many cases, but an important overlap exists between the normal and the affected group. The latter means that a diagnosis per patient on the G-ERG is often not possible. The reason for overlapping is that the decrease in the G-ERG is not caused by the macular degeneration only. Cones of the whole retina contribute to the photopic ERG. The number of cones in the 5° foveal area is only 110.000 (POLYAK 1941), in a 16° macular area only 650.000, while the total number of cones is 7 million. In this respect, cones in the 10° macular area might contribute very little to the G-ERG. Even if a 10° macular ERG is applied, the results are disappointing, although some differences can be seen. Such a result is also reported by BIERSDORF & DILLER (1969), using a 20° local central ERG.

The bad results, using M-ERG and M-VECPs, are probably due to the fact that lowered responses can be caused by a macular degeneration itself or by an eccentric fixation. Fixation is often difficult in patients with a lowered visual acuity. Therefore, we examined patients' fixation by the ophthalmoscope very carefully before the electro-ophthalmological examination. New techniques such as a TV-monitor used in the electroretinotopography (AARTS et al. 1973) may provide the solution for this problem.

The VECPs are mainly a reflection of the central part of the visual field (VAN HOF et al. 1960, RIETVELD et al. 1965, DE VOE et al. 1968).

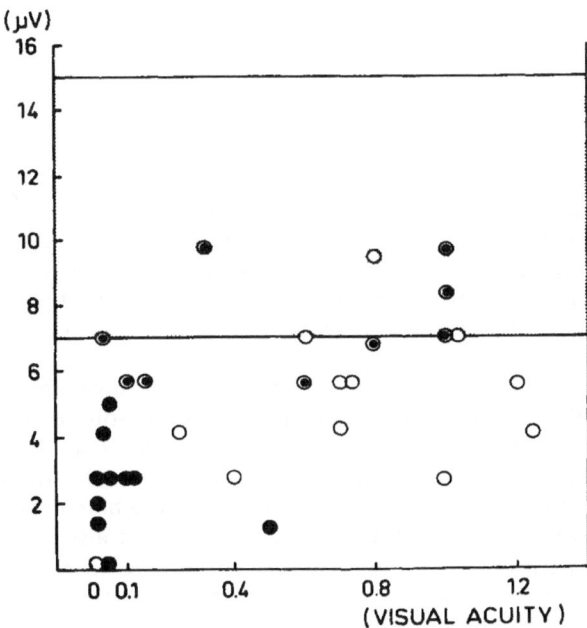

Fig. 7. M-VECP and visual acuity. For the symbols, refer to figure 5.

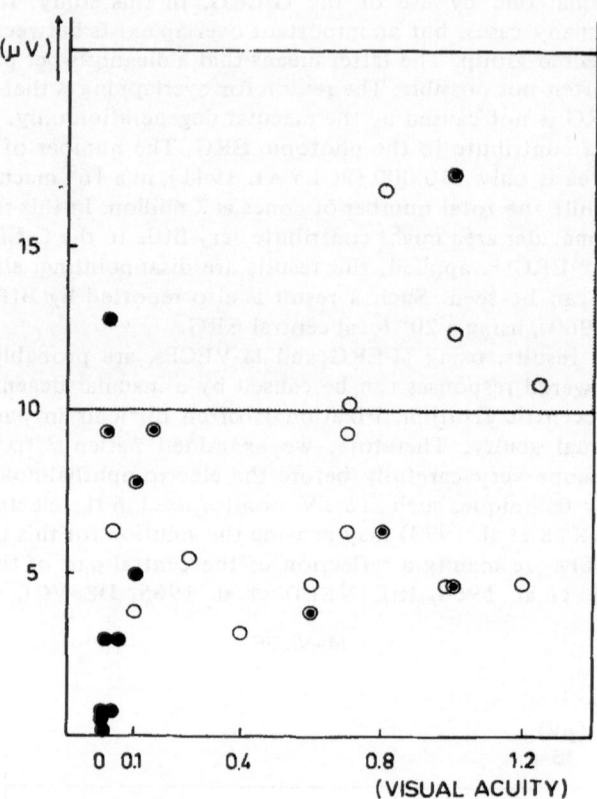

Fig. 8. P-VECP and visual acuity. For the symbols, refer to figure 5.

From this point of view, if the central part of the retina is deteriorated, it might be expected that the G-VECPs should be lowered. The results, however, prove this not to be the case. There are no essential differences between both groups. Even when the 10° M-VECPs is used, there is still a large overlapping zone between both groups, although clear differences can be observed.

The existence of an overlapping zone is not astonishing, since not only variation in the electro-ophthalmological results is found, but also in ophthalmoscopic findings, visual acuity and visual field. Therefore, it might be understandable that some pathological patients belong to the normal group. Furthermore, the amplitude of the VECPs also show much variation, even in the normal subjects (DE HAAS 1972). This should also be taken into account in the pathological group. The reason may be, that it is very difficult to analyse VECPs quantitatively. This difficulty is also present in the P-VECPs, although they represent a more accurate index of macular function (BEHRMAN, NISSIM & ARDEN 1972, SOKOL 1972). SOKOL, using a checkerboard pattern stimulus, too, could differentiate between a macular degeneration and a normal subject. The discrepancy between his results and ours might be due to the different conditions of the set-up. He used a checkerboard subtending 14 minutes, its rate of check being 16 per second. In this study, a 1° checkerboard was used, the rate being 4 per second.

As to the question of whether any relation exists between psychophysical and funduscopic examination on the one hand and the electro-ophthalmological results on the other hand, we expected at least some correlations between the height of the electrical responses and the visual acuity, except for the G-ERG. The results, however, were unsatisfactory. Only in the P-VECPs is a correlation observed, and still there are some exceptions. Again our 1° checkerboard may explain the discrepancies. Smaller squares have to be used.

SUMMARY

In conclusion it may be deduced that 1) it is difficult to differ a senile macular degeneration from a normal group based on the ERG and VECPs. Some differences are observed in the M-ERG, M-VECP and P-VECP. 2) there are almost no significant correlations between the amplitude in the ERG and VECPs obtained by flash stimuli and the visual acuity as well as the visual field. Only in severe disciform types, very often low responses are observed. 3) there are some correlations between the magnitude of P-VECPs and the visual acuity.

REFERENCES

AARTS, W.M.C., HENKES, H.E., LITH, G.H.M. VAN & MEININGER, J.: A stimulator for electroretinotopography. In: Proc. 11th Iscerg Symposium, Bad Nauheim 1973; ed. by E. DODT and J.T. PEARLMAN. Docum. Ophthal. Proc. Ser. 4: *329-335* (1974).

ARDEN, G.B. & BANKES, J.L.K.: Foveal electroretinogram as a clinical test. *Brit. J. Ophthal.* 50: *740* (1966).

ARMINGTON, J.C., TEPAS, D.I., KROPFL, W.J. & HENGST, W.H.: Summation of retinal potentials. *J. ophthal. Soc. Amer.* 51: *877-886* (1961).

BANKES, J.L.K.: The foveal electroretinogram. *Trans. ophthal. Soc. U.K.* 87: *249-262* (1967).

BEHRMAN, J., NISSIM, S. & ARDEN, G.B.: A clinical method for obtaining pattern visual evoked responses. In: The visual system: Neurophysiology, biophysics and their clinical application; Proc. 9th Iscerg Symposium, Brighton 1971; ed. by G.B. ARDEN, p. *199-206*. New York, Plenum Press, 1972.

BIERSDORF, W.R. & DILLER, D.A.: Local electroretinogram in macular degeneration. *Amer. J. Ophthal.* 68: *296-303* (1969).

DEVOE R.G., RIPPS, H. & VAUGHAN Jr., H.G.: Cortical responses to stimulation of the human fovea. *Vision Res.* 8: *135-147* (1968).

DIETERLE, P.: Electrorétinogramme et sénescence. *Ophthalmologica* 143: *296-299* (1962).

FRANÇOIS, J., VERRIEST, G. & ROUCK, A. DE.: Les fonctions visuelles dans les dégénérescences tapéto-rétiniennes. *Bibl. Ophthal.* 43: *1-86* (1956).

FRANÇOIS, J., VERRIEST, G. & ROUCK, A. DE.: L'électro-oculographie en tant q'examen fonctionnel de la rétine. *Bibl. Ophthal.* 49: *1-67* (1957).

FRANÇOIS, J., & ROUCK, A. DE.: Combined electroretino-encephalography in macular disease. In: Clinical electroretinography; Proc. 3rd Iscerg Symposium, Illinois

1964; ed. by H.M. BURIAN and J.H. JACOBSON, p. *289-297*. Oxford, Pergamon Press, 1966.

GASS, J.D.M.: Drusen and disciform macular detachment and degeneration. *Arch. Ophthal.* 90: *206-217* (1973).

GLIEM, H.: Das Electro-oculogram. Abhandlungen aus dem Gebiete der Augenheilkunde, Band 40. Leipzig, Thieme, 1971.

HAAS, J.P. DE.: An electro-ophthalmological study of affections of the optic pathway. Thesis Rotterdam. Den Haag, Junk, 1972.

HENKES, H.E.: Electroretinography in circulatory disturbances of the retina. III. Electroretinogram in cases of senile degeneration of the macular area. *Arch. Ophthal.* 51: *54-66* (1954).

HOF, M.W. VAN., HOF-VAN DUIN J. VAN & RIETVELD, W.J.: Enhancement of occipito-cortical responses to light flashes in man during attention. *Vision Res.* 6: *109-111* (1966).

JACOBSON, J.H., BASAR, D. & KORNZWEIG, A.L.: Spectro-differential electroretinography in macular disease. *Amer. J. Ophthal.* 42: *199-205* (1956).

JAYLE, G.E., BOYER, R. & AUBERT, L.: Étude de différents tests fonctionnels électro-rétinographiques sénile grave. *Ann. d'Oculist.* 192: *561-571* (1959).

KRILL, A.E.: The electroretinographic and electrooculographic findings in patients with macula lesions. *Trans. Amer. Acad. Ophthal. Otolaryng.* 70: *1063-1083* (1966).

LITH, G.H.M. VAN. & HENKES, H.E.: The local electric response of the central retinal area. In: Advances in electrophysiology and -pathology of the visual system; Proc. 6th Iscerg Symposium, Erfurt 1967; ed. by E. SCHMÖGER, p. *163-170*. Leipzig, Thieme, 1968.

LITH, G.H.M. VAN. & HENKES, H.E.: The relationship between ERG and VER. *Ophthal. Res.* 1: *40-47* (1970).

LITH, G.H.M. VAN., MEININGER, J. & MARLE, G.W. VAN.: Electrophysiological equipment for total and local retinal stimulation. In: 10th Iscerg Symposium, Los Angeles 1972; ed. by J.T. PEARLMAN. Docum. Ophthal. Proc. Ser. 2: *213-218* (1973).

MERIN, S. & AUERBACH, F.: Involvement of the central and peripheral retina in macular degenerations as reflected by the ERG. In: Textbook of the fundus of the eye; ed. by A.J. BALLANTYNE & I. MICHAELSON. Edinburgh, Churchill, 1973.

NAGATA, M., YAMANE, T., TAKATA, H., YANO, T. & HOSHINO, A.: Studies on photopic ERG of the human eye. *Acta. Soc. ophthal. Jap.* 66: *1614-1673* (1962).

NIEMEYER, G.: Elektroretinographie bei Maculadegenerationen. *Graefes Arch. Ophthal.* 177: *39-51* (1969).

PERDRIEL, G., SOUSSEN, G., DESBORDES, P. & LEBIANC, M.: Physiopathologie des ondes a de l'électrorétinogramme. *Bull. Mém. Soc. Fr. Ophtal.* 77: *77-84* (1964).

PERDRIEL, G.: Explorations fonctionelles et électrophysiologiques au cours des dégénérescences maculaires séniles. *Arch. Ophtal. (Paris)* 29: *877-880* (1969).

POLYAK, S.L.: The retina. Oxford, University Press, 1941.

RIETVELD, W.J., TORDOIR, W.E.M., HAGENOUN, J.R.B. & DONGEN, K.J. VAN.: Contribution of foveo-parafoveal quadrants to the visual evoked response. *Acta Physiol. Pharmacol. Neerl.* 13: *340-347* (1965).

ROUHER, F., SERPIN, G. & SOLE, P.: Un classement électrorétinographique des dégénérescences maculaires séniles. *Bull. Soc. Ophtal. Fr.* 66: *812-819* (1966).

RUEDEMANN, A.D. & NOELL, W.K.: The electroretinogram in central retinal degeneration. *Trans. Amer. Acad. Ophthal. Otolaryng.* 65: *576-594* (1961).

RUEDEMANN, A.D.: The electroretinogram in degenerative diseases. In: Electrical responses of the visual system; ed. by S.J. FRICKER. *Intern. Ophthal. Clinics* 9: *1005-1023* (1969).

SOKOL, S.: An electrodiagnostic index of macular degeneration. *Arch. Ophthal.* 88: *619-624* (1972).

STANGOS, N., REY, P., MEYER, J.J. & THORENS, B.: Averaged ERG responses in normal human subjects and ophthalmological patients. In: Symposium on electroretinography; Proc. 8th Iscerg Symposium, Pisa 1970; ed. by A. WIRTH, p. *277-304*. Pisa, Pacini, 1970.

STANGOS, N., SPIRITUS, M. & KOROL, S.: ERG et EOG dans les affections maculaires dégénératives. *Arch. Ophtal. (Paris)* 32: *277-290* (1972).

ZETTERSTRÖM, B.: Some experience of clinical flicker electroretinography in various eye diseases. *Acta Ophthal.* 42: *144-164* (1964).

SOME RESULTS ON MATHEMATICAL
ANALYSIS OF DYNAMIC ERG

C. BORGHI, M. CORDELLA, S. LETTIERI,
M. MAIONE & L. PROSPERI

(Parma, Italy)

1. INTRODUCTION AND METHODS

There is no uniformity for the interpretation of the plots obtained by means of conventional ERG techniques, especially from a quantitative standpoint, since a lot of different interpretations arise from different ways of measuring both the times (abscissae) and the amplitudes appearing in the ERG signals. For instance, the amplitudes of the ERG plots are measured sometimes (BURIAN, 1967) from the lowest point of the wave preceeding that one we observe, whilst a number of other researchers use as a zero point for the amplitudes the isoelectric line (SOLE, ALFIERI & SERPIN 1966), defined as the line drawn by the instrument when no signal input is feed in from the patient's eyes. In the present paper we will follow this second method, for the reason that we will be able to derive out of it some physical meaning.

Here we are only dealing with dynamic ERG plots, obtained by means of the standard classical methods already described by JAYLE et al. (1965) and JACOBSON et al. (1966), with some improvements of ours, as stated below.

The electrodes we used, are those of BURIAN & ALLEN (1954).

The stimuli are obtained with a conventional photostimulator (Vescovini Model 481), and duration is about 10 msec. Actually, a stimulus is a flash radiation entering in an hemispherical bowl (50 cm diameter) through a circular hole (10 cm diameter) on the upper top of the bowl, where different filters (white, red, blue) may be settled. The same bowl may be illuminated, either continuously or not, by means of two lamps, with different coloured filters, whose diffused radiation is used for light adaptation. These lamps are located near the widest lower section of the bowl, and are fed by alternating current. The intensity of illumination near each of the lamps is about 1500 lux, but at the place of the patient's eyes that intensity is reduced to 300 lux. The intensity emitted by the flash is 3 joule.

A Wratten-Kodak red Filter, model W K 92, for 646 manometer wavelenght with 36% transmittance shields the emitted stimulus directly on the source.

The recording was performed by means of a DC-AC Vescovini Preamplifier mod. 381, with a time constant of 0.3 sec. (vs. the 0.2 sec duration of the ERG). Any high frequency in the response was cut off by a low-pass filter.

The output response is preamplified, then fed into an Average Signal

Analyser, Hewlett Packard mod. 5840 A. As a function of the time, the averaging was obtained by means of 32 scannings, after 1, then 5, then 10 finally 15 minutes of darkness adaptation. The averaged data are supplied to the electronic memory of the device, and they may always be visible by display, also for photographic purposes, if needed. They may also be printed on conventional XY plotter. (Fig. 1)

An analog to digital conversion is also performed in order to have the numerical description of the ERG plot directly measured and printed and eventually recorded in the memory of the instrument for successive uses.

2. THE ALL–OR–NONE REPRESENTATION OF THE ERG'S WAVES.

An inspection of a large number of ERG diagrams shows a standard shape like that drawn in Figs. 1 and 2, that is the components or waves usually labelled a, b_1 and b_2. We take also into account the negative deflection after the b complex, if any. The absolute maximum we label, "k". For simplicity's sake it will be called the k wave. We will disregard the c waves, because with our recording methods it turns out to be inconstant and unclear (JAYLE et al. (1965). Very frequently (BRUNETTE 1972) all the waves a, b_1 b_2 and k

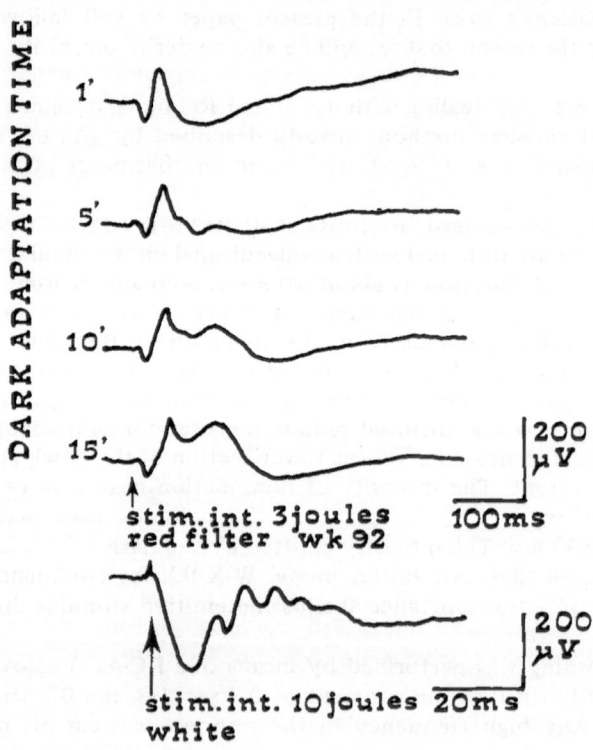

Fig. 1. An example of the ERG.

118

are far from a near wave form, but a certain number of more or less high wavelets are superimposed to the principal terms.

For every wave there is a latency, a duration and an amplitude of the principal terms, as well as wavelength and the amplitude of the wavelets. We will consider as a measure of the latency, the time interval, (in msec) between the starting point A =0 of the a wave and the starting of the considered wave.

In the present paper we deal with the research for a mathematical model of these ERG diagrams, which permits a standardized array of numbers whereupon we may work all the required investigations.

We will not introduce any physiological justification for our model, at once, accepting the ERG plots as a matter of facts to be mathematically analized. However, mathematics offers several known and available methods for a numerical representation of given plots, including all the methods based on the use of a set of orthogonal functions or polynomials, for example those called after the Cebyshef, the Bessel functions, and especially the widely used Fourier analysis (FRITZ et al. 1972). But, however elegant and efficient these methods may be, most of them are subject to the serious criticism that in many cases it appears rather difficult to establish a meaningful correspondence between the so found "harmonics" and some physiological event or component in the phenomena under study.

For this reason, in the present paper we try to represent the ERG plots as a sum of *waves* or *components*, whose general shape is sketched in Fig. 3. According to the suggestion of one of us, this represents phenomena subject to an "all-or-none" law, which is characteristic for a great number of physiological behaviours. This way, we use a representation whose physiological credibility is assured, without introducing any physiological explanation.

The mathematical representation of a diagram like that of fig. 2 is

(0.1) $\qquad W = w\,L\,(A)\,(1 - e^{-\lambda't})\,e^{-\lambda''t}$

where w is an amplitude characteristic for one wave, e is the base of the

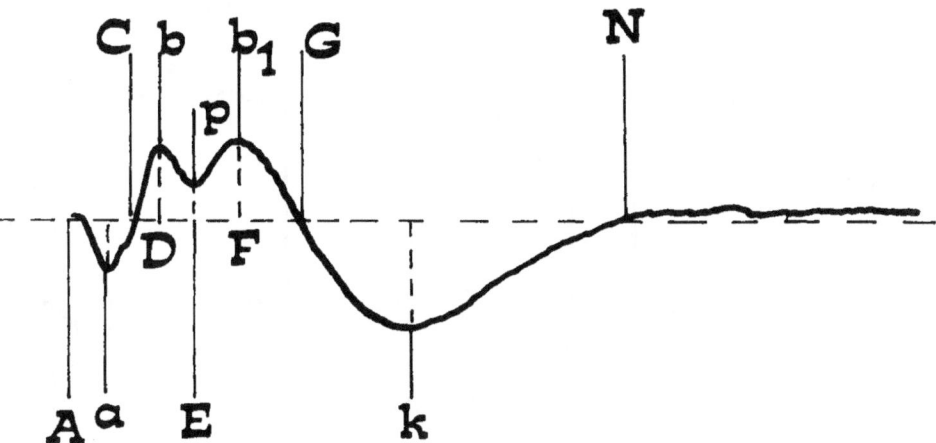

Fig. 2.   A particularly schematic ERG (Cordella).

natural logarithms, λ' and λ'' are two *time constants* (dimensioned as sec^{-1}), whereas L is a discontinuous factor defined by

$$(0.2) \qquad L(A) = \begin{cases} 0 \text{ for } t - A \leqslant 0 \\ 1 \text{ for } t - A > 0 \end{cases}$$

The form (0.1) represents the principal mode of the ERG waves, disregarding the already mentioned wavelets superimposed over them. Apart from the latency L, a physical model suggested by this form is the total radioactivity of a sample composed by an active mother whose radioactive constant is λ', decaying into another, "daughter", radioactive element whose constant is λ'', when $\lambda' \gg \lambda''$.

A more impressive model is given by Electronics, as shown in Fig. 4. A positive signal +S feeds the capacitor C_S through a rectifier and the resistor

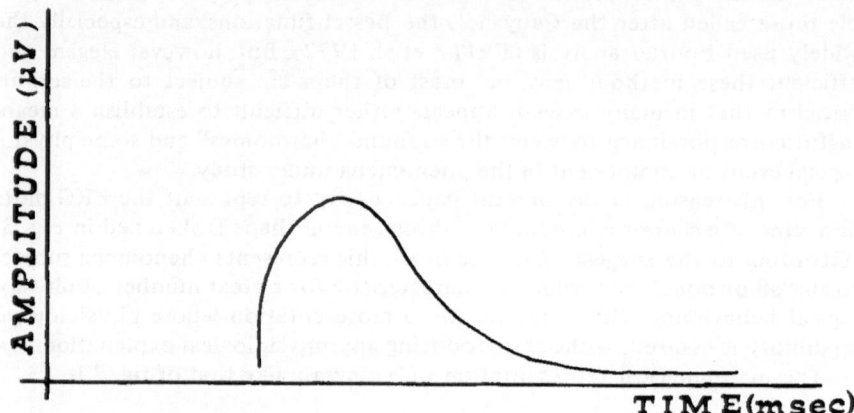

Fig. 3.   An "all-or-none" pulse.

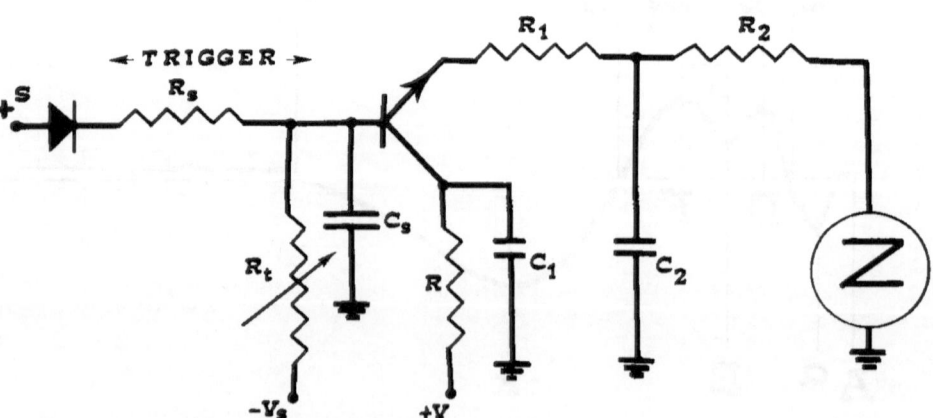

Fig. 4.   An electronic model for the source of the pulse.

120

R_S. The capacitor C_S was previously charged negatively by the polarization source $-V_S$ through the potentiometer R_t. The negative potential given to C_S blocks any passage of current through a triode. But the positive potential due to the signal, if any, diminishes the polarization negative potential on C_S till it vanishes and eventually becomes slightly positive. Then the triode begins to discharge the energy stored on the capacity C_1 by the source (positive) V. This way it appears that all of the device before the triode acts as a *trigger*. After the triggering, the energy stored previously on C_1 charges the capacity C_2 through the resistance R_1. The resistor R is rather large, so that the potential on C_1 is not sensibly modified during the discharge by the source $+V$, whilst the resistor R_1 is not too large. When the potential on C_2 is sufficiently large, for the beginning of the current through the Zener transistor Z, the energy already stored on C_2 flows through both R_1 and R_2, whereas the energy of C_1 flows only through the resistance R_2. In this model, it appears that the time necessary for the signal S to trigger the current to flow through the triode simulates the *latency*, whilst the amplitude and the principal form of any ERG signal is due to a potential energy already stored in some chemistry of the retina, in the same way as the amplitude and the principal term of the current through Z depends on the energy stored in the two successive capacitors C_1 and C_2, as well as on the resistance R_1 and R_2.

Our method consists in giving at once an approximate evaluation of the parameters of a single wave of the ERG, giving a linearized representation of the all-or-none wave as a triangle (Fig. 5), disregarding the O.P. or wavelets, in a first approximation. Then the assembly of the waves takes the form

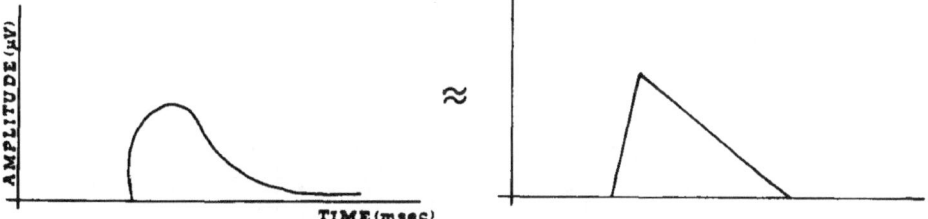

Fig. 5.   A "true" and an "approximate" pulse.

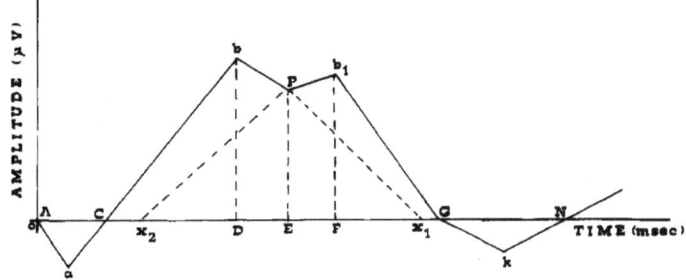

Fig. 5 bis.   A linearized ERG plot with its parameters.

sketched in Fig. 5 *bis* where also the symbols of the experimental data are given. The capital letters are the abscissae (in msec); the small letters are the ordinates, including the p ordinate of the point where b_1 and the b_2 waves are intersecting. Thereafter, we calculate the areas and the true heights, of the four waves. The data are A = O; C, D, E, F, G, N, a, b, p, b', k. These data are recorded on a board card (Fig. 6).

3. THE FIRST ELABORATED DATA

For the *a* and *k* waves there is no problem. Since their areas are respectively

$$(1) \qquad S_a = \frac{1}{2} C a \qquad\qquad (A = 0)$$

$$(2) \qquad S_k = \frac{1}{2} (N - G) k$$

Some assumptions must be made in order to have both the areas S_1, S_2 and the "true" heights b_1 and b_2 as well as the latency X_2 of the b_2 wave and the end X_1 of the b_1 wave. For this purpose we calculate the total area of the figure [C b p b' G] that is

$$(3)$$
$$\beta = \frac{1}{2} \left\{ (D-C)\,b + (E-D)\,(b+p) + (F-E)\,(b' + p) + (G-F)\,b' \right\} =$$
$$= \frac{1}{2} \left\{ (E-C)\,b + (F-D)\,p + (G-E)\,b' \right\}$$

E. R. G.

t	A	C	D	E	F	G	N	a	b	p	b1	k
1'		2153	3768	3844	5960	6152	22608	7974	11088	0	2772	3157
5'		2153	3768	6805	7997	10266	27222	6006	14014	4774	6160	7854
10'		2153	3768	6805	5155	12767	28376	6006	17171	12320	12874	9240
15'		2153	3768	6690	7766	12688	28376	6622	21560	15092	14563	12012

t	X1	X2	b1	b2	Sa	S1	S2	Sk	S	s1,2
1'	30,67	38,44	110,88	27,72	858,72	1005,90	251,48	2597,58	4713,68	0,25
5'	38,31	38,44	127,82	57,72	582,72	1314,43	328,43	1886,48	4312,07	0,22
10'	32,68	29,40	84,74	50,72	373,50	765,49	505,30	2111,00	3755,90	0,66
15'	33,58	29,40	87,04	18,42	373,50	825,71	272,63	0	1471,85	0,13

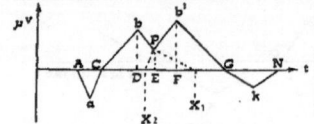

Fig. 6. A fac-simile of a card board.

122

and we assume that the "true" heights of b_1 and b_2 waves are $b_1 \leqslant b$; $b_2 < b'$, as well as the respective bases $(X_1\text{-}C)$, $(G\text{-}X_2)$, so that

(4) $\qquad \beta = S_1 + S_2$

Thus we may write

(5.0) $\qquad S_1 = \beta - gb'/(b+b')$

$\qquad\qquad S_2 = \beta - gb/(b+b')$

that is S_1 is β detracted a parcel proportional to the height b' of S_2, $g/(b+b')$ being a proportionality function. The same for S_2. Hence, with (5.0) one has $g = \beta$, whence

(5) $\qquad S_1 = \beta\, b/(b+b')$

$\qquad\qquad S_2 = \beta\, b'/(b+b')$

For the true heights b_1 and b_2 we assume

(6) $\qquad b_1 = b - b'p/(b+b')$

$\qquad\qquad b_2 = b' - bp/(b+b')$

because $b_1 = b$ and $b_2 = b'$ when $p = 0$ and $(b+b') - (b_1 + b_2) = p$, that is p is interpreted as the difference between the sum of the observed and the true heights.

The latency X_2 of the b_2 wave is comprised between the abscissae E and C, being $X_2 = E$ when $p = 0$. Hence we assume

(7) $\qquad X_2 = C + (E\text{-}C)\, b/(b+p)$

$b/(b+p)$ being the parcel of $(E\text{-}C)$ to be added to C and giving $X_2 = E$ for $p = 0$. The end X_1 of b_1 wave is deduced from the area S_1 written in the form

$$S_1 = \frac{1}{2}\, (X_1\text{-}C)\, b_1$$

that is

(8) $\qquad X_1 = C + 2S_1/b_1$

This way we have the array of first elaborated data:

$$X_1\ X_2\ b_1\ b_2\ S_a\ S_1\ S_2\ S_k$$

$$S = S_a + S_1 + S_2 + S_k; \qquad S_{21} = S_2/S_1$$

These are collected with the original data on a board card (Fig. 6).

4. THE CALCULATION OF λ''

Now, for the waves a, b_1, b_2, k, we define the parameters L, T_1, S_o according to the following schema

	a	b_1	b_2	k
L =	a	b_1	b_2	k
T_1 =	$\frac{1}{2}$ C	(D-C)	(F-X_2)	$\frac{1}{3}$ (N-G)
S_0 =	S_a	S_1	S_2	S_k

The meaning of L and S_0 is obvious, whereas T_1 means the difference between the abscissae of the maximum and the latency of the same wave. For a wave we took $T_1 \approx \frac{1}{2}$ C, whilst for the k wave $T_1 \approx \frac{1}{3}$(N-G), from observational evidence on the ERG plots.

Now, let us take our mathematical model (0.1) of a wave and calculate the "true" area

(9) $$S_0 = \int_0^\infty w(1 - e^{-\lambda't}) e^{-\lambda''t} \, dt = w/ \left[\lambda'' (1 + U) \right]$$

where λ' and λ'' and w are supposed to be complex:

(10) $$\lambda' = \lambda'_1 - i\lambda'_2 ; \lambda'' = \lambda'' - i\lambda'' \quad w = w_1 - iw_2 ; U = \lambda''/\lambda'$$

Since S_0 is real, we will take only the real part of the result. We will compare this way (9) with the approximated values calculated before.
Likewise the culminating time T_1 is calculated with

$$\frac{\partial}{\partial t} \left[(1 - e^{-\lambda't}) e^{-\lambda''t} \right] = 0$$

whereas the culminating amplitude L is obtained by putting T_1 instead of t in (0.1). Hence, we have the system

(11) $$S_0 = w/ \left[\lambda'' (1 + U) \right]$$

(12) $$T_1 \lambda' = \log (1 + \frac{1}{U})$$

(13) $$L = w/ \left[(1 + U)(1 + \frac{1}{U})^U \right]$$

From (11) we have $w = S_0 \lambda'' (1 + U)$ and from (12)

(12) $$U T_1 \lambda' = \log (1 + \frac{1}{U})^U . \text{ Hence}$$

(14) $$\lambda'' T_1 = \log (1 + \frac{1}{U})^U$$

$$\lambda'' S_0/L = (1 + \frac{1}{U})^U$$

124

whence

(15) $\qquad \lambda'' T_1 y = \exp(\lambda'' T_1)$

with

(16) $\qquad y = S_0/(LT_1)$

Separating in (15) the real from the imaginary part we have

(17) $\qquad \begin{cases} \exp(\lambda_1'' T_1) \cos(\lambda_2'' T_1) = \lambda_1'' T_1 y \\ \exp(\lambda_1'' T_1) \sin(\lambda_2'' T_1) = \lambda_2'' T_1 y \end{cases}$

Putting

(18) $\qquad x = \lambda_2'' T_1$

the sum of the square of the two sides, and their division give

(19) $\qquad \lambda_2''/\lambda_1'' = \tan x$

(20) $\qquad y = \dfrac{\sin x}{x} \exp\left(\dfrac{x}{\tan x}\right)$

Eq. (20) is the *first transcendental equation* in the unique unknown x, since y is experimentally given. Its solution has been found by means of a computer CDC 6600. The result must be foreseen because sinx and tangx are periodical functions, and y is always positive. Thus is explained the im-

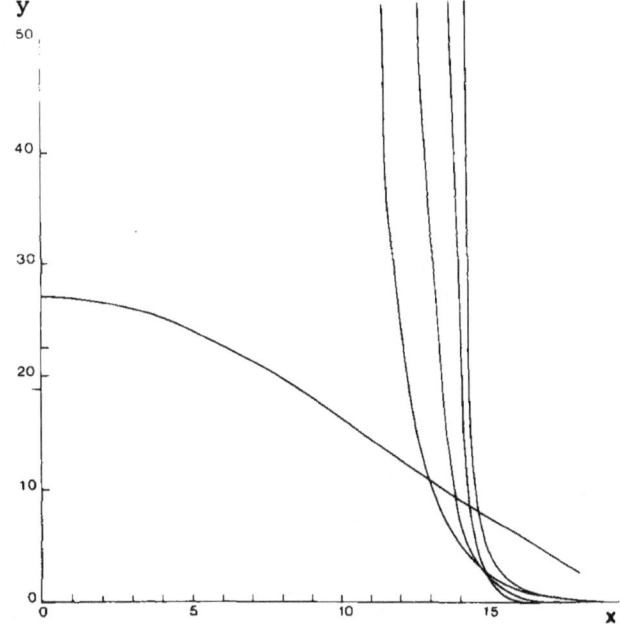

Fig. 7. Plot of x *vs.* y as solution of eq. (20).

125

portant result that to every given value of y correspond several discrete values of x (fig. 7, 8, 9).

Therefore to every y corresponds a set of values x_i, which gives two correlated sets of $(\lambda_2'')_i$ and $(\lambda_1'')_i$, namely

(21.1) $(\lambda_2'')_i = x_i/T_1$

(21.2) $(\lambda_1'')_i = \dfrac{1}{T_1} x_i/\text{tang } x_i$

5.   THE CALCULATION OF λ'

The values of λ' and λ'' are linked together by eq. (12) written in the form

(12) $\exp (\lambda' T_1) - 1 = \lambda'/\lambda''$

Putting

(22) $J = \exp (\lambda' T_1)$

and with (10), eq. (12) gives

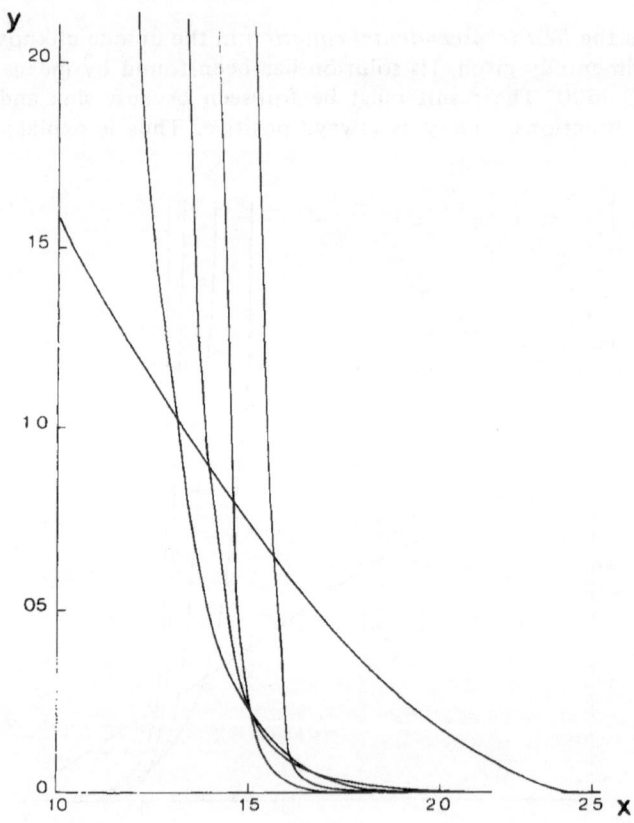

Fig. 8.   The same as in fig. 7 at minor scale.

126

$$(\lambda_1'' - i\lambda_2'') \left[(J \cos \lambda_2' \, T_1 - 1) - i J \sin \lambda_2' \, T_1 \right] = \lambda_1' - i\lambda_2'$$

Separating the real from the imaginary parts one obtains:

(23) $\quad\begin{cases} \lambda_1'' \, J \cos \lambda_2' \, T_1 - \lambda_2'' \, J \sin \lambda_2' \, T_1 = \lambda_1' + \lambda_1'' \end{cases}$

(24) $\quad\begin{cases} \lambda_2'' \, J \cos \lambda_2' \, T_1 + \lambda_1'' \, J \sin \lambda_2' \, T_1 = \lambda_2' + \lambda_2'' \end{cases}$

Putting for (19), with (21.1),

(25) $\quad\begin{cases} \lambda_1'' = M \cos x \\[4pt] \lambda_2'' = M \sin x \end{cases} \qquad M^2 = \lambda_1''^{\,2} + \lambda_2''^{\,2} = \dfrac{1}{T_1^2} \left(\dfrac{x}{\sin x} \right)^2$

adding the squares of both sides of (22) and (24) and dividing the same sides we obtain, with (25), the system

(26) $\qquad (\lambda_1' + \lambda_1'')^2 + (\lambda_2' + \lambda_2'')^2 = J^2 \, M^2$

(27) $\qquad \text{tang}\,(\lambda_2' \, T_1 + x) = (\lambda_2' + \lambda_2'')/(\lambda_1' + \lambda_1'')$

From (26) one has

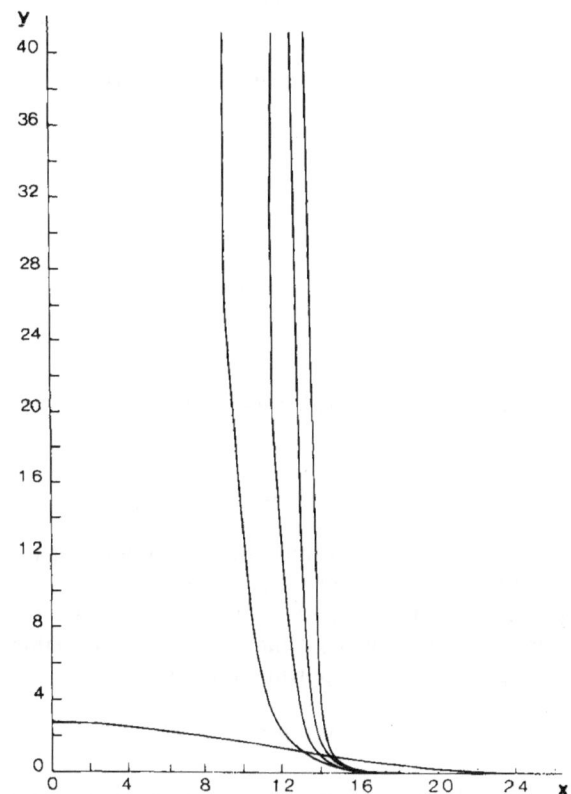

Fig. 9.   The same as in fig. 7 at a small scale.

127

(28) $$\lambda_2' = \left[J^2 M^2 - (\lambda_1' + \lambda_1'')^2 \right]^{\frac{1}{2}} - \lambda_2''$$

Substituting (28) into (27), this becomes

(29) $$(\lambda_1' + \lambda_1'')\, \mathrm{tang} \left\{ T_1 \left[J^2 M^2 - (\lambda_1' + \lambda_1'')^2 \right]^{\frac{1}{2}} \right\} = \left[J^2 M^2 - (\lambda_1' + \lambda_1'')^2 \right]^{\frac{1}{2}}$$

or for (22), we have the second transcendental equation

(30) $$\left(\log J + \frac{x}{\mathrm{tang}\, x} \right)^2 \sec^2 \sqrt{ J^2 \frac{x^2}{\sin^2 x} - \left(\log J + \frac{x}{\mathrm{tang}\, x} \right)^2 } = J^2 \frac{x^2}{\sin^2 x}$$

where the unique unknown is J. Also this equation may be resolved numeri-
cally by means of a computer, for every given value of a. The periodicity of
the function $\sec^2$ justifies the result according which to a given value of x
correspond several values of J. When x_i is known, the corresponding values
J_{ij} are also known, as well as the values λ_1' and λ_2', that is

(31.1) $$(\lambda_1')_{ij} = \frac{1}{T_1} \log J_{ij}$$

(31.2) $$(\lambda_2')_{ij} = \frac{1}{T_1} \left[J_{ij}^2 \frac{x_i^2}{\sin^2 x_i} - \left(\log J_{ij} + \frac{x_i}{\mathrm{tang}\, x_i} \right)^2 \right]^{\frac{1}{2}}$$

6. THE CALCULATION OF w AND W

Since $w = S_0 (\lambda' + \lambda'')$, we have

(32) $$w_1 = S_0 (\lambda_1' + \lambda_1''); \quad w_2 = S_0 (\lambda_2' + \lambda_2'')$$

Thus a total wave is the real part of W as already said, and it is

(33) $$W = \left\{ w_1 \left[1 - e^{-\lambda_1' t} - 2 \left(\sin^2 \frac{\lambda_2' t}{2} - e^{-\lambda_1' t} \sin^2 \frac{\lambda_2' + \lambda_2''}{2} t \right) \right] - \right.$$
$$\left. - w_2 \left[\sin \lambda_2'' t - e^{-\lambda_1' t} \sin (\lambda_2' + \lambda_2'') t \right] \right\} e^{-\lambda_1'' t}$$

7. THE OSCILLATORY POTENTIALS

An inspection to the hitherto obtained results shows that the form (33), of
an ERG wave contains a principal term of the form $w_1 (1 - e^{-\lambda_1' t}) e^{-\lambda_1'' t}$,
plus a waving, small amplitude term which reminds the form of the oscil-
latory potentials, although the legitimacy of such a possible identification
needs a wider comparison with experimental data.

8. THE SPECTRA OF λ' AND λ''

But maybe the most important result is that the parameter y experimentally measured determines a spectrum of discrete values of x_i, that is of λ_1''

128

and λ_2'', as well as a ar more complicated spectrum of discontinuous values J_{ij}, that is of λ_1' and λ_2'. This result is consistent with the observed existence of levels in retinal, whose flash photolysis paths have been described by E.W. ABRAHAMSON and S.M. JASPER (1972). Nonetheless, the immediate evidence of our results is that in the formation of the ERG there is a production of either substances or states, in two steps, whose inverse mean lives are λ_1' and λ_1'' which have a discontinuous spectrum of values like that of a fine structure (Fig. 10). Experimental evidence for more detailed conclusions, is the aim of further work.

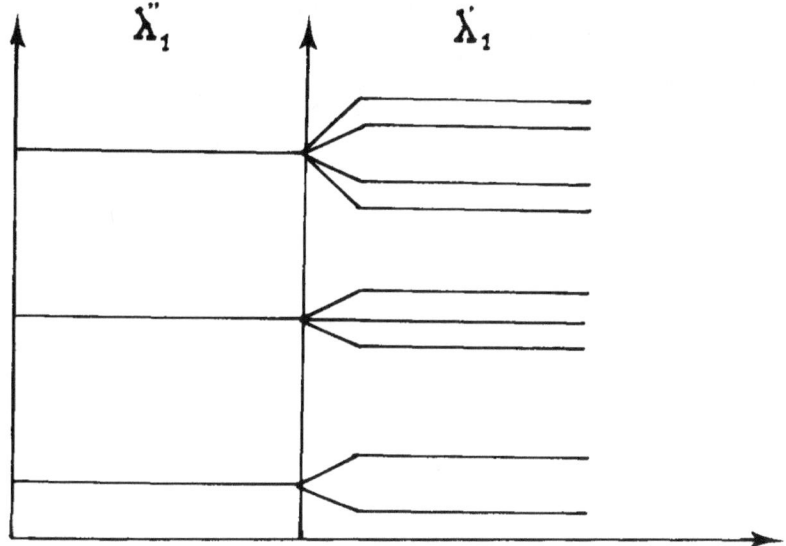

Fig. 10.   A "fine structure" model.

9.   ACKNOWLEDGEMENTS

The A.A. are deeply indebted to profs. C. GIORI and A. CALABRESE — Inst. of Physics of the Univ. of Parma, for their unvaluable collaboration in programming and executing the calculations with a CD 6600 computer.

SUMMARY

The ERG is linearized in an approximate form measurable by a number of experimental data. The same ERG is also assumed to be the sum of four "all-or-none" pulses defined by two decay constants and an amplitude. A mathematical comparison made by means of a computer shows that these decay constants and the amplitudes have discrete components.

BIBLIOGRAPHY

BURIAN, H.M., The ERG in Strabismic Ambliopia, *Docum. Ophthalm.* 23, 232 (1967).
SOLE, P., ALFIERI, R. & G. SERPIN, ERG and functional ambliopia, in the Clinical

Value of Electroretinography, ISCERG, Symp., Gent, 1966, Karger, Basel/N.Y., 1908, p. 127-132.

JAYLE, G.E., BOYER, R.L. & J.B. SARACCO, L'électrorétinographie, Paris, Masson, 1965, p. 481 et suivantes.

JACOBSON J.H., HIROSE T. & A.B. POPKIN, Independence of the oscillatory Potentials in Photopic and Scotopic b-waves of the human E.R. Grain, in The Clinical Value of ERG, ISCERG, Symp., Gent 1966, p. 8-19.

BURIAN H.M. & L. ALLEN, A speculum contact lens electrode for ERG, *Electroencephalography Clinical Neurophysiology* 6, 509 (1954).

See Ref. (3), P. 48 ss.

BRUNETTE J.R., Double a-waves and their relationship to the oscillatory potentials, *Investigative Ophthalmology* 11, 199 (1972).

FRITZ K.J., STEINHOFF J., HIRATA A., BUFFUM D., GILBERT N.G. & A.M. POTTS, Computer processing of the Visual Evoked Response, Docum. Ophthalm. Series X, ISCERG Symposium Los Angeles 1972, vol. 2, p. 145-161.

ABRAHAMSON E.W. & S.M. JASPER, Photochemistry of the vision, in Handbook of Sensory, vol. VII/1, Springer, Berlin 1972, p. 28-32.

CALCULATION OF GLARE EFFECT

An example of interaction of mathematical modeling
and experimental research

J. SCHULZE & H. BRÖDNER

(Dortmund, Germany)

ABSTRACT

Quantification of biological processes is a fundamental task of physiological research. For that, mathematical modeling is a very efficient aid. Pure mathematics are of less value for biological interpretation. It must be verified that the theoretical function fits not only a small amount of empirical data but the whole course of the biological process. In case of any uncertainty, especially in borderline values, additional experiments have to be performed to get more numerous and better measuring points to describe the empirical function and to correct the model, if necessary. Another point, to prove the validity of the model is to look at what happens with the theoretical function in case of extrapolation out of the experimental range. This must not lead to meaningless or absurd values in biological sense. In the following report the development of the investigation on readaptation course after dazzeling will be described in such a manner, alternating stepwise between performing new experiments and correcting the model. Finally, the usefulness of a good model and facilitation of experimentel work by its application will be explained.

Quantification of biological processes is a fundamental task in physiological research as well as in clinical examination. It enables us to control the effectiveness of therapeutic treatment or to observe the stability or progressive nature of a disease. We feel that one reason for the relatively minor importance of the ERG in ophthalmological examinations up to now, is that we have only a very rough classification of ERG instead of a more sophisticated quantitative interpretation.

Much work has been done during the last decade to solve this problem, but unfortunately without a great deal of influence on routine clinical electroretinography. One reason for that is that it makes a considerable difference, wether one is working under the good conditions of a well equiped research laboratory or in a troublesome clinical environement.

Mathematical modeling can be helpful both to gain a better understanding of scientific results and to introduce research methods into a clinical routine. Our aim is to demonstrate the interdependence of modeling and experimental research, because modeling without correction by purposeful experiments is frequently misleading.

In our studies on the readaptation of the retina after glare represented by the growth of the b-amplitude we obtained many readaptation curves showing a clear and systematic dependence on the intensity of the glare stimulus (Figure 1). But we are still missing a method to compare the different curves, their slopes and courses quantitatively. This is a necessary prerequi-

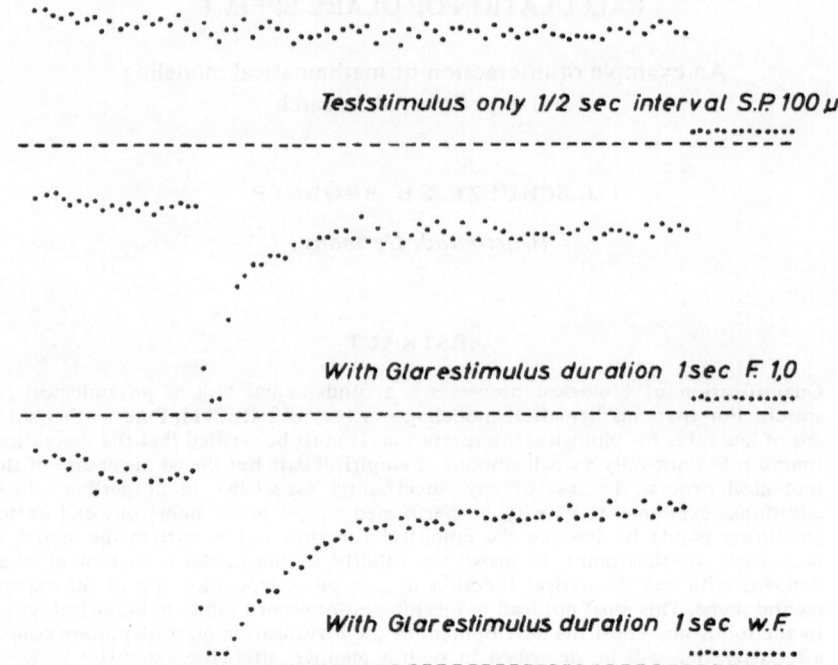

Fig. 1. The middle and lower trace show two readaptation curves, elicited by two different glare stimuli. Uppermost trace represents a control registration without glare. Each point represents the average of ten measured b-amplitudes. The time between two points is half a second.

site in evaluating the relationship between the glare stimulus and the readaptation course. In addition, the knowledge of this relationship allows us to determine normal reactions and their boundary conditions and to discriminate pathological cases.

Generally, the first step to describe an empirical curve is to try a curvefitting with a polynomial. This is of advantage with regard to the mathematical handling of such a function, e.g. differentiation, integration or any other mathematical manipulation and leads to a better understanding of the time course or the interpendence of the parameters measured. In some cases, especially when a satisfactory approximation requires a polynomial of higher order (10th or 15th degree) this method is less helpful, because it gives only another type of description of the collected data, but does not lead to an understanding of the mathematical function describing the biological process. We met with this problem when we attempted to analyse the timecourse of readaptation by a polynomial curve-fitting method.

The next step would be the approximation of the empirical curve by an exponential function which is a type very common in biology, especially in growth processes — and readaptation means an increase of sensitivity from a lower level caused by the glare stimulus. Since we found that this could not be achieved by using a single exponential function, we tried to combine two exponential functions considering that either two types of receptors or two types of reactions, namely the dark and light adaptation, exist in the retina which can be represented by two e-functions. We succeeded in obtaining theoretical functions which agreed very well with the empirical data (Figure 2). But frequently we found intersections of both curves and it was impossible to determine the link between both functions even with large computer programs. Determination of the link, however, is a relevant pre-condition in determining the parameters of each function and enables us to compare the readaptation courses quantitatively. Further experiments show-ed that the transition from very flat to extremely bent curves was continu-ous (Figure 3) and this combined with the unavoidable variation of biologi-cal data, may be the cause for the failure of this method. At this point we had no more theoretical aspects to try further mathematical methods. Ob-viously, testing various selected functions randomly would be a hazard. So we started a completely different method without theoretical premise. We tried to obtain a curve fitting by an analog computer. This is not too complicated but very time-consuming unless either a very big analog computer or a real hybrid computer are available, since the coefficient potentiometers must be turned and corrected until an optimal curve fitting is obtained. Some of the

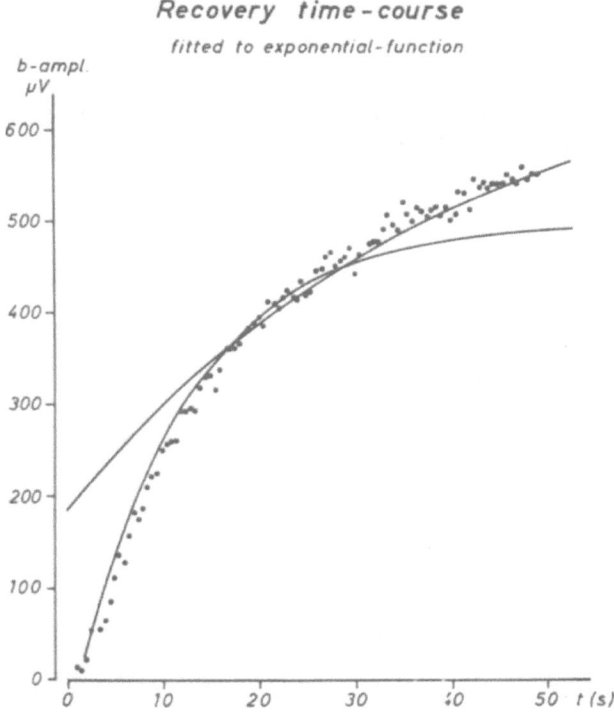

Fig. 2. Fitting the empirical data by two e-functions. From the beginning up to the 20th second best approximation by the more bent curve. From 20th to 30th second to the end better approximation by the flat curve. Note the two intersections between the e-functions.

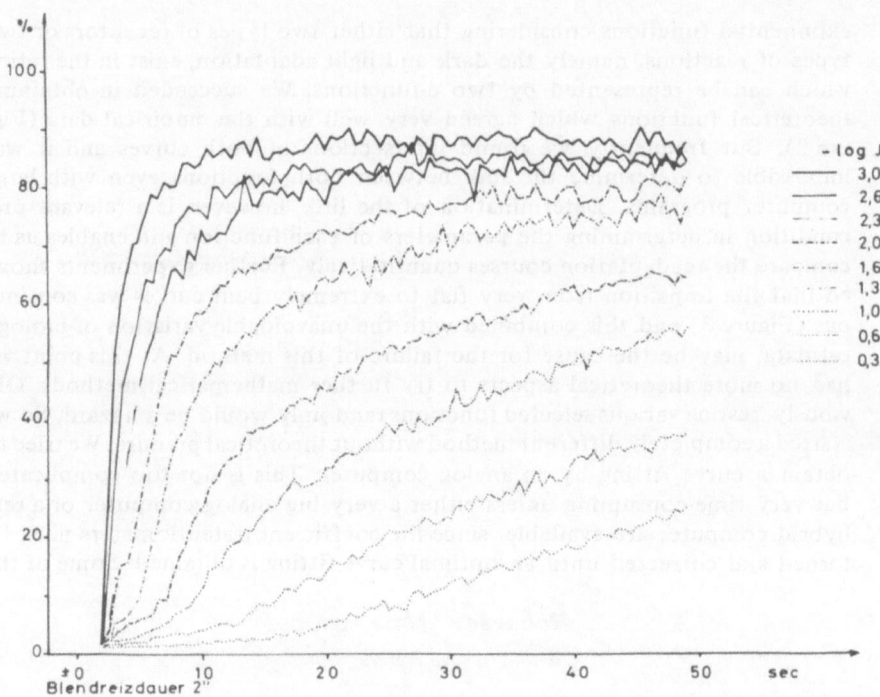

Fig. 3. Group of readaptation curves obtained with glare stimuli of constant duration but stepwise increasing intensity for about three log units.

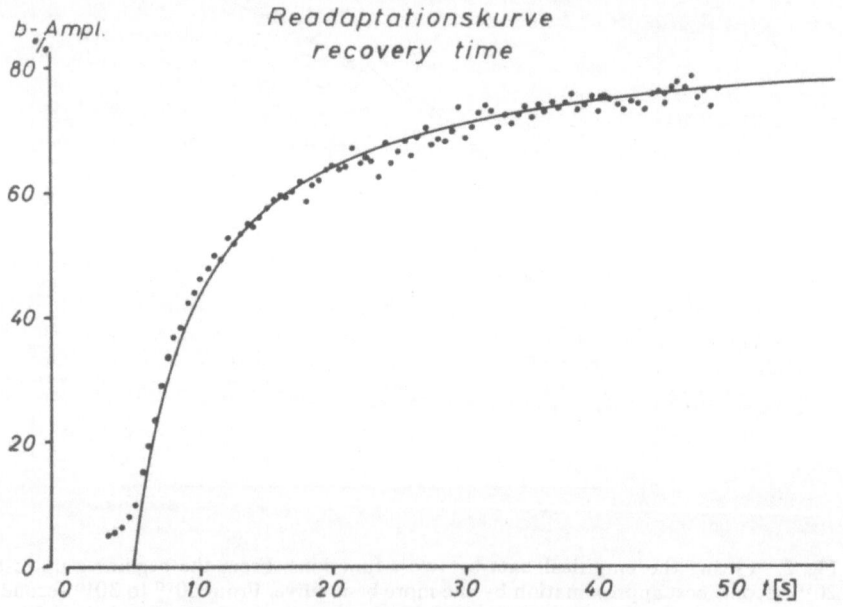

Fig. 4. Recovery time course fitting by hyperbola equation. Note the systematical deviation of the first five empirical data from the theoretical function.

coefficients become zero and then the whole term is skipped out of the equation.

Retransformation of the analog computer program to mathematical terms results in the equation for the approximation detected experimentally. This procedure shows that a simple hyperbola fulfills our conditions, and in fact, many experimental recovery curves can be quantitatively described by the parameters of a hyperbola (Figure 4). However, there are two problems left:

1) At the end of the recovery curve the calculated values are usually slightly higher than the experimental data and, according to the hyperbola equation, by extrapolation out of the measured region the values must grow and approximate infinity. From a biological point of view this method has therefore some disadvantages, because the amplitude of the measured potential can never reach values higher than before glare stimulus.

2) Some of the recovery curves did not start at the origin of the ordinates but later in time. This means that they are shifted to the right of the x-axis. We therefore must add a dead-time or delay term to the hyperbola equation. This, however, makes the hyperbola enter the fourth quadrant with values lower than zero, which is in strict contrast to any biological sense, because whatever occurs in a biological system, a response smaller than no-response can never be obtained. So the hyperbola has to be cut arbitrarily at the intersection with the x-axis. The question arises as to what really happens during the dead time, and, additionally, what does it really mean to speak of an 'estinguished ERG'. During this first period an ERG could not be detected with our equipment. To answer these question experiments had to be

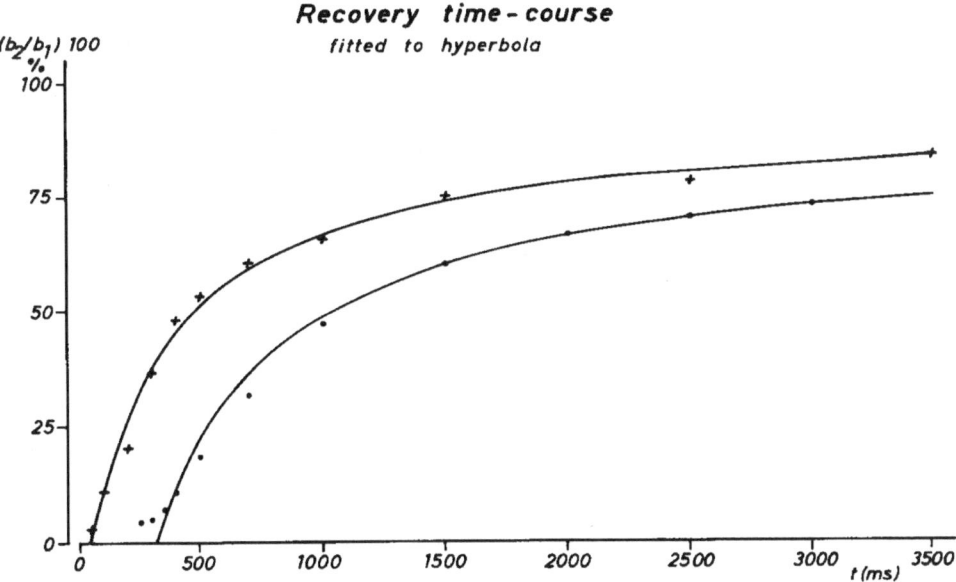

Fig. 5. Two different recovery curves. In the upper trace a sufficient approximation by a hyperbola. The lower curve shows the typical discrepancy between empirical data and calculated function.

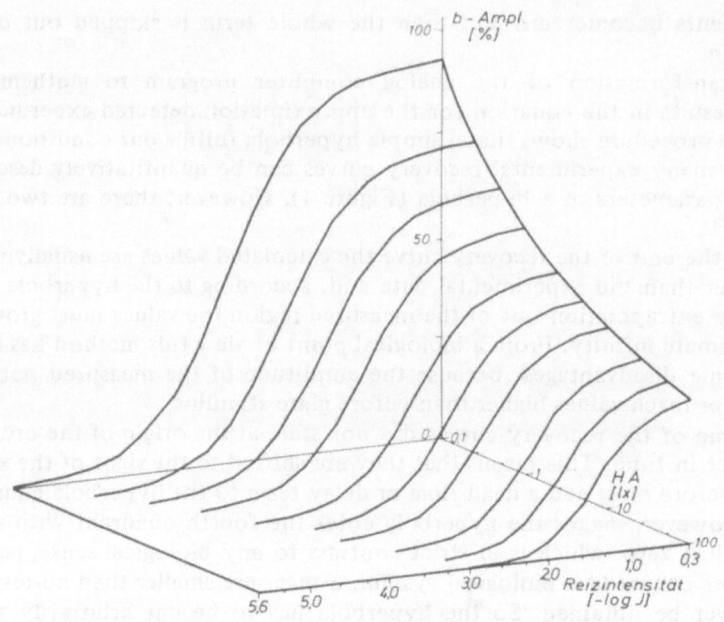

Fig. 6. Three dimensional model of the reaction of the retina (b-amplitude) depending on the test-flash-intensity and the stage of adaptation.
x-axis: test-stimulus intensity in log. units
y-axis: relative amplitude of b-wave
z-axis: intensity of background illumination in log. units.

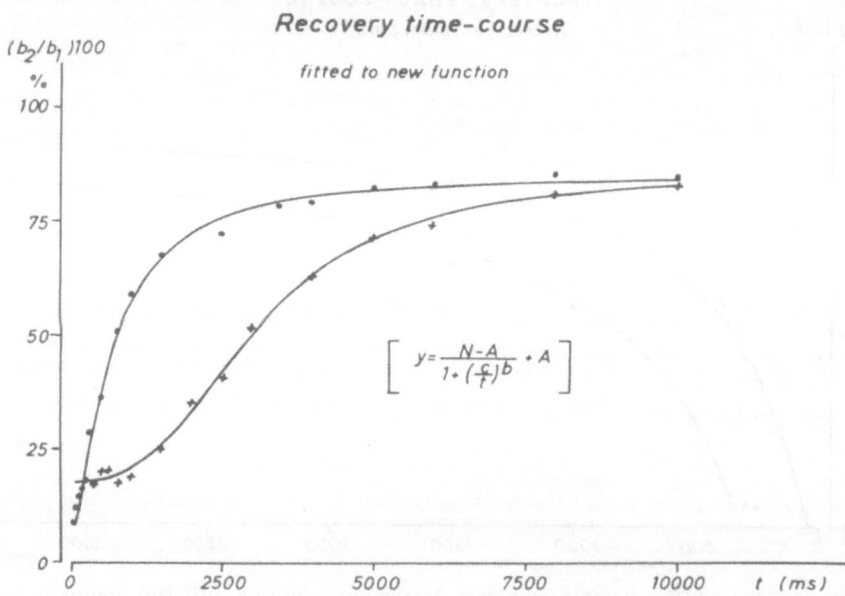

Fig. 7. Two kinds of readaptation curves. Both correctly fitted by the theoretical function, calculated from the new equation similar to a logistic function.

performed, because modeling or mathematical considerations could not solve the problems. So we studied the ERG elicited by a stimulus intensity which was gradually lowered down to extremely low intensities. We obtained well configurated ERGs of an amplitude of half a microvolt or even less. Of course, the signal had to be averaged several hundreds of times. This means that the term 'extinguished ERG' must be used with some criticism, because in some cases the loss of ERG may be caused by an insufficiency of the equipment or method rather than by a real breakdown of the biopotential production of the retina.

Some figures show that in the early beginning of the readaptation curves several points deviate from the ascending slope of readaptation curve and fall in the dead time mentioned above. This might have different causes. Firstly, the earliest potentials after glare stimulation are very small. Inaccuracies may therefore occur when they are measured and disturbances may contribute to measure a pseudopotential. Secondly, the earliest few ERGs conincide frequently with the descending slope or the c-wave of the large ERG elicited by the glare stimulus itself, and this may also cause erroneous measurements. But finally the measurements can be quite correct because one must consider that a glare stimulus, which is not too strong, does not 'extinguish' the ERG but diminishes it to a fraction of its initial value. We therefore performed a series of experiments with weaker glare stimuli and found the latter opinion was right. Consequently, we conclude that the hyperbola approximation fits only a small group of readaptation curves and cannot be used as a general rule (Figure 5). Meanwhile we have developed a model describing the behaviour of the b-wave in dependence on the stimulus intensity and the adaptation degree. This model is based on some sigmoidal functions (Figure 6). Of course, the model represents a static test and it is quite different from the dynamic process of readaptation. If readaptation would be a process linear in time, the readaptation curve could be described by a perpendicular cross-section through the model in parallel to the adaptation axis, but since obviously it is nonlinear, a profile more or less curved will result. However, a theoretical basis combining both models seems to be possible. We tried to derive a new equation similar to those describing the static model. In some way it is similar to the logistic function and in that another type of growing function. The problems seem to be solved now to some extent. Control experiments have shown that the new formula fits both types of readaptation curves, those with a sharp and steep start and those with a minor slope in the beginning (Figure 7). Now, what it is the philosophy behind such studies beyond the theoretical aspects and the incitation of new research problems? It has been shown that a formal description or simple analysis of a readaptation curve requires many measuring points, about 50 to 60, and that the examination is very time-consuming. We performed such experiments in both animals and human volunteers and it is quite clear that such a method cannot be used in clinical routine, especially, as the procedure must be repeated five or ten times to obtain a smooth curve by averaging. But an equation derived from a well-proven model enables us to calculate the whole course of a curve from a few points measured, and for this reason we hope that, at some time or other, readaptation measurements will be added to clinical retinography.

PRELIMINARY ATTEMPT AT A DIGITAL PROCESSING OF THE ELECTRO–OCULOGRAM (EOG): APPLICATION TO A SPATIO–TEMPORAL TIME AND SPACE ANALYSIS OF SACCADIC EYE MOVEMENTS DURING FREE SEARCH[1].

J.F. BAILLON[2] & N. LESEVRE[3]

(Paris, France)

I. INTRODUCTION

In our Laboratory we have been working for some years on electrophysiological signal processing, in particular in the time domain and applied mainly to the digital electro-encephalogram (REMOND & RENAULT 1972, FINDJI et al. 1973, 1974).

The following study is a first attempt at a digital processing of the electro-oculogram (EOG) with an application to a spatio-temporal analysis of saccadic eye movements during free search.

One knows indeed the extent to which various parameters which characterize eye movements recorded by EOG are complex and difficult to measure with precision from the analog signal. It is in order to answer the needs of several electro-oculographists working in the field of neuro-psychological or psycho-physiological problems of oculomotricity and visual perception — especially when dealing with the problems of strategy of visual exploration — that this study has been undertaken (REMOND et al. 1957, LESEVRE et al. 1959, JEANNEROD et al. 1967, 1968, LHERMITTE et al. 1966, 1971, LEVY-SCHOEN 1969, CHEDRU et al. 1973 etc ...).

METHODOLOGY

a) EOG recordings[1]

The horizontal and vertical eye movements have been recorded with DC amplifiers on two separate channels (X and Y) according to the electro-oculographic method described by JEANNEROD et al. (1966). The coding of events appears on a third 'technical' channel (Fig. 1: upper part). The X and Y potentials were relayed to an oscilloscope where they were combined in XY and appeared in the form of a vecto-oculogram. The recordings were made simultaneously on paper and on magnetic tape. The EOG was filtered analogically in order to eliminate high frequencies above 200 HZ.

The experimental conditions during a typical EOG recording were as

---

1. This computer study has been obtained from EOG data recorded at the Laboratoire de la Vision of the Unité INSERM de Neuro-psychologie (Pr. LHERMITTE) by M. LEBLANC and Mlle PEYNET whom we wish to thank for their help.
2. Ingénieur C.N.R.S.
3. Maitre de Recherche INSERM.

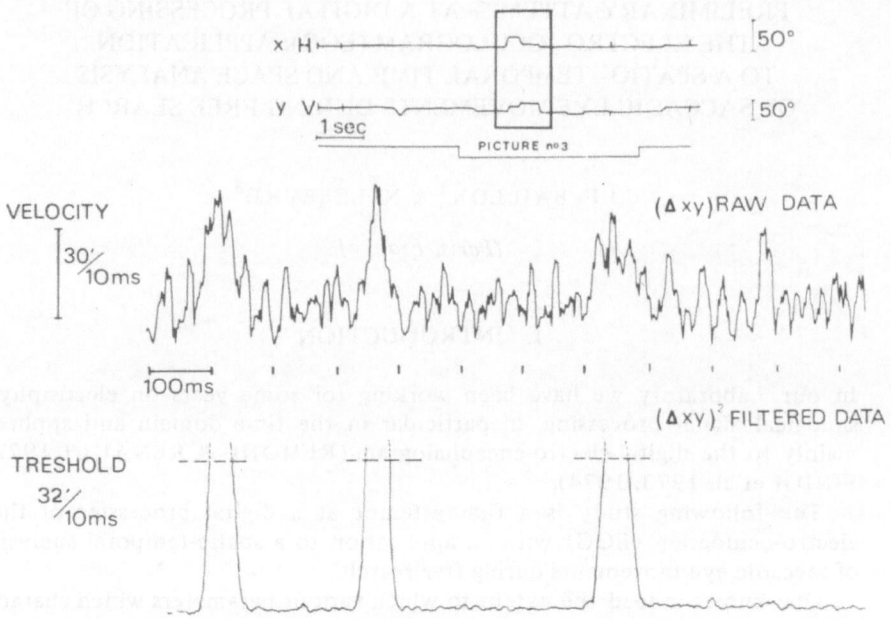

Fig. 1. *Upper part*: Recording of the analog EOG (H: Horizontal eye movements, V: Vertical movements) and the technical channel.
Middle part: Raw digital data which corresponds to the 1.100 ms analog data framed on the EOG recording shown above. In ordinate, each point of this curve represents, every 2 ms (sampling rate), the sum of all the displacements during 5 successive points in abcissa, that is during 10 ms.
Lower part: In ordinate, each point represents the square of the displacements during 10 ms after having filtered the XY data (moving average on 10 points). The threshold indicated here is that chosen to define the beginning and the end of a saccadic movement (see text).

follows: The subject was seated in front of a screen subtending a visual angle of 70 ° on the horizontal axis and 40 ° on the vertical one.

Calibration of eye movements was obtained by asking the subject to perform eye movements in various directions of 20 ° on the vertical plane and 35 ° on the horizontal one: that is, going from a point situated at the center of the screen to a luminous point located at the middle of the four sides of the screen.

A series of 11 pictures were then shown to the subject, the presentation time being 4 seconds for some of them and 8 seconds for others.

In the interval between the successive pictures the subject was asked to fixate on a red point located in the middle of the screen. This red point disapeared when the picture appeared and came back again as soon as the picture disappeared. At the onset of each slide the subject was asked to explore the picture as well as he could and to come back to the red fixation point at the end of each presentation.

b) Computer processing

For this computer study we have utilized the EOG data obtained from four normal subjects. The analog-digital conversion of the two EOG channels and of the 'technical channel' was achieved at a frequency of 500 samples per second (1 sample every 2 ms). The digital data was then processed by computer (B.G.E. M. 40) in the following way:
— First of all, taking into account the calibration of eye movements obtained in the way we have just described, the data obtained from each subject was corrected so that a given angular displacement of gaze in X or Y would correspond to the same numerical value for all the subjects.
— The next problem we were faced with was a problem of 'pattern recognition': the definition of a saccadic eye movement has been made from the curve of velocity of each saccade (Fig. 1: middle curve). This velocity was measured on 5 samples, and represents the amplitude of eye displacements during 10 ms (Fig. 1 middle curve).

In order to eliminate noise, in particular 50 cycle, the raw data was then filtered with a moving average on 20 ms. This filtered data was then squared in order to increase contrast (Fig. 1 lower curve). On this filtered and squared data, a *threshold* was then chosen in order to define a 'saccadic movement'. In the case of this work the threshold is 32' displacement during 10 ms (Fig. 1).

The beginning and the end of a saccadic movement is thus measured on this curve, at the level of this threshold. Any other values could of course have been chosen for this threshold, according to the electrophysiological data one had to deal with.

COMPUTER RESULTS

Various types of representation of this EOG digital data have been obtained by program in order to immediately visualize the various space and time parameters of oculomotor patterns occurring during visual perceptive activity, as well as the relationships between these parameters.

Many other sorts of visual representations of EOG digital data are possible, depending on the problem the electro-oculographist has to deal with.

The following outputs, obtained on a digital plotter, shown in Fig. 2, 3, 4 and 5 have been achieved to respond to the following questions:

a) How does a subject look at a given picture (Fig. 2)

On the upper part of Fig. 2 the vecto-oculogram of a normal subject looking at a car has been superimposed on the picture. The successive eye movements of the subject are shown with their own amplitude and direction, starting from the fixation point (marked O) and coming back to this same point at the end of the exploration (marked E).

This vecto-oculogram is obtained from digital data after having corrected the amplitude according to the calibration values and filtered the 50 c/s with the moving average filter. It is very similar to the analog vecto-oculo-

141

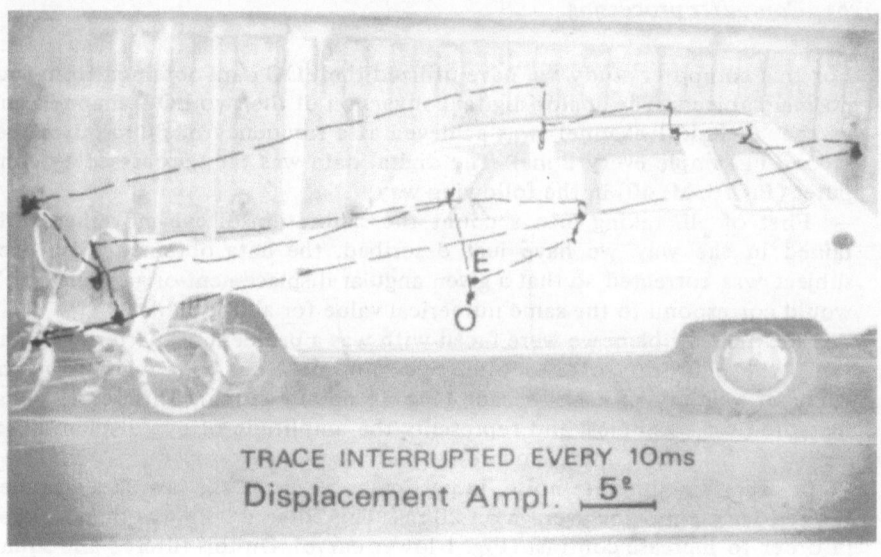

TRACE INTERRUPTED EVERY 10ms
Displacement Ampl. 5⁰

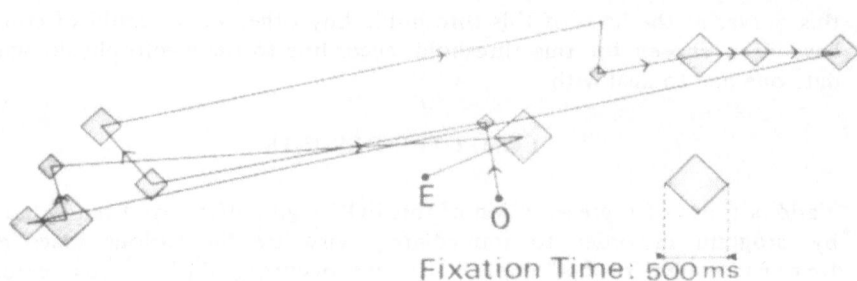

Fixation Time: 500 ms

Fig. 2. *Upper part*: Vecto-oculogram obtained on filtered digital data (moving average on 20 ms), for subject A looking at picture 6.
Lower part: Only the fast displacements (defined as indicated Figure 1) are represented here by straight lines: the intervals between two successive saccades (fixations) are represented by square diamonds the width of which is proportional to their duration.

gram which appears on the oscilloscope. It has taken into account the whole data: that is, all movements which occur during the recording without any criteria of threshold. Besides, there is in this vecto-oculogram no information about the duration of each successive fixation. The time scale is only given in this case by interruptions in the lines indicating the displacements, which occur every 10 ms.

A second step has been to present a vecto-oculogram after having made a choice amongst these movements by keeping only the saccadic movements as defined by our threshold criteria; besides in this new vecto-oculogram we

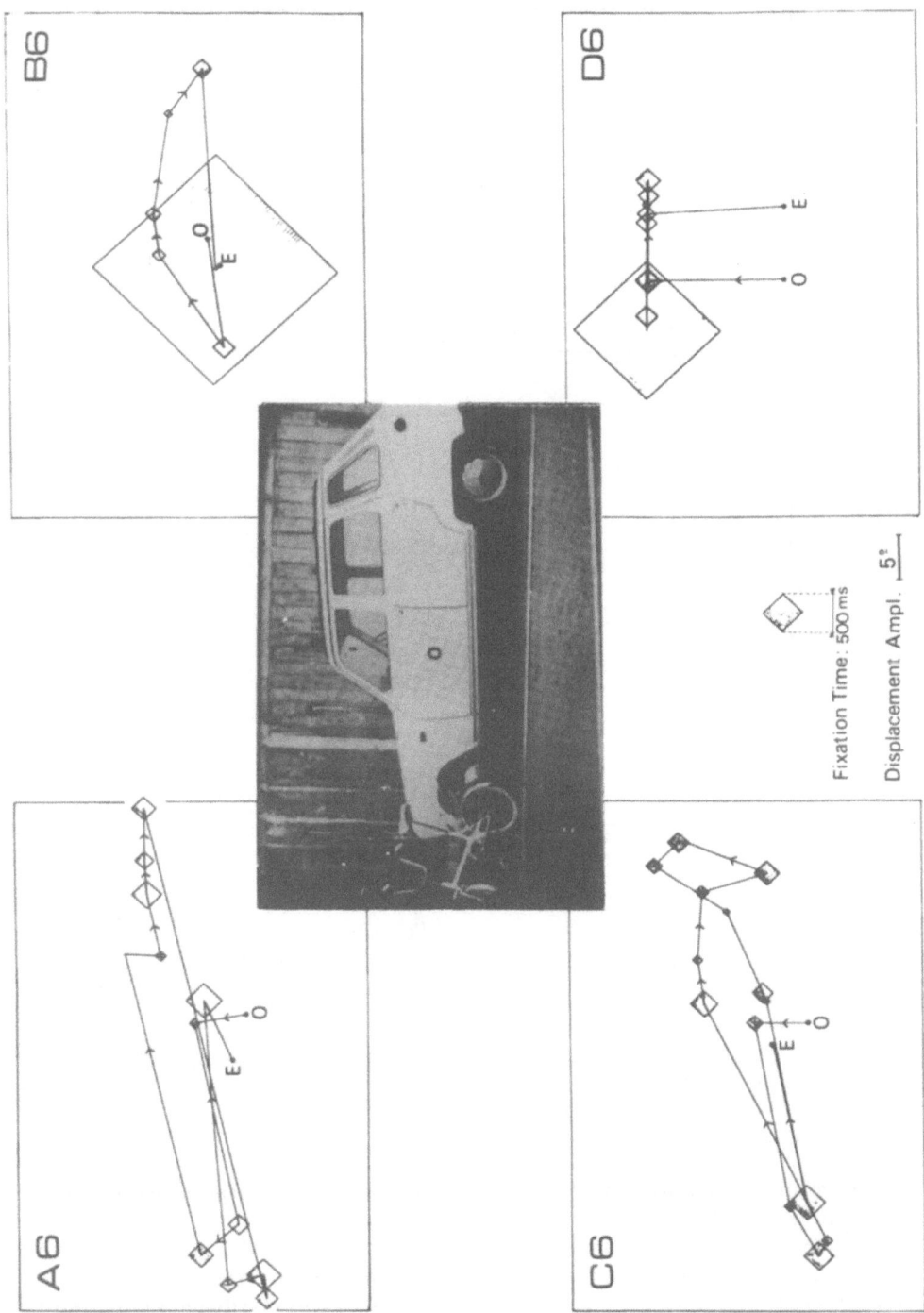

Fig. 3. Exploration of picture 6 by four different subjects.

143

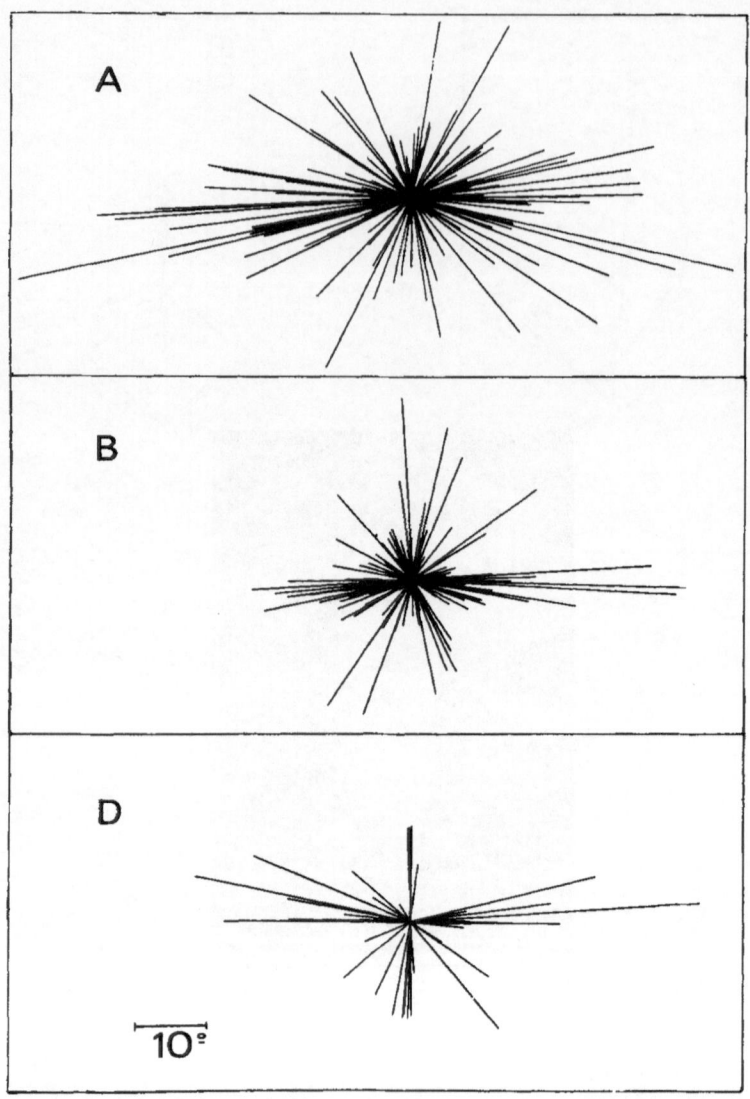

Fig. 4. Representation, for three subjects, of all the fast displacements as a function of their direction and size. All the saccades achieved during the presentation of the 11 slides have been drawn from the same origin.

have included information about the duration of each successive fixation (lower part of Fig. 2).

In this space and time representation (lower part of Fig. 2), each time interval between two successive saccades — that is, each fixation occurring on a precise location of the picture — is represented by a square diamond the width of which is proportional to its duration. Theoretically, the beginning (O) and the end (E) of the exploration ought to merge into one another. The distance between these two points (O and E) is due to various 'artefacts' coming from insufficient calibration, head movements, wrinkling of the forehead, base line shift etc. etc. ... These arte⁴acts — which vary according to the method used for recording eye movements — could of course be eliminated or at least corrected by program, insofar as they can be defined and measured with enough precision by the electrooculographist. But this is the next step, which we have not come to yet.

b) What kind of inter-individual scanning differences can be seen? (Fig. 3)

In Fig. 3 the digital space and time scanning representation of four different normal subjects looking at the same picture is shown. The differences are immediately evident: some people make many small movements and short fixations (subject C); others do not really explore, but stay a long time on one particular part of the picture (This is the case of subject D who told us afterwards that he knew this picture by heart and had great difficulty in really exploring it).

The way people look at pictures depends, of course, on what on what they are asked to do. Intra or inter-individual differences in eye movement organization can only be studied correctly if the required task is well defined. In this case, the kind of information that gives this space and time representation may be very useful for clinical examination of hemianopias, cases of unilateral inattention or various forms of visual and spatial agnosia.

c) What is the preferential direction of gaze? (Fig. 4)

In Figure 4 all the saccadic movements obtained during the whole session of 11 pictures have been represented for 3 different subjects, with their own amplitude and direction and all starting from the same point. This type of representation — which allows one to detect immediately the existence of a preferential direction of gaze — seems to be an interesting tool when dealing with pathological cases.

d) Is there any relationship between the duration of fixations and the amplitude of saccadic movements? (Fig. 5)

Mathematical correlations can of course be calculated from the digital data, but in many cases it might be useful to visualize these relations before and after having done the calculus. A visual representation of digital EOG data, helpful in studying the relationships between the duration of a given fixation and the amplitude of the preceding or following saccade, is shown in Fig. 5.

CONCLUSION

Other methods of data processing and other computer outputs could have been chosen, depending on the problem one had to deal with. These computer realizations have just been given as an example of what can or could be done in the domain of electro-oculography and in order to stress the various

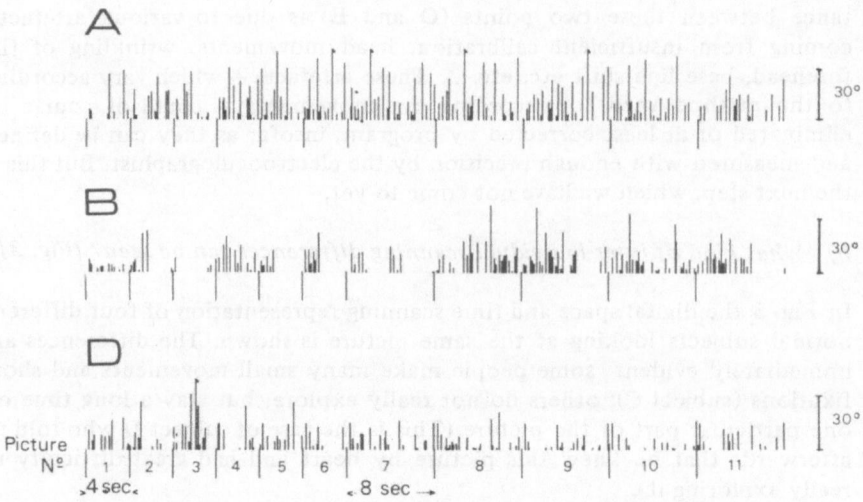

Fig. 5. Fast displacements during exploration of the whole series of pictures for three different subjects. The vertical lines are proportional to the size of the displacements and the intervals between them are proportional to the duration of the fixations.

difficulties which still have to be overcome before this type of E.O.G. data processing becomes 'functional', practically useful for clinical purposes.

First of all, in order to get a more precise representation of the position of the eye in time and space while a subject is looking at a picture, a more sophisticated calibration method ought to be utilized which would take into account not only the various directions of eye movements but also the position of the eye at the onset of each movement.

On the other hand — and this is probably the most difficult part to handle — a better definition and measure of electrophysiological 'artefacts' should to be given in order to try and correct them by computer. Good computer results can only be obtained from 'good' electrophysiological data. This truism needs to be especially emphasized in the case of electro-oculographic data. Indeed, many difficulties are inherent in this method based on the changes of the corneo-retinal potential. For instance, those due to the lack of homogenity of the potential field around the eyes and on the surface of the whole face have to be made more precise before further steps can be taken. This will only be possible through a continuous dialogue between electrophysiologists and specialists in signal processing.

SUMMARY

A reliable method for analyzing exploratory saccadic eye movements during free search would be of great help to workers in the field of neurophysiological or pathological problems of visual perception. Indeed, one knows the extent to which various parameters characterising eye movements recorded by electro-oculography (EOG) are complex and difficult to measure with precision from the electrophysiological signal.

In order to answer the needs of several electro-oculographists interested in visual perceptive activity and oculomotricity, the authors have tried to develop this analysis by computer on the EOG signal recorded in the following situation: After calibration of the vertical and horizontal eye movements amplitude, the subject is asked to look at a series of pictures, each picture being presented for 4 or 8 seconds, and to return to a fixation point between two pictures.

Preliminary results obtained by computer are shown: 'wave form' recognition, spatio temporal representation of fixations and saccadic movements, classification of these movements as a function of their duration, amplitude, direction etc ... which enables various statistical studies.

These computer data are discussed in relation to the normal and pathological oculo-motor and visual problems posed.

REFERENCES

CHEDRU F., LEBLANC M. & F. LHERMITTE — Visual searching in normal and brain-damaged subjects (contribution to the study of unilateral inattention). Cortex, IX, 94-111 (1973).

FINDJI F., RENAULT B., BAILLON J.F. & A. REMOND — Premiers résultats d'une methode d'étude statistique originale du signal EEG considéré comme une succession de demi-ondes. Rev. Neurol. 3, 3, 304-309 (1973).

FINDJI F., RENAULT B., BAILLON J.F. & A. REMOND — A mimetic method of automatic EEG Analysis: principle and first results. 1 st world Conference on Medical Informatics, Stockholm, In Press (1974).

JEANNEROD M. — Déplacements et fixations du regard dans l'exploration libre d'une scène visuelle. Progr. Ophtal. 19, 52-99 (1968).

JEANNEROD M., GERIN P. & J. ROUGIER — Enregistrement bidimensionnel des mouvements et des pauses oculaires. 1966. Rev. Oto-Neuro-Ophtalm. 38, 51-53 (1966).

JEANNEROD M., MONIER F., REVOL M. & P. GERIN — Intérêt de la vecto-oculographie dans l'étude des troubles de la structuration perceptive. Rev. Neurol. 117, 1, 332-336 (1967).

LESEVRE N., GABERSEK V. & A. REMOND — Diagnostic électro-oculographique des hémianopsiques. Rev. Neurol. 3, 101, 248-253 (1959).

LEVY-SCHOEN A. — L'étude des mouvements oculaires. Ed. Dunod, Paris, p. 261 (1969).

LHERMITTE F., CHAIN F., ARON D. & A.M. MONTARAL — Recherche sur le mouvement du regard dans un cas d'agnosie visuelle. Rev. Neurol. 114, 6, 409-420 (1966).

LHERMITTE F. & F. CHAIN — Données préliminaires sur les mouvements du regard en pathologie cérébrale. In: La Fonction du Regard — Colloque INSERM, édité par A. DUBOIS-POULSEN, G.C. LAIRY & A. REMOND. Paris 315-341 (1971).

REMOND A., LESEVRE N. & V. GABERSEK — Approche d'une sémiologie électrographique du regard. Rev. Neurol. 96, 6, 536-546 (1957).

REMOND A. & B. RENAULT — La théorie des objets électrographiques. Rev. EEG, Neurophysiol. 2, 241-256 (1972).

TIME CONSTANT OF THE DECAY
PROCESS OF BOTH ERG AND VER
AT THE OFF-SET OF STIMULATION

LUCIA RONCHI & GIUSEPPE MOLESINI

(Florence, Italy)

SUMMARY

After the cessation of a sinusoidally modulated stimulus, the ERG response is found to continue, in the form of a damped oscillation (the time constant of the decay process being of the order of 1 sec) with the same frequency as the primary stimulus (3.7 Hz).

The cortical response also seems to continue and to decay slowly (the time constant being of the same order as that of the VER). However, no counterpart of this effect is found when applying the multivariate analysis leading to the estimate of eigenvectors of various average cycles after the Off-set of the light stimulus.

The off-set of the visual system, that is, the response to the cessation of illumination, has been recorded at any stage across the visual pathway. Let us consider first the ERG response. For a general view of the controversies concerning its existence and its dependence on the state of adaptation and on the duration of previous stimulation, we refer to JAYLE et al. (1965). In the case where the eye is presented with a jump of luminance (say, a negative step), the response or end-effect represents a measurement of the d.c. level of the retina (TROELSTRA, 1964; BIERSDORF & ARMINGTON, 1957). It consists of a downward deflection, dropping to zero within no more than a quarter of a second. On the other hand, after the off-set of a sequence of flashes, the end response is found to be more complicated and to exhibit a number of wavelets (DODT, 1951; BEST & BOHNEN, 1957, NAGATA & TAKATA, 1962).

At the cortical level, the off-effect of the VER consists of a negative deflection (HARTER, 1971), followed by a small scalp-positive wave. The off-response is extinguished within about 0.2 sec. Abstraction is made here from conditioning effects, taking place under peculiar conditions of stimulation (limp technique) leading to responses of endogenous origin (JOHN, 1967; MORREL et al. 1960; BARLOW et al. 1967).

At the level of sensation, a number of psychophysical data have been recorded within the first 50 msec after the off-set of a light stimulus (SPERLING, 1965; IKEDA, 1965; RASHBASS, 1970, BOYNTON, 1972), that is, during the course of the lingering primary image (LE GRAND, 1948) and before the occurrence of the so-called Hering after-image (BROWN, 1965).

Let us recall that there is a controversy about the existence of a dark interval between the cessation of the light sensation outlasting the stimulus and the occurrence of the after-image. There seems to be a relation between the duration of the flash and the pattern of subsequent events (MILLER, 1966).

The sensory consequences of the off-effect have been dealt with by various authors (PIRENNE, 1957; ASHER, 1957; LIECHTENSTEIN & BOUCHER, 1960). The dependence of the amplitude of the drop of luminance on the off-effect has been recorded for the ERG response (SCHWEITZER & TROELSTRA, 1966; RONCHI 1960; BROOKS & HUBER, 1972). A model common to all the outputs is being sought for (BIRD & MOWBRAY, 1973).

The present paper deals with both ERG and VER responses to a sinusoidally modulated light. The question is set what happens at the off-set of the stimulus, that is, when the time modulation ceases and the eye is presented with a steady field (whose luminance equals the average level of the previous stimulus).

It is hard to predict what we should expect, on the basis of the previous findings obtained with negative steps of luminance or with a sequence of square pulses of light. In fact, as LEVETT (1970) remarks, a jump of illumination involving an infinite rate of change is likely to cause the retina of establish operations much faster than in the case of sinusoidal stimuli.

APPARATUS AND METHOD

The subject is seated in a screened cage. One electrode is applied in the corneal bulge of the contact lens, the indifferent electrode is on the forehead. In this way ERG is recorded. The occipital potential is recorded from the scalp, the active electrode being on the right hemisphere, $2\frac{1}{2}$ cm above

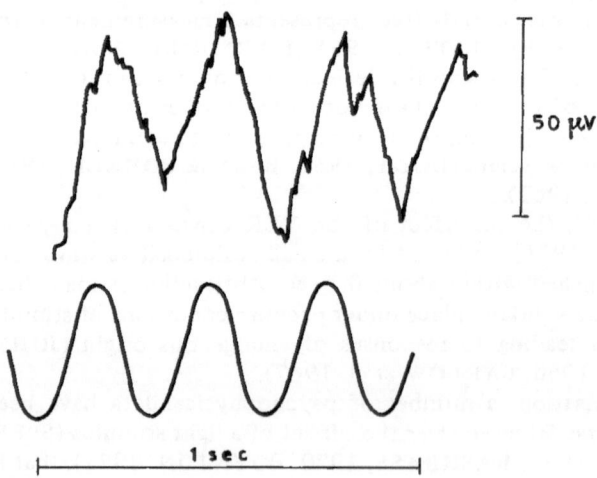

50 µv

1 sec

Fig. 1.   ERG response to a sinusoidally modulated stimulus.

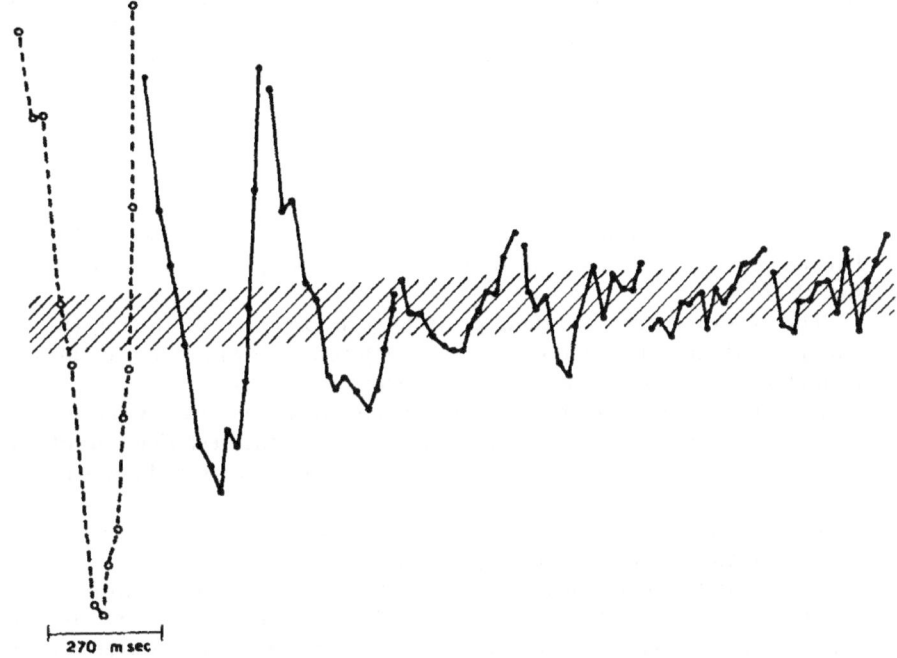

Fig. 2a. Average ERG response before the offset (broken line) and average tracing after the offset. The dashed area represents the noise.

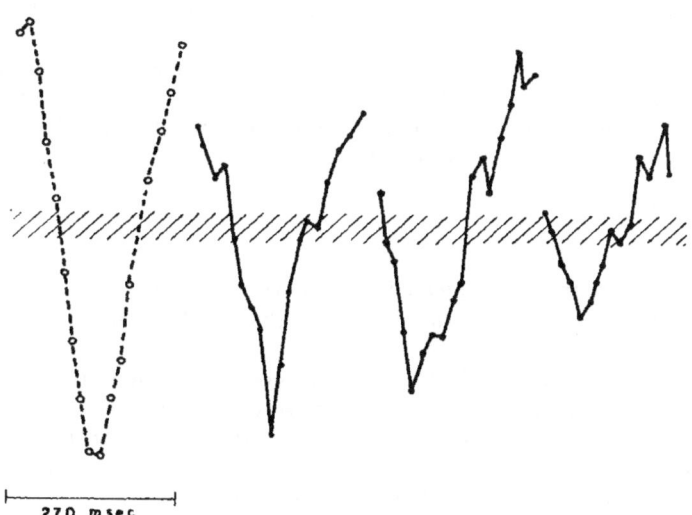

Fig. 2b. As for Fig. 2a), but for a different session.

151

the inion, 3 cm from the midline. The indifferent electrode is on the ear-lobe, the contralateral one being earthed.

The test field consists of a circular patch, subtending at the eye 9 deg. diam. It contains a circular grating (J. Bessel's function), the spatial frequency of which is 10 cpd, the spatial modulation 90%. The light is sinusoidally modulated in time, the modulation depth being 90%, the frequency 3.7 Hz in some sessions, 5 in others.

Responses are recorded with the aid of a pen writing system (OTE Mod. E 8 a), the bandpass being 1-75 Hz. In some sessions also the Hewlett Packard Signal Analyser 5480 A is used, the preamplifier being the Tektronix 88111A.

The recorded trace is then projected, in order to attain the suitable enlargement, and then is digitized (for each response wave the ordinates are read at a number of time points varying from 16 to 25).

Prior to each session the observer pre-adapts his eyes to the darkness for 20 min. and then, to the average luminance of the test field (4 nit) for 5 min. The surround covering the greatest part of the visual field is kept at this same luminance.

Five young adult experienced observers took part in the experiment, in repeated sessions throughout the past year.

At the beginning of the session, the subject was presented with the signal and the responses were recorded. After a few minutes of exposure, the time varying stimulus was interrupted by means of an electronic shutter, and the level passed from the peak of the sinewave to the average level, which, thereafter, remained steady. Sixteen to twenty interruptions were distributed at random across a 30 min. lasting session.

EXPERIMENTAL FINDINGS

Fig. 1 shows the ERG response to a 3.7 Hz stimulus. Fig. 2 a shows the average of the data recorded soon before and soon after the cessation of the sinusoidally modulated stimulus. Twenty portions of the baseline, recorded at different times across the same session, under the same experimental conditions, were put together to obtain these data. Fig. 2b refers to another session. The dashed area represents the amplitude (S_{lim}) of the just detectable signal estimated in terms of equation 1):

$$1) \qquad S_{lim} = 2 \frac{S.D.}{\sqrt{N}}$$

where S.D. is the estimate of the mean Standard Deviation of various samples of 20 digitized data and 2 is the assumed value of the signal-to-noise ratio.

Fig. 3 shows the average cortical evoked response recorded from the scalp before the off-set and soon after it, respectively. Sample numerosity is 16. These data are in line with those produced by HARTER (1971). The question arises now what happens after the time interval corresponding to the first "cycle" of light stimulus, spent in the darkness.

As is shown in Figures 4 a) and b), there is evidence of a sort of damped oscillation of the tracing which, after 1 or two seconds, drops within the dashed area representing the amplitude of the just detectable signal (eq. 1).

DISCUSSION

Our ERG data show a sort of continuation of the response after the off-set of the sinusoidally modulated stimulus. By fitting the data recorded in a number of different sessions to an equation of the type:

2) $Y(t) = K\ e^{-t/\tau}\sin(2\pi ft+\varphi)$

where f is the frequency of the primary stimulus, the time constant τ of the decay process is found to vary within wide limits say, 300 through 1200 msec) when passing from one session to another. The modal value is 600 msec. The correlation coefficient of the best fit is no less than 0.80.

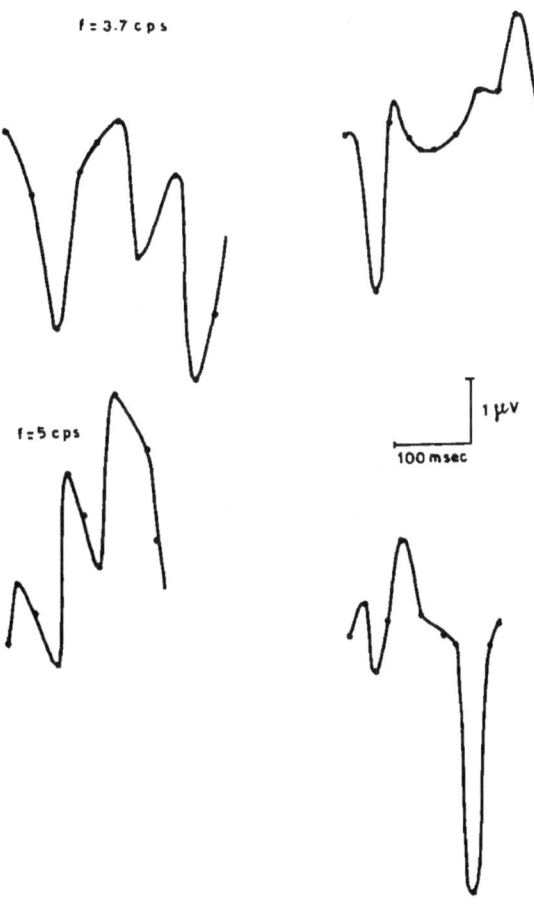

Fig. 3. Cortical responses to a sinusoidally modulated stimulus before and after the offset of the cyclical stimulus. Label denotes the frequency.

153

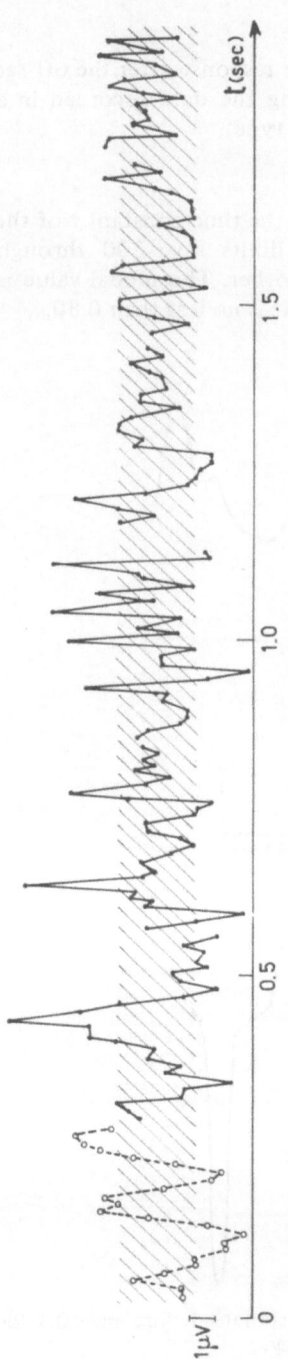

Fig. 4a. Average VER before the offset (broken line) and average tracing after the offset. The dashed area represents the noise.

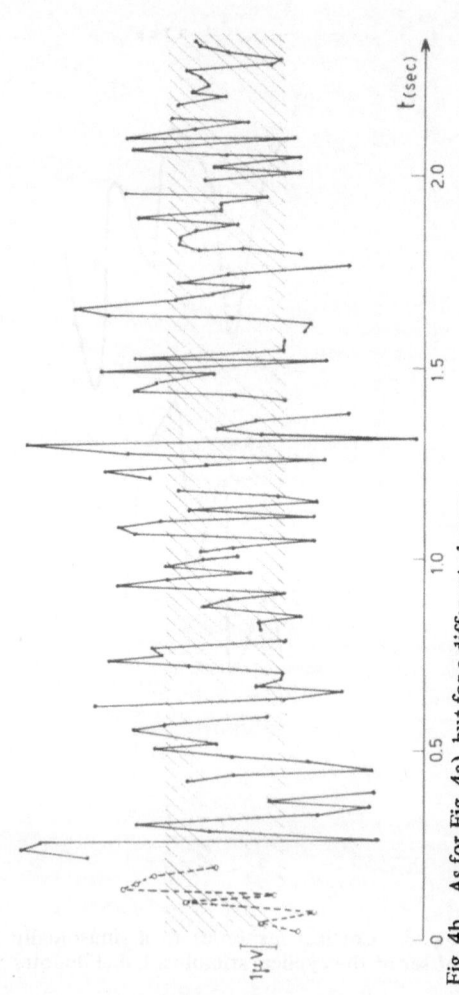

Fig. 4b. As for Fig. 4a), but for a different observer.

This behavior might be represented in terms of TROELSTRA & SCHWEITZER's physical model (1966). Their multiplier is now replaced by a mixer, followed by an amplifier which, in turn, is follwed by a low-pass filter. The output of this filter is fed back to the mixer. The existence of this non-passive feedback network might find its counterpart in some suggestions made by a number of authors, on the basis of data recorded in quite different experiments (FEINSOD et al., 1971 a) and b); RONCHI, quoted by JAYLE et al. 1965).

Let us consider now the cortical response. The time constant, estimated with the aid of eq. 2) by making reference to the maximum peak-to-peak amplitude, is found to be 1100 msec, the correlation coefficient of the fit being 0.9. This agreement with the ERG data is unexpected. In fact, the majority of the record lies within the noise level. Apparently, the noise is so large because of the limited number of summations used, sixteen. Now, the correlation between the responses obtained by averaging 16 single trial data and that with, say, 110 data, is rather high, for our subjects (no less than 0.8). In turn, it did not seem worthwhile to increase the number of interruptions beyond 16 (sometimes even 20), throughout the same session, nor to combine the data recorded in different sessions.

Next, we applied the multivariate analysis leading to the eigenvectors (SIMONDS, 1963; SAUNDERS, 1973). Fig. 5 (left portion) shows the mean response to a cycle of the light stimulus, and the two first vectors, accounting for the greatest part of the total variance (74% and 14%, respectively). The most variable point seems to be the positive peak occurring in the neighborhood of 100 msec. Now, after the off-set of the sinusoidal stimulus, the maximum variance accounted for by the first vector does not exceed 50%, whatever the order number of the cyclus considered, as is shown in Fig. 6, where the percentage of the total variance accounted for by the main vectors is displayed. Note that some of the first four vectors, when plotted as a function of time show a double-peaked behavior, resembling an oscillation with a frequency of 10 Hz. The percentage of variance accounted for by this component attains even 50%, around 1 sec after the off-set. The question arises whether this source of variability is due to a sort of alpha activity (Fig. 5, right portion) or if we are faced with a sort of persistence of the rectified component of the response evoked by the light stimulus (whose frequency is 5 Hz), by invoking SPEKREIJSE & VAN DER TWEEL model (1966). Note that the subjects taking part in the present experiment are of low alpha type (RONCHI et al. 1971).

CONCLUDING REMARKS

After the cessation of a sinusoidally modulated light stimulus, the ERG response seems to continue, in the form of a damped oscillation, whose frequency is the same as that of the primary stimulus. The time constant of the decay process is of the order of 1 sec. The question arises whether these residual oscillations are actually in the direct chain of events leading to sensation, or whether the response is an epiphenomenon of some sort. Also at the cortical level, there is a damped oscillation after the off-set of the stimulus. The order of magnitude of the time constant of this decay is of

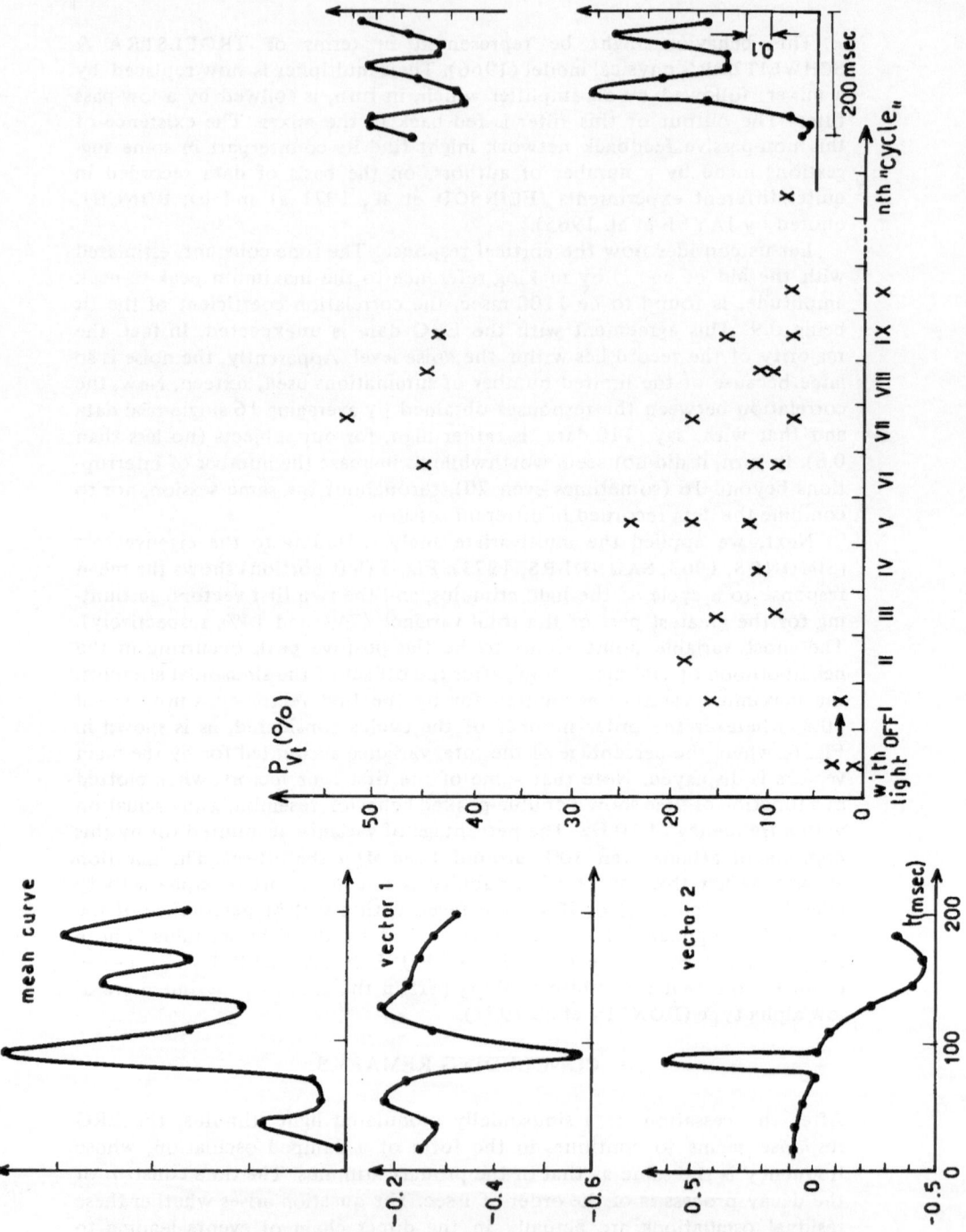

Fig. 5. Outcome of the multivariate analysis. Left portion: The average response and the first two vectors Right portion: The percentages of total variance accounted for by α-like components, more-or less shifted in phase from one another, at various cycles before and after the offset.

156

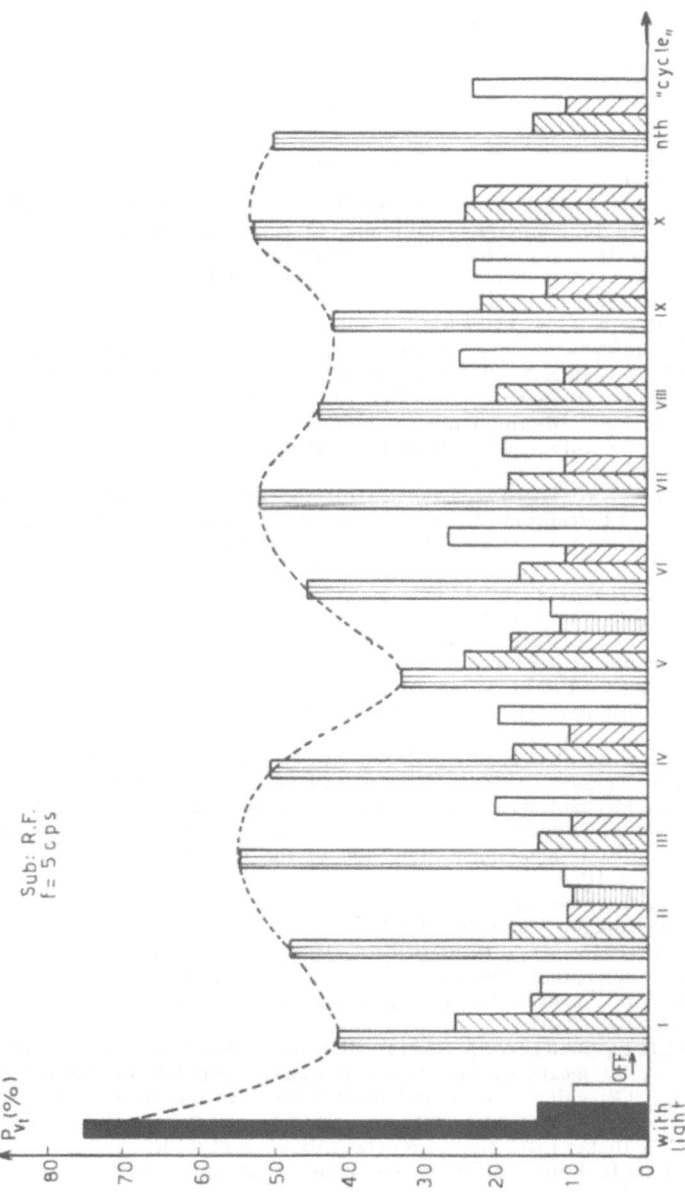

Fig. 6. The percentage of total variance accounted for by the first vectors and (empty space) by the residual ones, for various cycles.

the same order of magnitude as that of ERG. However, the majority of response features drop below the noise level. The multivariate analysis leading to the estimate of eigenvectors indicates that the greatest part of total variance of the actual response to light is accounted for by a given vector. This is no longer the case after the cessation of stimulation. Further experimental data are needed in order to establish whether the pattern of electrical events following the cessation of light constitute a non functional correlate to the actional mechanism of informational analysis.

REFERENCES

ASHER, M.F. Off-effect giving rise to a sensation of blackness. *J. Physiol. (Lond.)* 137, *48* (1957).

BARLOW, J.S., MORREL, L. & F. MORREL, Some observations on evoked response in relation to temporal conditioning to paired stimuli in man. Trans. int. Coll. *Bratislava Acad. Sci.*, *11-14* sept. 1965 (1967).

BEST, W. & X. BOHNEN, Ueber den Off-Effekt in ERG des Menschen-Graef. *Arch. Ophthal.* 158, *568* (1957).

BIERSDORF, W.R. & J.C. ARMINGTON, Responses of the human eye to sudden changes in the wavelength of stimulation. *J. Opt. Soc. Am.* 47, *208* (1957).

BIRD, J.F. & G.H. MOMBRAY, Analysis of transient visual sensations above the flicker fusion of frequency. *Vision Res.* 13, *673* (1973).

BOYNTON, R.M. Discrimination of homogeneous double Pulses. In: Handbook of Sensory Physiology, JAMESON, D. & HURVICH, L.M. Eds., Vol. VII/4, Springer, Berlin (1972).

BROOKS, B. & C. HUBER, Evidence for the role of the transient neural "off-response" in perception of light decrement: a psychophysical test derived from neuronal data in the cat. *Vision Res.* 12, *1291* (1972).

BROWN, J.L. Afterimages. In: Vision and Visual Perception, GRAHAM C.H. Ed., Wiley, New York, p. 479 (1965).

DODT, E. (1951) Cone ERG by flicker. *Nature*, 168, *738*.

HARTER, M.R. Visually evoked cortical responses to the on- and off-set of patterned light in humans. *Vision Res.* 11, *685* (1971).

HECK, J. Der off-Effekt im menschlichen ERG. *Acta Physiol. Scand.* 40, *113* (1957).

IKEDA, M. Temporal summation of positive and negative flashes in the visual system. *J. Opt. Soc. Am.* 55, 1527 (1965).

JAYLE, G.E., BOYER, R.L. & J.B. SARACCO, L'Electroretinographie-Bases Physiologiques et Données Cliniques. Masson et Cie, Paris, Vol. I (1965).

JOHN, E.R. Mechanisms of Memory. Ac Press, New York, pp. 354 and 418 (1967).

LE GRAND, Y. Optique Physiologique, Ed. de la Rev. d'Opt. Paris, Vol. II (1948).

LEVETT, J. Non linear-linear transition in the frog intraretinal electroretinogram. *Vision Res.* 10, 1347 (1970).

LEVETT, J. Linear-nonlinear-linear transition as a function of frequency in the retinal response to light. *Vision Res.* 12, 1301.

LIECHTENSTEIN, M. & R. BOUCHER, Minimum detectable dark interval between trains of perceptually fused flashes. *J. Opt. Soc. Am.* 50, 461 (1960).

MILLER, N.D. Positive after-image following brief high intensity flashes. *J. Opt. Soc. Am* 56, 802 (1966).

MORRELL, F., BARLOW, J. & M.A. BRAZIER, Analysis of conditioned repetitive response by means of the average response computer. In: Recent Advances in Biological Psychiatry, Grune and Stratton Inc. U.S.A. (1960).

NAGATA, M. & H. TAKATA, Off-responses of human eye and their significance in the photopic flicker ERG. Newsletter (ISCERG) 3, 4 (1962).

PIRENNE, M.H. Retinal off-units and human visual acuity. *J. Physiol. (Lond.)* 137, 48 (1957).

RASHBASS, C. The visibility of transient changes of luminance. *J. Physiol. (Lond.)* 210, 165 (1970).

RONCHI, L. Negative electrical off-responses of the human retina. Atti fond. G. Ronchi, 15, 515 (1960).

SAUNDERS, R.Mc D. Eigenvectors of the sensitivity to variations across the human central fovea- *Vision Res.* 13, 182 (1973).

SIMONDS, J.L. Application of characteristic vector analysis to photographic and optical response data. *J. Opt. Soc. Am.* 53, 968 (1963).

SPEKREIJSE H. & J.H. VAN DER TWEEL, Flicker and noise. Suppl. Vision Res. N° 1 (Proc. Int. Iscerg Symp.), p. 275 (1966).

SPERLING, G. Temporal and spatial visual masking. *J. Opt. Soc. Am.* 55, 541 (1965).

TROELSTRA, A. Non-linear system analysis in Electroretinography. Inst. for Perc. RVO-TNO, Soesterberg, The Netherlands (1964).

TROELSTRA, A. Harmonic distortion in the frog's ERG and its possible relation to differences in latencies. *Vision Res.* 11, 403 (1971).

TROELSTRA, A. & N.M.J. SCHWEITZER A model for the scotopic electroretinographic system. In: Studies in Perception, Festschrift dedicated to M.A. BOUMAN, Inst. for Perc. RVO-TNO, Soesterberg, The Netherlands (1966).

Authors' address
Prof. Lucia Rositani Ronchi and Dr. Giuseppe Molesini
Istituto Nazionale di Ottica
Largo Fermi 6, Arcetri, 50125 Florence
Italy

STATISTICAL DISCRIMINATION BETWEEN VISUAL EVOKED RESPONSES ACCORDING TO PHOTOSTIMULUS WAVELENGTH

RINALDO ALFIERI* & MARIE-HÉLÈNE BASSANT**

(Clermont-Ferrand, France)

I. STATEMENT OF THE PROBLEM

With the experimental conditions, usually applied for recording human visual evoked responses (VERs), it is not possible to obtain a univocal and perfectly reproducible waveform with monochromatic light of different wavelength. This may be understood, if we realize, that: 1) recording electrodes on the scalp are placed widely apart from the electrogenerating areas (edges of calcarine fissure); 2) the number of summations, performed, is limited to 100 (comfort of the patient); 3) a low photopic luminance is used (sensitization of pathological responses through juxtaliminal monochromatic photostimulation).

In order to avoid the 'constraints' inherent to experiments with human beings, we have recorded VERs in animals. The electrodes were placed directly on the primary area of the visual system in the occipital lobe.

In view of the variability in waveform, we assessed the VERs according to the 'all or nothing' method, thus limited to the appearance or non-appearance of a response. Through this approach we established (ALFIERI & SOLÉ, 1971; ALFIERI, RIGAL & SOLÉ, 1972):
1) an electrophysiological semiology of photoreceptors: a. in red monochromatic light the electroretinogram (ERG-r) explores the photopic function, i.e. the cones as a whole (multiple, early, stationary waves during dark adaptation following dazzling: a-, e- and b_1-waves): α. in red monochromatic light the visual evoked response (VER-r) explores the conduction of the central macular bundle of the optic nerve, representing the function of the central cones. Their activity cannot be examined with the ERG, as their number is too small as compared to that of the peripheral cones. In the VER, on the contrary, the cortical projection of the macula is preponderant in comparison with the retinal periphery; β. in blue monochromatic light the visual evoked response (VER-b) explores the conduction of the peripheral bundles of the optic nerve, i.e. the peripheral cones. Their activity conceals that of the rods of which the cortical projection is too deep for the electrode placed on the scalp; b. in blue monochromatic light the electroretinogram

* Department of Biomathematics, Faculty of Medicine, P.O. Box 38, 63001 Clermont-Ferrand Cedex (France).
** Health Protection Department, Atomic Energy Commission, P.O. Box 6, 92260 Fontenay-Aux-Roses (France).

(ERG-b) explores the scotopic function, i.e. the rods (a single, delayed, evolving wave during dark adaptation after dazzling: b_2-wave);

2) an electrophysiological nosology of retinopathies: a. Photopic retinopathy: α) central only: ERG-r Λ ERG-b Λ $\overline{\text{VER-r}}$ Λ VER-b, where Λ represents the logical conjunction (AND), while the bar overlining an examination indicates a pathological result. The expression stated above corresponds to a disturbance of the visual evoked response alone in red monochromatic light; β) global: ERG-r Λ ERG-b Λ $\overline{\text{VER-r}}$ Λ $\overline{\text{VER-b}}$, where $\overline{\text{VER-r}}$ indicates that the central cones are damaged while $\overline{\text{ERG-r}}$ Λ $\overline{\text{VER-b}}$ indicates a damage to the peripheral ones. b. Scotopic retinopathy: ERG-r Λ $\overline{\text{ERG-b}}$ Λ VER-r Λ VER-b: this shows that rod lesions appear only in the ERG. c. Combined retinopathy: α) peripheral only: ERG-r Λ $\overline{\text{ERG-b}}$ Λ VER-r Λ $\overline{\text{VER-b}}$; VER-r shows that the macula is unimpaired; β) global: $\overline{\text{ERG-r}}$ Λ $\overline{\text{ERG-b}}$ Λ $\overline{\text{VER-r}}$ Λ $\overline{\text{VER-b}}$; we may ultimately obtain complete electric silence;

3) a Boolean notation of results: by attributing the value 1 to a normal result and 0 to a pathological one, the various retinopathies considered above are individualized by a four-digit binary number as follows: merely central photopic retinopathy 1101; global photopic retinopathy 0100; scotopic retinopathy 1011; merely peripheral combined retinopathy 0010; global combined retinopathy 0000; this notation technique ensures an exhaustive enumeration of every possible case and is particularly suited for entry in a computer data file.

However, we attempted to make fuller use of the visual evoked responses instead of the two-valued logic (all or nothing); but in view of the highly variable results obtained for a single individual at various times and in order to avoid a subjective evaluation of the morphology of the electrical tracing, *we objectively determined statistical parameters for the responses recorded* in relation to the wavelength of the stimulus.

II. PROCEDURE

A. VER-recording (see fig. 1)

Our experiments were done with Burgundy fawn-coloured rabbits. Metal electrodes are planted on a permanent basis; they are short, in contact with the cortex, and placed on the surface of visual areas. Pupils are dilated (with atropine). Photostimulation is performed with flashes of a 0.5 Hz frequency. Schott interferential filters are used, either red (maximum transmission at 650 nm with a 14 nm band-pass) or blue (maximum transmission at 450 nm or 410 nm with a 9 nm band-pass). VERs are tape-recorded (bandpass: 250 Hz), then sampled by a HC26 Intertechnique analog-to-digital converter (512 points for each VER at a 250 μs sampling pace, i.e. analysis duration: 128 ms), and then summed (20 to 100 sweeps); the output data are analog on graphic recorder and digital on punch tape (8-moment IBM code).

It must be noted that our sampling frequency (4000 Hz) is much higher than the design frequency called for by SHANNON's theorem (500 Hz = 2 x 250 Hz).

B. Statistical analysis of VERs

From punch tapes data are transferred to punch cards, then processed in an IBM 360-20 computer by means of a program providing us with the following data of each averaged VER: the histogram of the amplitudes, the corresponding mean m and the standard deviation s, the variation coefficient $v = \dfrac{s}{m}$, as well as Fisher's skweness coefficient

$$\gamma_1 = \left[\frac{M_3^2}{M_2^3}\right]^{\frac{1}{2}} \quad \text{and kurtosis coefficient}$$

$$\gamma_2 = \frac{M_4}{M_2^2} - 3, \text{ where } M_r \text{ is the r-order centred moment.}$$

Further details on biopotential recordings, performed with planted electrodes and statistical analysis programs, may be found in MARIE-HÉLÈNE BASSANT's thesis (1969) and in the paper published by COURT's team which also includes an important bibliography (COURT, 1972).

III. RESULTS

The tables presented on figures 2 and 3 show the results of VERs recorded in red and blue monochromatic light, respectively. From left to right are listed: the identification number (no.), the number of sweeps (p), the mean (m) and the standard deviation (s) of amplitudes in arbitrary units, the variation coefficient (v) and fisher's skewness (γ_1) and kurtosis (γ_2) coefficients.

In order to avoid any restrictive assumption on the distribution of v, γ_1 and γ_2, we compared them by means of a distribution-free test: the median test.

A. Comparison of variation coefficients

Let us arrange in ascending order the v of red and blue VERs, underlining the red ones:

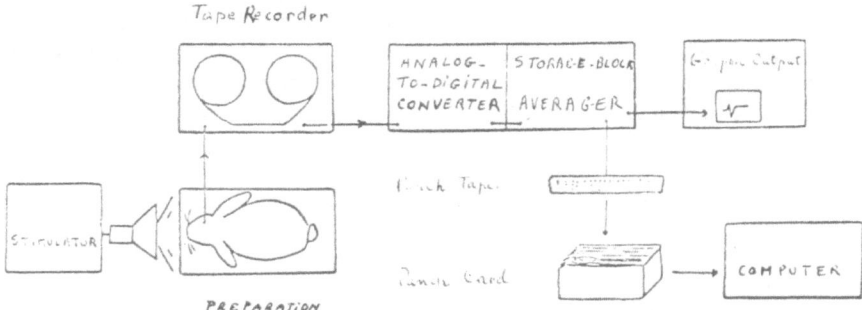

Fig. 1. Experimental system

no.	p	m	s	v	γ_1	γ_2
6	50	7703.24	184.62	0.024	− 1.61	8.44
7	50	7601.63	275.07	0.036	− 2.00	6.93
8	50	7015.41	739.81	0.105	− 1.40	0.49
9	50	7318.49	544.73	0.074	− 1.41	0.94
10	50	7445.45	527.33	0.070	− 2.72	5.89
15	50	6852.81	786.14	0.114	4.79	12.63
16	50	6664.19	461.42	0.069	0.40	0.62
17	100	13135.50	452.92	0.034	0.94	2.79
24	50	5710.25	1194.30	0.209	7.76	24.08
25	50	6126.41	914.72	0.149	5.63	16.42
26	50	5931.48	1546.30	0.260	2.64	4.14
27	50	7015.41	739.81	0.105	2.80	7.19

Fig. 2.   Red VERs (See text for legend).

no.	p	m	s	v	γ_1	γ_2
18	100	13751.97	1764.16	0.128	1.15	− 0.10
19	100	12628.64	1174.51	0.093		
20	100	13441.59	1493.47	0.111	− 0.02	− 1.85
21	100	12395.65	2179.83	0.175	0.04	− 1.67
28	100	5590.07	1265.16	0.226	2.42	5.17
29	50	4995.34	1351.61	0.270	1.16	2.76
30	50	6214.02	1272.97	0.204	1.96	1.87
31	50	5585.68	1312.24	0.234		
32	20	2321.92	515.72	0.222		
33	50	6233.34	1331.00	0.213		
34	50	5618.16	1074.08	0.191		

Fig. 3.   Blue VERs (See text for legend).

0.024 *0.034* *0.036* 0.069 *0.070* 0.074
0.093 *0.105* *0.105* 0.111 *0.114* 0.128
0.149 0.175 0.191 0.204 *0.209* 0.213
0.222 0.226 0.234 *0.260* 0.270

The median of both samples (red v_s and blue v_s) is $\tilde{v} = 0.128$.

Now we shall test the null hypothesis according to which the medians $\tilde{v}_r$, of red v_s, and $\tilde{v}_b$, of blue v_s, are equal; we shall replace these unknown medians which are assumed to be equal by $\tilde{v}$, and we shall determine, for each sample, the observed numbers of values smaller than or equal to $\tilde{v}$ and of values higher than $\tilde{v}$; we obtain the following table on which the expected numbers are given between brackets (i.e. those which would correspond to $\tilde{v}_r = \tilde{v}_b = \tilde{v}$).

	red v_s	blue v_s
$\leqslant \tilde{v}$	9 (6)	3 (5)
$> \tilde{v}$	3 (6)	8 (5)

Let us now test χ^2 as to compare the two separate distributions:

$$\chi^2 = \frac{(9\text{-}6)^2}{6} + \frac{(3\text{-}6)^2}{6} + \frac{(3\text{-}6)^2}{6} + \frac{(8\text{-}5)^2}{5} = 6.30$$

The value obtained enables us to rule out the null hypothesis with a risk of 1.3%. This gives evidence to the existence of a statistically significant difference between variation coefficents corresponding to red VERs and those corresponding to blue VERs.

B.   Comparison of Fisher's skewness coefficients

We shall proceed as we did for variation coefficients; we obtain in succession:

$$
\begin{array}{cccccc}
-2.72 & -2.00 & -1.61 & -1.41 & -1.40 & -0.02 \\
0.04 & 0.40 & 0.94 & 1.15 & 1.16 & 1.96 \\
2.42 & 2.64 & 2.80 & 4.79 & 5.63 & 7.76 \\
\end{array}
$$

$$\tilde{\gamma}_1 = \frac{0.94 + 1.15}{2} = 1.05$$

	red γ_{1S}	blue γ_{1S}
$< \tilde{\gamma}_1$	7 (6)	2 (3)
$> \tilde{\gamma}_1$	5 (6)	4 (3)

The expected numbers are smaller than 5 but higher than 2. We shall calculate a corrected χ^2 through Yates' methode:

$$\chi_c^2 = \frac{(|7\text{-}6|\text{-}0.5)^2}{6} + \frac{(|5\text{-}6|\text{-}0.5)^2}{6} + \frac{(|2\text{-}3|\text{-}0.5)^2}{3} + \frac{(|4\text{-}3|\text{-}0.5)^2}{3} = 0.25$$

The value obtained does not enable us to rule out the null hypothesis (the risk would be 61.7%): hence, there is no statistically significant difference between Fishers's skewness coefficients corresponding respectivaly to red and blue VERs.

C.   Comparison of Fisher's kurtosis coefficients

The process used here, is similar to the preceding one (sect. B); we obtain successively:

$$
\begin{array}{cccccc}
-1.85 & -1.67 & -0.10 & 0.49 & 0.62 & 0.94 \\
1.87 & 2.76 & 2.79 & 4.14 & 5.17 & 5.89 \\
6.93 & 7.19 & 8.44 & 12.63 & 16.42 & 24.08 \\
\end{array}
$$

$$\tilde{\gamma}_2 = \frac{2.79 + 4.14}{2} = 3.47$$

	red γ_{2s}	blue γ_{2s}
$< \tilde{\gamma}_2$	4 (6)	5 (3)
$> \tilde{\gamma}_2$	8 (6)	1 (3)

$$\chi_c^2 = \frac{(|4-6|-0.5)^2}{6} + \frac{(|8-6|-0.5)^2}{6} + \frac{(|5-3|-0.5)^2}{3} + \frac{(|1-3|-0.5)^2}{3} == 2.25$$

The value obtained does not enable us to rule out the null hypothesis (the risk would be 13.4%): hence, there is no statistically significant difference between Fisher's kurtosis coefficients corresponding respectively to red and blue VERs.

IV. CONCLUSIONS

This first statistical approach, once completed, will make it possible to differentiate between VERs induced by a red monochromatic photostimulation and VERs induced by a blue monochromatic one, since the histograms of their amplitudes give:

1°) a statistically significant difference at the 5 per cent level for variation coefficients: for the 12 red VERs their mean is $\tilde{v}_r = 0.104$, and for the 11 blue VERs, $\tilde{v}_b = 0.188$.

2°) a non-statistically significant difference at the 5 per cent level for Fisher's kurtosis coefficients; their mean is $\overline{\gamma}_{2r} = 7.55$ for the 12 red VERs and $\overline{\gamma}_{2b} = 1.03$ for the 11 blue VERs. Likewise, a non-statistically significant difference is found between Fisher's skewness coefficients, of which the mean is $\overline{\gamma}_{1r} = 1.32$ for the 12 red VERs and $\overline{\gamma}_{1b} = 1.12$ for the 6 blue VERs.

The numerical results stated may be literally expressed as follows: 'The histogram of red VERs amplitudes is usually less dispersed ($\tilde{v}_r < \tilde{v}_b$) and leptokurtic ($\overline{\gamma}_{2r} > \overline{\gamma}_{2b}$) compared with the histogram of blue VERs amplitudes; also, distributions are asymmetrical and the frequency is higher for high amplitudes (γ_{1r} and $\gamma_{1b} > 0$)'.

To explain these differences the following hypothesis may be put forward: in red stimulation the cones alone (in small numbers in rabbits) are excited, while in blue stimulation the rods (in large numbers) are excited, hence a platykurtic histogram of amplitudes reflecting a much higher number of responses; besides, the order relation between $\tilde{v}_r$ and $\tilde{v}_b$ tallies with the one existing between γ_{2r} and γ_{2b}. The asymmetry noted indicates non-Gaussian distributions; this conclusion implies that the receptive cells which respond to the stimulus are not independent of one another; it is highly likely an interaction exists between these neurons.

We still have to increase the number of analyzed VERs so as to determine distributions and thus define confidence intervals for the parameters which have been selected as exploratory criteria.

REFERENCES

ALFIERI, R. & SOLÉ, P. Electrorétinographie et recueil des potentiels évoqués visuels: exploration fonctionnelle des voies optiques. *Trace 5: 354-362* (1971).

ALFIERI, R., RIGAL, DANIELLE & SOLÉ, P. Electrophysiological nosology (ERG and VER) of retinopathies. In: Symposium on electroretinography; Proc. 8th ISCERG Symp., Pisa 7-12 Sept. 1970, pp. 305-313. Pisa, Pacini (1972).

BASSANT, MARIE-HÉLÈNE. Contribution à l'étude de l'analyse statistique de l'activité électrique spontanée. (Thèse de sciences de 3ème cycle, Paris, 1969).

COURT, L. et al. Analyse mathématique de l'activité électrique cérébrale spontanée. In: Actualités neurophysiologiques (9ème séries), pp. 53-93. Paris, Masson (1972).

DYNAMIC ELECTRORETINOGRAPHY IN MONOCHROMATIC LIGHTS AND FLUORESCENCE ELECTRORETINOGRAPHY IN LEMURS

RINALDO ALFIERI*, GEORGES PARIENTE[†]** & PIERRE SOLÉ***

(Clermont-Ferrand and Brunoy)

ABSTRACT

By means of electroretinographic techniques, using Lemur mongoz, we have been able to demonstrate: on the one hand, the existence of a dual system of cones and rods in the retina (we found an α-point during a dynamic electroretinogram made with a yellow monochromatic light); on the other hand, a possible fluorescent effect (we obtained a response with ultra-violet photostimulation) which can explain why these animals have an excellent vision under scotopic conditions. They may indeed possess a tapetum lucidum with fluorescent riboflavine.

INTRODUCTION

By applying monochromatic photostimulation and summation of the electroretinographic responses, we could already demonstrate the dualism of the retina in man (ALFIERI & SOLÉ, 1968). VAN NORREN & PADMOS (1971) use this electroretinographic method in Macaque. Our method of fluorescent electroretinography (ALFIERI & SOLÉ, 1969) is characterized by the use of an ultra-violet (364 nm) photostimulus. Under these conditions, the electrical response is absent, since ultra-violet photons have no effect in man. If, however, endocular tissues are impregnated with a fluorescent substance, ultra-violet photons are changed into efficient photons of longer wavelength, resulting in an electroretinogram.

We have applied these technical procedures in *Lemur mongoz* (fig. 1), a prosimian primate from Madagascar, to demonstrate the existence of a dual system of cones and rods in the retina, and to find an explanation for the very good scotopic vision of these animals (see GRAVELINE et al., 1967, for an electroretinogram in the nocturnal Galago).

Firstly, we have to make clear which is the position of prosimians among other primates, and why Malagasy Lemurs are particularly interesting to be examined. They are an essential stage in primate evolution, an animal closely related to an ancestor of both man and apes. We can find this meaning in the word prosimian, in contradiction to the later-simians. Geo-

* Department of Biomathematics, Faculty of Medicine, P.O. Box 38, 63001-Clermont-Ferrand, Cedex (France).
[†]** Department of General Ecology, Museum National d'Histoire Naturelle, 4, avenue du Petit Château, 91800 Brunoy, Cedex (France).
*** Department of Ophthalmology, Faculty of Medicine, P.O. Box 38, 63001 Clermont-Ferrand, Cedex (France).

graphically, Madagascar was separated from Africa and Asia, leaving on it a primitive stock of nocturnal and small prosimians (PETTER, 1962). As a result, prosimians were totally cut off from the rest of the world (PETTER et al., 1975. In press). As a consequence, the Malagasy Lemurs have occupied every ecological place available. This evolution led to a variety of animal forms, such as very small nocturnal species (*Microcebus*) or very big and diurnal species (*Propithecus* and *Indri*) (ORDY & SAMORAJSKY, 1968). Many intermediate forms, mostly crepuscular, can also be found. When man reached Madagascar, only about 2000 years ago, he completely disturbed the fragile biological balance (a special fauna in a very peculiar

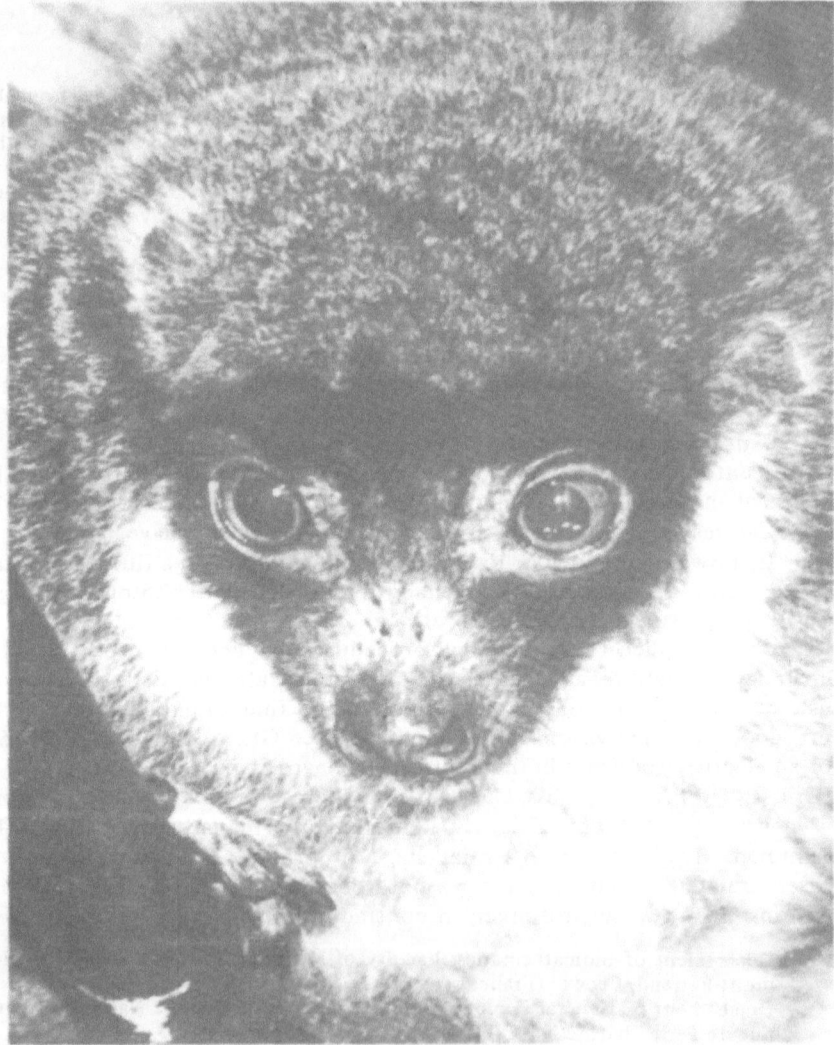

Fig. 1. *Lemur mongoz*. (Photograph of G.F. PARIENTE).

biotope). *Lemur mongoz*, studied here, belongs to a diurnal species. He shows different levels of activity during the day, with a strong maximum at sunset. Therefore, we may assume that this animal can see rather good in dim light, the more since it is living in trees in the Ankarafantsika forest, near the city of Majunga. It is a rare species threatened with extinction. ROHEN & CASTENHOLTZ (1967) showed by histological examination the great variability of retinal structures in a few species of Lemurs. At the moment all we know about the retina of *Lemur mongoz* is by fundus photography. In figure 2 no foveal zone can be seen, but the convergence of the blood vessels draws a perfect macular area. There is no real pigmentation; we can see a faint shine on the fundus. This aspect is quite different from the fundus of more diurnal Lemurs, although the general morphology of all these species is very close.

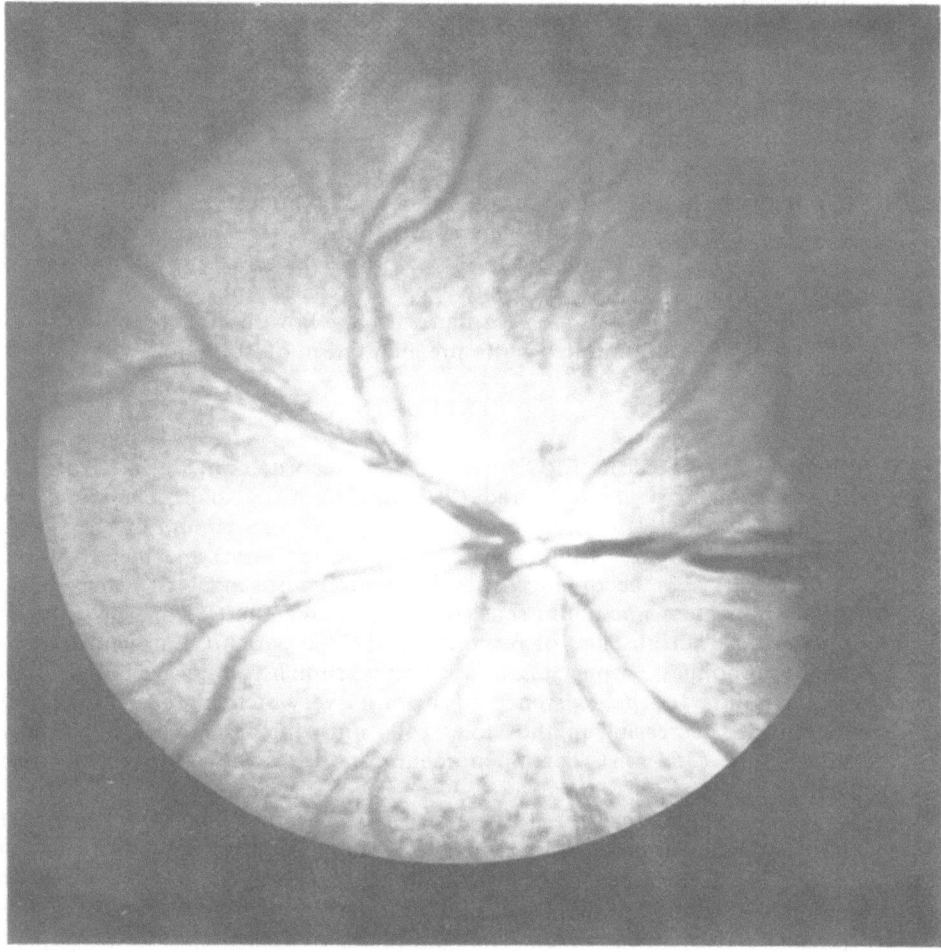

Fig. 2. Fundus photograph of *Lemur mongoz* eye: no fovea can be seen in this zone, but the convergence of the blood vessels can be noted.

METHODS

The *Lemur mongoz* were awake, did not get any pre-medication and were kept in hand during the recording period. The active electrode is placed on the anaesthetized cornea, being specially adapted by Dr. Lumbroso. The indifferent electrode is a needle placed through the skin of the frontal area in the midline. Both pupils are dilated (mydriaticum). Photostimulation is obtained by xenon-flashes at a frequency of 4 Hz (Epiphote apparatus), using interference filters (Schott), of which the specifications can be found in the table.

colour	wavelenght nm	maximal transmission %	band-pass nm
ultra-violet	364	39	9
violet	407	35	9
blue	450	40	9
yellow	553	44	11
orange	589	40	10
red	658	50	14
red	707	40	15

To improve the signal to noise ratio a computer (Art 1000 S.A.I.P.) is applied. The physical parameters are as follows: time constant 0.2 s; band-pass 250 Hz; analysis duration 200 ms; number of sweeps: 50 in static electroretinography and 200 in dynamic electroretinography.

The dynamic ERG's are recorded with a yellow monochromatic stimulus (553 nm) after a 6-minutes white pre-adaptation of 3000 lux.

RESULTS

Figure 3 shows static ERG's. They were recorded with stimuli of wavelengths ranging from deep red (707 nm) to ultra-violet (364 nm) from retinas, adapted to low photopic luminance. The maximum of the spectral sensitivity curve was found between yellow (553 nm) and blue (450 nm). This result is in accordance with behavioral tests made in other species, which indicate a maximum sensitivity in the green part of the spectrum. We also noticed an absence of response in the red part (707 nm and 658 nm) and a monophasic aspect of the responses (similar to b_2 wave in man). This result points to the existence of a retina very rich in rods. Finally, the amplitude, decreasing in the violet (407 nm), increased again in the ultra-violet zone (364 nm). This phenomenon indicates the existence of a peculiar mechanism.

In figure 4 we can see a dynamic ERG. The first recording (fig. 4: AE) was obtained immediately after the white adaptation light is turned of. There is no response. The two following recordings were made 4 and 6 minutes later. We observe a biphasic aspect of the response: b_1-wave (cones) and b_2-wave (rods). After 4 minutes of dark adaptation the b_1- and b_2-waves are of equal amplitudes. This point is called the electroretinographic α-point. At the 6th minute the b_2-wave is still increasing, but the b_1-wave is still perceptible, as a notch on the ascending part of the record-

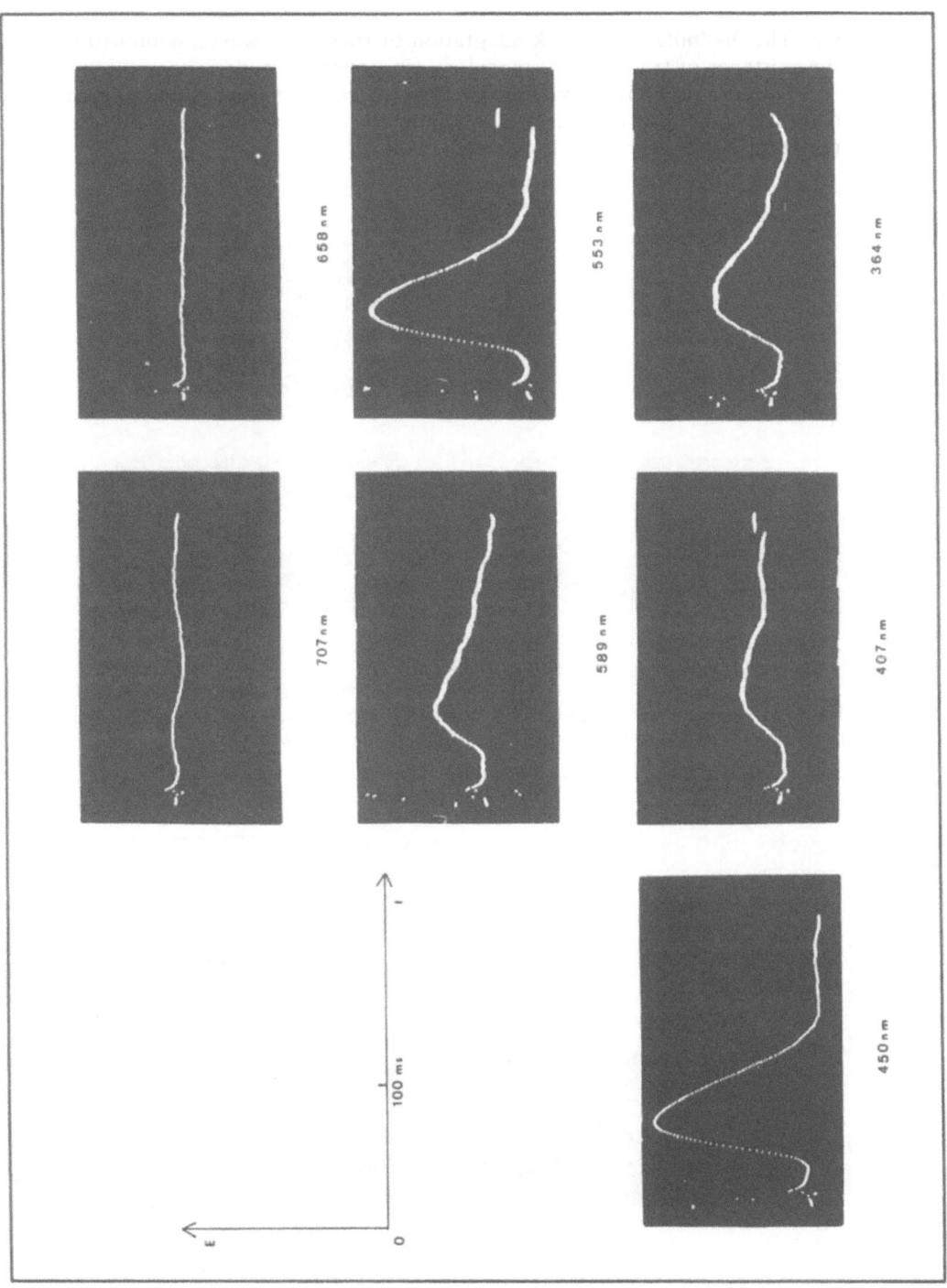

Fig. 3. Static electroretinographies in monochromatic lights from 707 nm to 364 nm.
E: potential; t: time.

ing. The dissimilarity in dark adaptation of these two waves, demonstrates the existence of two types of receptors, viz. cones and rods.

Figure 5 represents a dynamic ERG which has been obtained with monochromatic blue light (450 nm). The response is monophasic as a result of the preference of the rods for short wavelengths.

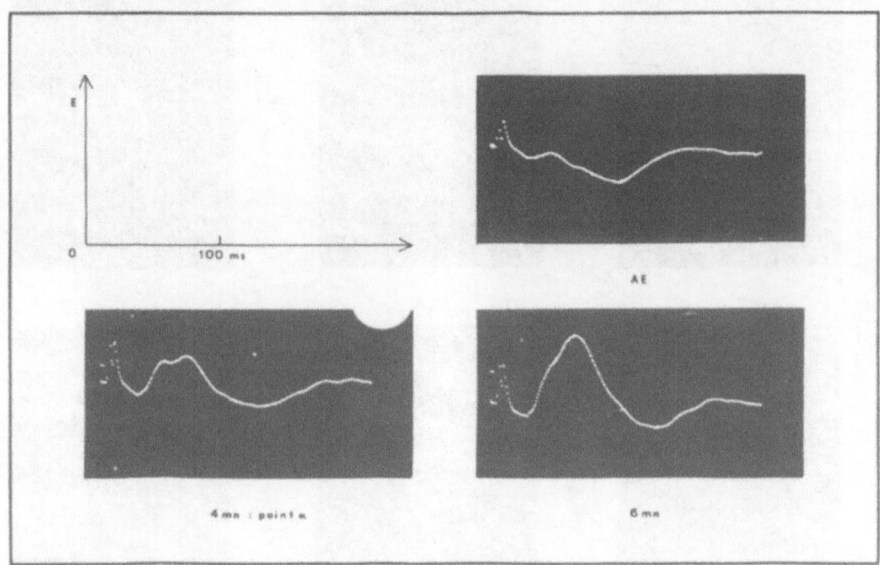

Fig. 4. Dynamic electroretinography in monochromatic yellow light (553 nm): α-point is at the 4th minute. E: potential; t: time; AE: after dazzle.

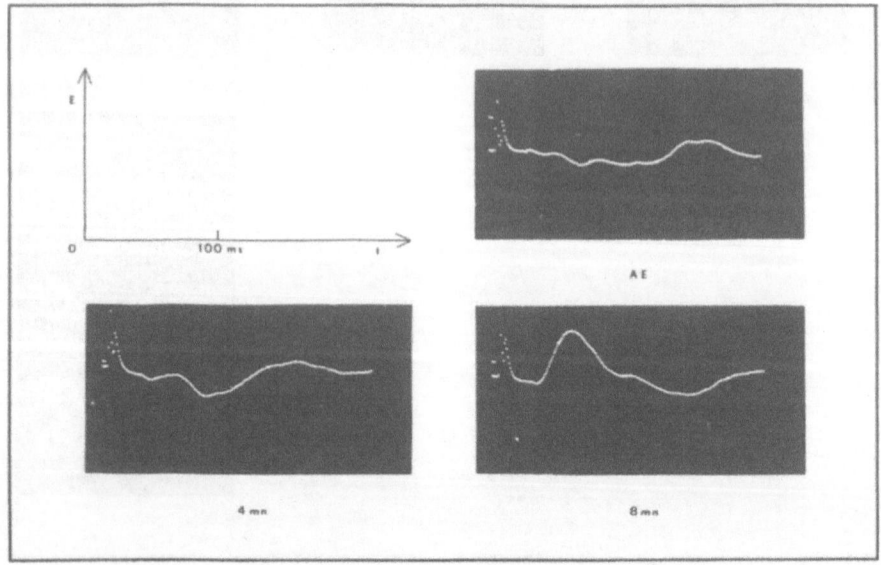

Fig. 5. Dynamic electroretinography in monochromatic blue light (450 nm): monophasic response. E: potential; t: time; AE: after dazzle.

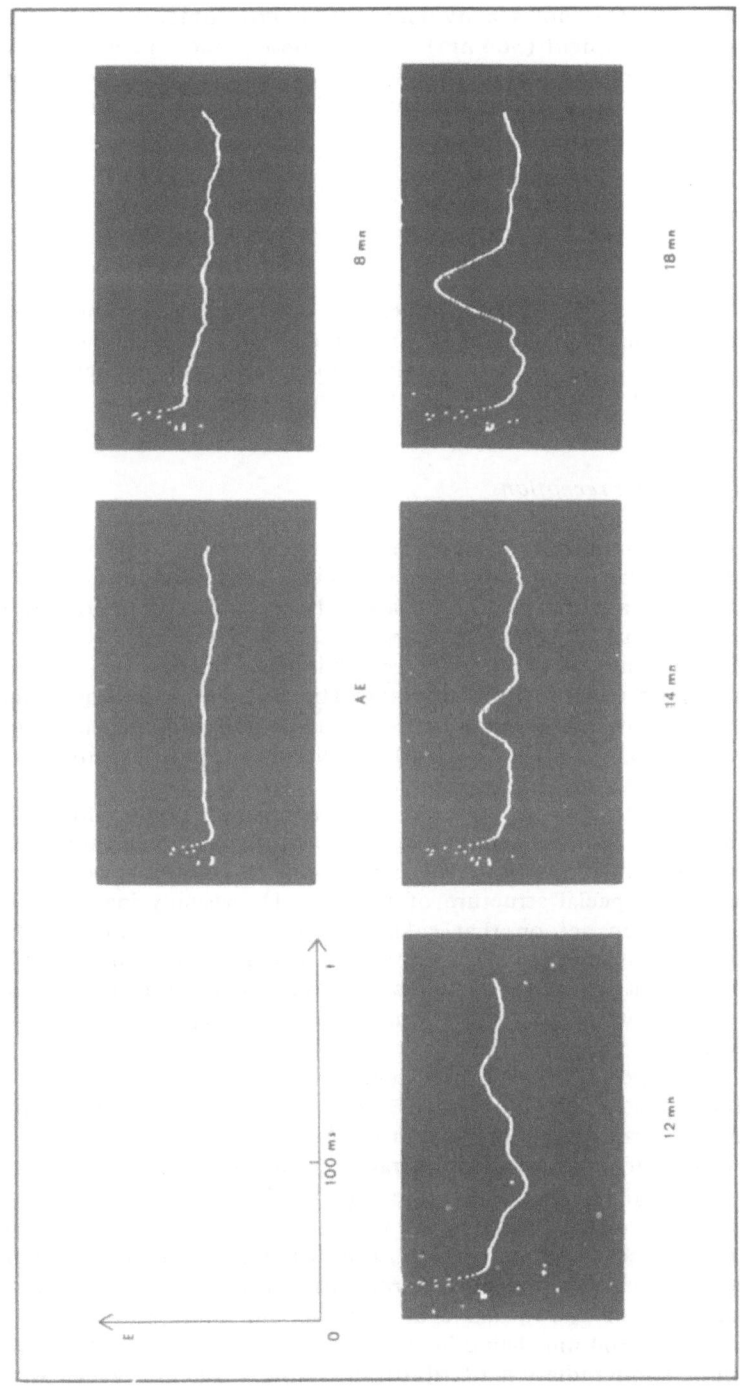

Fig. 6. Dynamic electroretinography in monochromatic ultra-violet light (364 nm): monophasic and late response. E: potential t: time; AE: after dazzle.

Figure 6 also shows a dynamic ERG, now obtained with ultra-violet monochromatic light (364 nm). The response is monophasic, deriving from the rod system. In addition, this response becomes marked only after a 14 minutes dark adaptation. This indicates that the amount of energy reaching the receptors is very low.

DISCUSSION

A.   Duality of the retina

The retina of *Lemur Mongoz* appears to be a dual one. Furthermore, retinographic examination makes the existence of a macula highly probable (fig. 2). By dynamic electroretinography with yellow light (fig. 4) we demonstrated conclusively the dual photoreceptor system by finding an α-point.

B.   Ultra-violet receptions

Lemur mongoz is able to perceive ultra-violet radiations as is shown by the response obtained in static retinography (fig. 3: 364 nm). This could be explained by admitting some ultra-violet absorption by the receptor photopigment. We hardly believe this hypothesis.

1.   On the one hand, with electrophysiological arguments: the electric response starts to increase from orange (fig. 3: 589 nm) reaches a maximum between yellow and blue (fig. 3: 553 nm and 450 nm) and then decreases in the violet (fig. 3: 407 nm). This looks like the typical monophasic absorption curve of a visual photopigment.

2.   On the other hand, for reasons of comparative physiology: like man, Lemurs are primates. Therefore, we may assume that their photopigment are not sensitive to ultra-violet. We may suppose that a fluorescent substance is present in a special structure of the eye. The visually inactive ultra-violet light may then act on that substance producing radiations with a good luminous efficiency. By this photonic change the luminous efficacy in lumen per watt would be increased and consequently the visual performance of these nocturnal species. We can support this hypothesis with the following facts:

1°:   Many species of nocturnal Lemurs and in some cases diurnal ones have a retinal tapetum lucidum (PARIENTE, 1970) and on the fundus picture of figure 2, we can see a faint shine in the *Lemur mongoz* fundus.

2°:   It has already been demonstrated on an African Lemur (*Galago crassicaudatus*) (PIRIE, 1959) that the tapetum lucidum is made of riboflavine (PEDLER, 1963). In addition, we found ourselves a substance, of which the absorption peaks are close to those of riboflavine in the tapetum of two other Malagasy prosimians (*Microcebus murinus:* fig. 7, and *Hapalemur griseus*). One of these peaks is at 370 nm. Our interferential filter happens to be just at 364 nm, being in the suitable range for excitation. Moreover, the fluorescent radiation of riboflavine is near 500 nm, which is probably the maximum of retinal sensitivity in this animal.

   Our hypothesis thus implies the presence of an oculary structure with a fluorescent substance in *Lemur mongoz*. The energetic efficiency of the photonic conversion from 364 nm to 500 nm is low. This could explain the long dark adaptation period, required to obtain a definite ERG response (fig. 6). Any fluorescent effect in the lens would be much to weak to act on the retina through the vitreous body. PIRIE (1959), DARTNALL et al. (1965) and SILVER (1966) already assumed the incidence of such an effect on visual performance at a low level of light. We suppose that our experiments can be considered as an objective proof of their hypothesis. This hypothesis concerning a fluorescent effect is not contradictary to a possible absorption of the ultra-violet photopigment in light. As shown before, we have strong doubts about the possibility of such phenomenon. The two processes probably overlap in the blue zone, since one of the riboflavine absorption peaks is at 445 nm, while our interferential filter is precisely at 450 nm. This would explain the relatively strong response recorded with this short wavelength (fig. 5).

CONCLUSION

What we know of *Lemur mongoz*, both from the point of view of an ecological and chromosomic study tends to show this animal as a rather primitive Lemur (RUMPLER & ALBIGNAC, 1970). To be sure, his social abilities are obviously less evolved than those of close species. Similarly, he is less prone to diurnal life, as could be expected from fundus photographs, which show an unpigmented fundus and no fovea, and from electroretinographic studies. The latter prove the existence of a dual retina (showing an α-point in the yellow). The cone response, however, is very small (none at

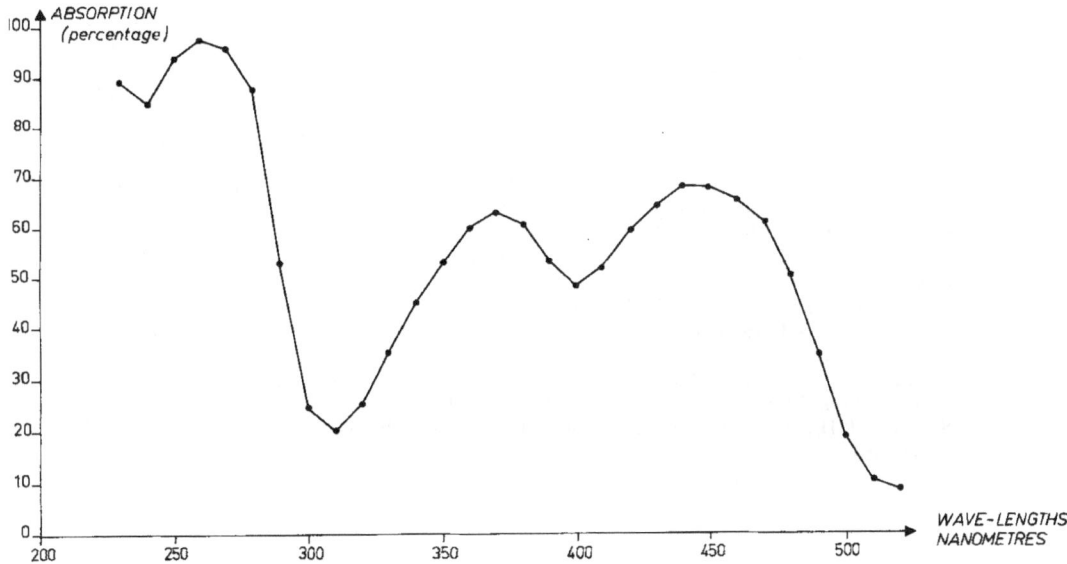

Fig. 7. Absorption curve of an extract from the tapetum lucidum of *Microcebus murinus*.

177

all in the red). The nocturnal vision is probably influenced by a fluorescent effect in aim light.

All these data give us a better understanding of *Lemur mongoz* in his relation with other prosimians and the process of his ecological adaptation in the Ankarafantsika forest.

ACKNOWLEDGEMENTS

We wish to thank Dr. LUMBROSO who made the special corneal lenses, and Mr. ROUAISSNEL and Mr. GIRAUD for their technical help with the recordings, and also Ms. GARDES and Mr. HEYDEL for their help with the drawings and pictures.

REFERENCES

ALFIERI, R. & SOLÉ, P.: Adapto-electroretinogram (AERG) in monochromatic light in man. In: The clinical value of electroretinography; Proc. 5th Iscerg Symposium, Ghent 1966; ed. by J. FRANCOIS, p. *215-220*. Basel, Karger, 1968.

ALFIERI, R. & SOLÉ, P.: On very short wave-length electroretinography: an original technique of diagnosis in infraclinical synthetic antimalarial retinopathies. In: Occupational and medicative hazards in ophthalmology; Proc. 3rd Congress Europ. Soc. Ophthal, Amsterdam 1968. *Ophtalmologica add. ad Vol.* 158: *661-668* (1969).

DARTNALL, H.J., ARDEN, G.B., IKEDA, H., LUCK, C.P. & ROSENBERG, M.E.: Anatomical, electrophysiological pigmentary aspects of vision in the bush-baby: an interpretative study. *Vision Res.* 5: *399-424* (1965).

GRAVELINE, J., BERT, J. QUÉRÉ, M., GODET, R. & COLLOMB, H.: L'électrorétinogramme chez un Lémurien nocture: le *Galago senegalensis*. *Ophtalmologica* 154: *143-150* (1967).

NORREN, D. VAN & PADMOS, P.: Spectral sensitivity of Macaque cones determined with an ERG method. *Vision Res.* 11: *1175-1177* (1971).

ORDY, J.M. & SAMORAJSKY, T.: Visual acuity and ERG-CFF in relation to the morphological organization of the retina among diurnal and nocturnal primates. *Vision Res.* 8: *1205-1225* (1968).

PARIENTE, G.F.: Rétinographies comparées des Lémuriens malgaches. *C.R. Acad. Sci. (Paris)* 270: *1404-1407* (1970).

PEDLER, C.: The fine structure of the tapetum cellulosum. *Exp. Eye Res.* 2: *189-195* (1963).

PETTER, J.J.: Recherches sur l'écologie et l'éthologie des Lémuriens malgaches. *Mém. Mus. Nat. Hist. Nat. (Paris)* 27: *1-146* (1962).

PETTER, J.J., ALBIGNAC, R. & RUMPLER, Y.: Les Lémuriens de Madagascar; ed. by R. PAULIAN. Paris, CNRS, Coll. Faune de Madagascar. To be published.

PIRIE, A.: Crystals of riboflavine making up the tapetum lucidum in the eye of a Lemur. *Nature* (London) 183: 985-986 (1959).

ROHEN, J.W. & CASTENHOLTZ, A.: Über die Zentralisation der Retina bei Primaten. *Folia Primat.* 5: *92-147* (1967).

RUMPLER, Y. & ALBIGNAC, R.: Evolution chromosomique des Lémuriens malgaches. *Ann. Univ. Madagascar* 12/13: *123-134* (1970).

SILVER, P.H.: Spectral sensitivity of a trained bush-baby. *Vision Res.* 6: *153-162* (1966).

BEHAVIOUR OF THE GANGLION CELLS
OF THE FROG'S RETINA SUBMITTED TO
A POLARIZING CURRENT:
AN IN VIVO STUDY

V. MAXIMOV, B. LIEGE & G. GALAND*

(Poitiers, France)

INTRODUCTION

In the frog's retina, the receptive fields of the ganglion cells are made of a central area (the excitatory receptive field or ERF) and of a peripheral area (the inhibitory receptive field or IRF). These two areas are antagonist: See GRUSSER & GRUSSER-CORNEHLS (1973). In order to explain this functional situation, it is necessary to ascribe great importance to the transverse cells of the retina: that is, the horizontal cells and the amacrine cells. In order to study this situation we have used the trans-retinal currents. These currents, or polarizing currents, are well known to alter the function of the retina. For instance, there are the subjective phosphenes (see BRINDLEY, 1970). How does a polarizing current work? This is one problem we have encountered in this study.

In the vertebrate retina, light stimulation provokes an hyperpolarization of the photoreceptors (see TOMITA, 1972). This hyperpolarization provokes a large hyperpolarization of the horizontal cells: it is the S-potential of L-type. This S-potential is elicited by the reduction of the release of a transmitter normally secreted in darkness by the receptor (see review: WITKOVSKI, 1971).

With polarizing currents, we have nearly the same phenomena. At the outer parts of the photoreceptors, a cornea-positive current provokes a depolarization: this is an outward current. At the level of the inner parts of the photoreceptors, this same current provokes an hyperpolarization: this is an inward current. This hyperpolarization provokes an important hyperpolarization of the horizontal cell.

So, a cornea-positive current provokes an hyperpolarization of all the horizontal cells of the retina: such a polarization simulates to a certain extent a light stimulation of the whole retina.

At the level of the receptive fields of the ganglion cells, and if there is a strong antagonism between ERF and IRF, the stimulation of both ERF and IRF by the polarizing current will evoke the response of the periphery; that is, an inhibition. With cornea-negative currents, the phenomena are reversed: we have the withdrawal of the IRF inhibition and the ganglion cell is activated.

Now, we shall try to apply these hypotheses at the level of the frog's retina.

* ERA CNRS No. 07-0624 (Neurophysiologie de la vision).

METHODS

This study has been made *in vivo*. General methods used have been already described earlier (LIEGE & GALAND, 1972; MORIN, GAILLARD, LIEGE & GALAND, 1974). Light stimuli are given at the level of a horizontal area, which is seen by the frog by means of a mirror. Polarizing currents are given by inter-ocular means. Unit responses are recorded at the superficial tectal level with micropipettes filled with Wood's metal. Sometimes, in order to stimulate only the central part of a receptive field, we used a horizontal screen to mask the moving target when the target is in the IRF.

RESULTS

Stimulation by a polarizing current

The results obtained with class IV cells are easy to interpret. The class IV cells are the *off* cells described by HARTLINE (1938). In practice, they have no inhibitory periphery (BARLOW, 1953). A cornea-positive current, simulating light stimulation, will evoke an inhibition of the cell. The end of the polarization activates the unit: it is an *off* effect. Such an activation appears only in darkness, because light inhibits the unit. With cornea-negative currents, the unit is activated and there is an *on* sustained discharge. This activity is controlled by the amount of ambient light and is maximal in darkness.

By itself, polarization does not affect the class I cells (sustained contrast detectors), nor those of class II (convexity detectors). Such effects are interpreted by the strong antagonism between the periphery and the center of the receptive fields of these cells. So, we meet the normal behaviour of these cells when they are stimulated by an *on-off* ambient light: these cells do not respond (MATURANA, LETTVIN, McCULLOCH & PITTS, 1960).

Stimulation with a moving target

When class I, II and III ganglion cells are stimulated with a moving target, there is an activation of the response when the cornea is negative, and an inhibition when it is positive.

Delayed response

When the retina is fully dark adapted, a flash of light evokes a discharge the latency of which is long: it is the delayed response (PICKERING & VARJU, 1967).

When the cornea is positive, there is an inhibition: the delayed discharge is shorter, its latency is longer, and its total number of spikes is smaller. When the cornea is negative, the phenomena are reversed (MAXIMOV, LIEGE & GALAND, 1973).

In order to understand the delayed response phenomenon, VARJU & PICKERING (1969) have made a model. There are two antagonistic components: an excitatory component E, and an inhibitory component H. They are added algebraically to produce a curve labelled R. This curve controls the response of the unit when it is above a threshold T. When there is a polarization, everything is as if the threshold T was altered: higher in positive cornea, and lower in negative cornea.

Polarization of class III cells

Next, we have to consider a particular situation: when a class III cell is submitted to a polarizing current. Class III cells are the *on-off* cells described by HARTLINE (1938). With a negative-cornea polarization, we get a sustained response. This sustained response is modified by the luminous level. When this level is too low (darkness) or too high, the unit does not respond.

Our initial hypothesis does not explain such a result. In the different functional cellular levels of the retina, *on-off* responses appear with amacrine cells (WERBLIN & DOWLING, 1969). The silence of an *on-off* ganglion cell during a sustained light stimulation may be explained in the following manner: An amacrine cells receives afferent signals from sustained *on* bipolar cells and from sustained *off* bipolar cells. *On* bipolar cells provoke a sustained depolarization of the amacrine cell; *off* bipolar cells provoke a sustained hyperpolarization. When these two signals are added together the polarization of the amacrine cell is not modified and the cell does not respond (TOYODA, HASHIMOTO & OHTSU, 1973). This balance is disturbed by polarizing currents. And, inside a narrow range of luminosity, an *on-off* cell may give a paradoxical sustained response.

CONCLUSION

MATURANA and his collegues have shown that a ganglion cell performs its operation whatever the luminosity level. Such a result can be found with polarizing currents. Apart from class III cells, polarizing currents do not modify the operation made by a ganglion cell. Polarizing currents only modify the inhibitory control that the periphery exerts on the central part of the receptive field. These results stress the importance of the role played by horizontal cells in the functional architecture of the ganglion cell receptive field.

RÉSUMÉ

Nous avons étudié in vivo, chez la grenouille, le comportement des cellules ganglionnaires de la rétine sous l'action d'un courant électrique de polarisation. En règle générale, on observe une inhibition en cornée positive et une activation en cornée négative. La polarisation seule est sans effet sur les cellules des classes I et II; en cornée négative, elle active les cellules des classes III et IV. Pour les classes I, II et III, la réponse au mouvement d'une cible noire sur fond blanc est augmentée en cornée négative et diminuée en cornée positive. En cornée négative, la latence des réponses retardées des unités des classes I, II et III adaptées à l'obscurité est diminuée, avec augmentation de la fréquence, de la durée et du nombre total de spikes de la décharge. En cornée positive, on a le phénomène inverse. Ces résultats sont interprétés en faisant intervenir le rôle des courants de polarisation sur les cellules horizontales de la rétine.

Acknowledgements. This work was supported in part by INSERM (CRL 73-1-103-8) and in part by CNRS (ATP: Physiologie et Pathologie de l'oeil). Address for reprints: G. GALAND, Laboratoire de Neurophysiologie, Faculté des Sciences, 86022-Poitiers-France.

REFERENCES

BARLOW, H.B. Summation and inhibition in the frog's retina. *J. Physiol. (London)*, 119, *69-88* (1953).

BRINDLEY, G.S. Physiology of the retina and visual pathway. Edward Arnold, London (1970).

GRÜSSER, O.J. & GRÜSSER-CORNEHLS, U. Neuronal mechanisms of visual movement perception and some psychophysical and behavioral correlations. In: Handbook of sensory physiology, VII/3: Central processing of visual information – A: Integrative functions and comparative data. Ed. by JUNG, R. pp 333/429. Springer Verlag, Berlin (1973).

HARTLINE, H.K. The response of single optic nerve fibres of the vertebrate eye to illumination of the retina. *Amer. J. Physiol.*, 121, *400-415* (1938).

LIEGE, B. & GALAND, G. Single-unit visual responses in the frog's brain. *Vision Res.*, 12, *609-622* (1972).

MATURANA, H.R., LETTVIN, J.Y., McCULLOCH, W.S. & PITTS, W.H. Anatomy and physiology of vision in the frog (Rana pipiens). *J. Gen. Physiol.*, 43, *Suppl.*, *129-176* (1960).

MAXIMOV, V., LIEGE, B. & GALAND, G. Influence de la polarisation rétinienne sur la réponse retardée des cellules ganglionnaires de la grenouille. *J. Physiol.*, (Paris), 67, *207A* (1973).

MORIN, G., GAILLARD, G., LIEGE, B. & GALAND, G. Réponses proprioceptives unitaires à l'abaissement de la mâchoire enregistrées dans le tronc cérébral de la grenouille. Interactions hétérosensorielles visuelles. *J. Physiol.*, (Paris) 68, *121-144* (1974).

PICKERING, S.G. & VARJU, D. Ganglion cells in the frog retina: inhibitory receptive field and long-latency response. *Nature*, 215, *545-546* (1967).

TOMITA, T. Light-induced potential and resistance changes in vertebrate photoreceptors. In: Handbook of sensory physiology, Vol. VII/2: Physiology of photoreceptor organs. Ed. by FUORTES, M.G.F. pp 483/511. Springer-Verlag, Berlin (1972).

TOYODA, J.I., HASHIMOTO, H. & OHTSU, K. Bipolar-amacrine transmission in the carp retina. *Vision Res.*, 13, *295-307* (1973).

VARJU, D. & PICKERING, S.G. Delayed responses of ganglion cells in the frog retina: the influence of stimulus parameters upon their discharge pattern. *Kybernetik*, 6, *112-119* (1969).

WERBLIN, F.S. & DOWLING, J.E. Organization of retina of the mudpuppy, Necturus maculosus – II: Intracellular recording. *J. Neurophysiol.*, 32, *339-355* (1969).

WITKOVSKI, P. Peripheral mechanisms of vision. *Ann. Rev. Physiol.*, 33, *257-280* (1971).

ERG PHOTOMETRY IN GOLDFISH BY THE
CRITERION RESPONSE METHOD

T.J.T.P. VAN DEN BERG & H. SPEKREIJSE

(Amsterdam, The Netherlands)

INTRODUCTION

In man, direct recordings can seldom be made from the various neural structures along the visual pathway, and in general only gross potentials can be derived. Of these the electroretinogram (ERG) is fairly easy to measure and has good reproducibility both in the same subject and among different subjects. This paper describes an application of ERG recordings to obtain insight into the spectral characteristics of the visual pigments.

The present investigation was initiated by a reported discrepancy in goldfish and carp (BURKHARD, 1966; REYNAULD, 1972; WITKOWSKY, 1973) between the electrophysiologically determined scotopic spectral sensitivity curves and the absorption spectra of the rod pigment, porphyropsin (MUNZ & SCHWANZARA, 1967; CRESCITELLI & DARTNALL, 1954). This contrasts with the findings in man, where the scotopic luminosity curves determined by psychophysical tests at absolute threshold or by means of spectrophotometric recordings (CRESCITELLI & DARTNALL, 1953) coincide.

It is generally accepted that such a close relationship also holds for electrophysiological data. However, these generally suprathreshold scotopic measurements can be influenced by the photopic system. This is also the case for the human psychophysical scotopic luminosity curve, which resembles the rhodopsin absorption curve only if the measurements are performed close to the absolute threshold. At higher, yet scotopic, criterion levels cone activity cannot be neglected, resulting at first in a broadening of the curve at the long wavelength side. It was therefore assumed by earlier investigators that the deviation (broadening) of the electrophysiological spectral sensitivity curves in goldfish could also be attributed to a cone contribution. None of them showed, however, experimental evidence for such an interpretation.

In this paper experiments will be described that were performed in order to ascertain whether cones are, indeed, responsible for the deviating scotopic sensitivity curve of goldfish. This is of importance since frequently spectrophotometrically determined absorption curves are used as keystones in the description of spectral properties of the visual system (WALRAVEN, 1962; JAMESON & HURVICH, 1968; SPERLING & HARWERTH, 1971). The topic of this paper can be condensed to the following three questions:

1. How may one recognize a cone contribution in a scotopic response?

2. What is the spectral sensitivity of the response that is initiated solely by the rods?

3. What is the relationship between the rod spectral sensitivity and the absorption curve of the rod photopigment?

METHODS

To obtain a measure for sensitivity at a given wavelength, the intensity of monochromatic light that elicited a criterion ERG response was determined. Normally, the monochromatic light was alternated 3 times per second with equally long dark/light intervals. The procedure used is similar to that of PADMOS & VAN NORREN (1972). The wavelengths of the stimulus could be changed continuously by use of a monochromator, while its intensity

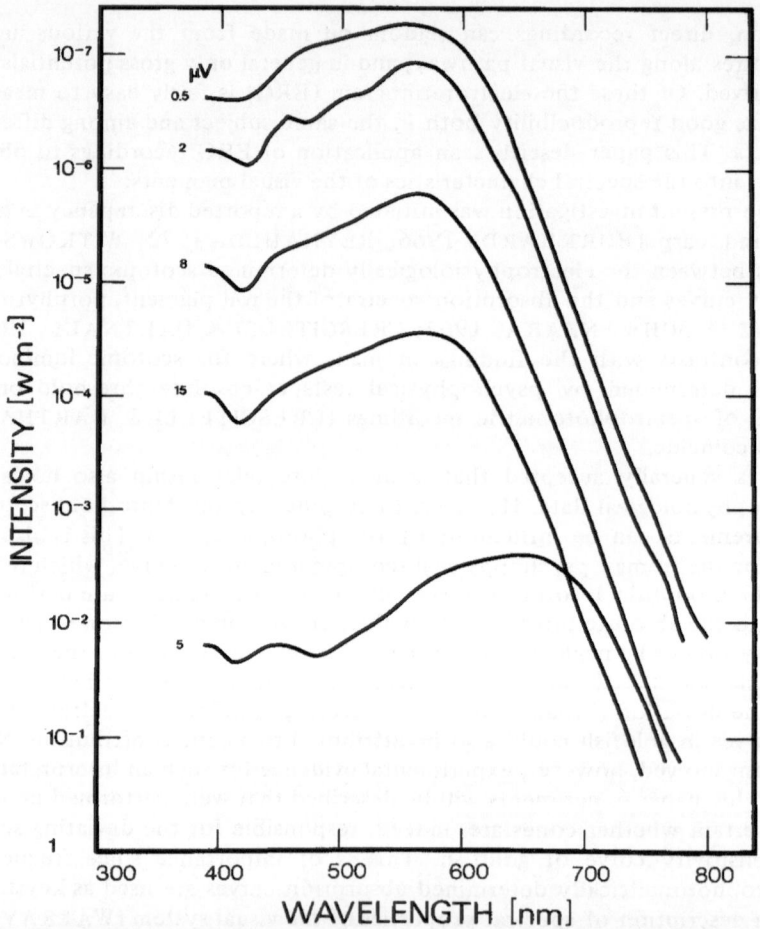

Fig. 1. Goldfish spectral sensitivity curves determined on the basis of a criterion response ERG. The amplitude criteria used are given at the left of each curve. The monochromatic stimulus was modulated 100% at 3 Hz, with equal light and dark intervals. The lowermost curve was obtained after light adaptation and is typical for the sensitivity of the photopic system. The shape of the scotopic spectral sensitivity curves remains invariant over an intensity range of almost 3 log-units.

was adjusted automatically to maintain a constant response. This has the advantage of avoiding sudden changes in the stimulus conditions, after which the retina has to adapt to the new level.

Instead of a periodically flickering light, the stimulus could also be a light that was modulated by gaussian noise that had a bandwidth of 0 to 50 Hz. In a linear system the cross-correlation function between response and stimulus is the impulse response which, by Fourier transformation, gives the amplitude (and phase) characteristics. The procedure followed to determine these characteristics is described in more detail by SCHELLART, SPEKREIJSE & VAN DEN BERG (1974).

The retina was homogeneously illuminated by a diffuser placed directly in front of the eye. Sensitivity is defined as the reciprocal of the corneal power necessary to evoke the criterion response. The ERG was recorded with a tapered platinum-iridium needle with a mean diameter of 75 μm which, except for the tip, was insulated with resin. It was inserted through the sclera to a depth of 3 mm behind the *ora serrata*. A platinum-iridium wire placed in the nostril ipsilateral to the stimulated eye served as a reference electrode.

RESULTS

The shape of the spectral sensitivity functions obtained on the basis of a constant response ERG can be a function of the criterion chosen. It is, therefore, necessary to measure this curve for various response criteria. Since the stimulus was always modulated at 100%, lower response criteria require lower intensities. In man the pure rhodopsin curve is only found when very low response criteria are used. However, in goldfish the choice of criterion level hardly influences the shape of the scotopic curves, as shown in Fig. 1. Over a scotopic intensity range of almost 3 log units and down to criteria as low as 0.5 μV, no change in the shape of the spectral sensitivity curve can be observed; although presumably a change would have occurred if systems with different absolute sensitivities and temporal properties were contributing to the response. Only at the highest criterion used (15 μV) the curve is slightly broadened at the red end of the spectrum. The bottom curve of Fig. 1 shows the photopic spectral sensitivity curve obtained with a criterion of 5 μV after light adaptation.

In accordance with the general assumption that the difference between electrophysiological scotopic sensitivity and absorption spectra is due to a contribution of the cone system, WITKOWSKY (1973) reports that the sensitivity to long wavelength stimuli can be lowered selectively by adaptation with a red light. The lower curves of Fig. 2 show the results of a chromatic adaptation experiment that we carried out in an attempt to substantiate this claim. Firstly, the scotopic spectral sensitivity curve was determined for a 4 μV criterion (drawn curve in Fig. 2). Next, the stimulus was set at 500 nm, where one expects the least contamination by the cone system and a criterion of 2 μV was chosen. The intensities of either a red (Wratten 25) or a green (Wratten 99) adaptation light were then adjusted so that the 500 nm stimulus elicited a 2 μV response at the same intensity that previously elicited a 4 μV response. The spectral sensitivity curves were redetermined in the presence of either the red or the green adapting light at intensities that reduced the 500 nm response to 2 μV. As can be seen in the bottom half of Fig. 2 (dashed and dotted curves), the presence of these adapting lights did not change the shape of the spectral sensitivity curves, although, if a red sensitive pigment was contributing to the response, one would expect the red light to selectively reduce sensitivity to long wavelength stimuli.

In the above adaptation experiment the wavelength of the adapting light was kept constant, and that of the stimulus varied. In case there is a restric-

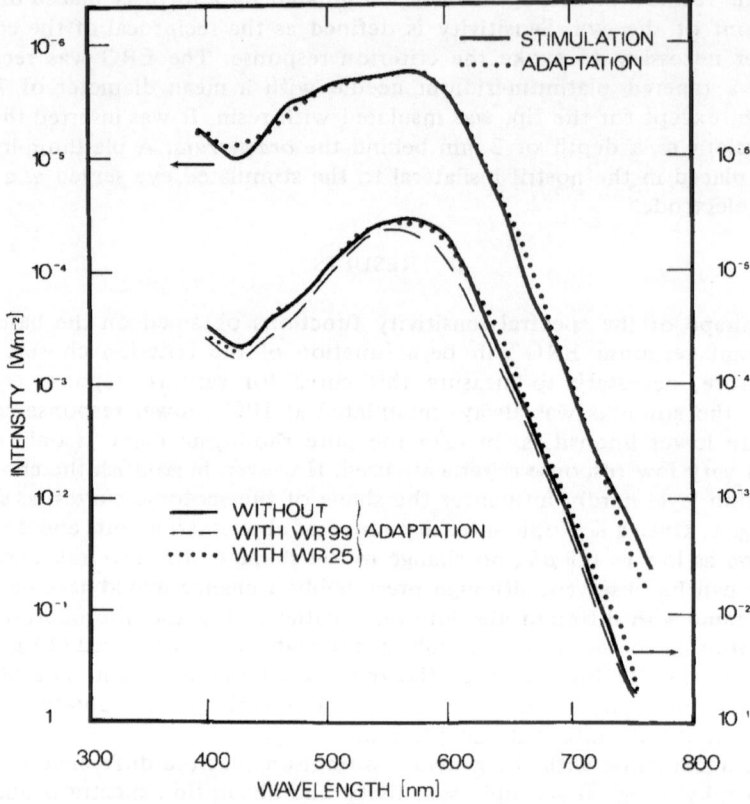

Fig. 2. The drawn lines represent the scotopic spectral sensitivity curves obtained from goldfish for ERG response amplitude of 4 μV (upper) and 2.7 μV (lower), respectively. The upper dotted curve was obtained by recording the ERG to a 500 nm stimulus, as a function of the wavelength of a monochromatic adapting field whose intensity was so chosen that the 500 nm stimulus resulted in a criterion response of 2 μV.
The dotted and dashed curves of the lower set were obtained by measuring the spectral sensitivity during adaptation with either a green (Wratten 99) or a red (Wratten 25) light, whose intensities were so chosen that either adapting field reduced the response to 1.8 μV. The lower set of curves is shifted downwards 1 log unit for clarity. The right vertical scale belongs to the lower curves, the left one to the upper curves. The two sets are from different goldfishes.

ted region in the scotopic spectral sensitivity curve where *no* contamination by the photopic system occurs, it can be advantageous to keep the stimulus wavelength fixed in such a region, and to vary the wavelength of the adapting light. Taking into account the shapes of the photopic and scotopic spectral sensitivity curves and of the porphyropsin absorption curve (peak wavelength 523 nm), the best choice wavelength for activating the rod system alone lies around 500 nm. By measuring the response to a 500 nm flickering light one can determine the intensity of an adapting light that is needed as a function of wavelength to adapt the rod system such that the response to the fixed 500 nm light is reduced by a given factor. If the 500 nm light indeed activates only the rod system, and if the adaptation of the rod system is not mediated through the cone system, then this recording will reveal the rod spectral sensitivity curve. The result of such an experiment is shown in the top half of Fig. 2. The drawn curve is the spectral sensitivity curve obtained without adaptation light for a criterion ERG amplitude of 2.7 μV. Then the 500 nm stimulus intensity of this curve was used as adaptation light, and a 500 nm stimulus intensity was chosen such that the adapting light suppressed the response with approximately a factor of 2. In this way, the total amount of light used in both the adapted and non-adapted situations were comparable to each other. With the intensity and flicker rate of the 500 nm stimulus fixed, the intensity of the adapting light was determined as a function of wavelength to reach the criterion response chosen. As is evident from the top half data of Fig. 2 (dotted curve) also in this case no change in the shape of the scotopic curve could be observed.

In the experiments described so far a cone contribution to the scotopic spectral sensitivity curve could only be observed indirectly, i.e. through a variation in the shape of the curve. Since, however, the flash responses of the cone and rod systems differ, a possible cone contribution can also be recognized directly by taking into account the shape of the response. This holds equally for the transfer characteristics which, for simplicity, might be thought to be the Fourier transform of the response to a short flash. A search for a cone contribution on the basis of response waveform can best be carried out in the frequency domain since the cone system responds to higher frequencies than the rod system. This difference in sensitivity with frequency forms an easy way to separate and recognize rod and cone contributions in the response.

The experiment was carried out as follows (Fig. 3): During the determination of the scotopic spectral sensitivity curve with the criterion response method (5 μV), the monochromator was stopped at a number of wavelengths and the modulation of the stimulus was changed from periodic (3 Hz) into Caussian noise modulation without change in mean intensity. Cross-correlation between the input noise and the ERG resulted in the 'flash' responses depicted near the corresponding wavelengths along the spectral sensitivity curve. The responses obtained at wavelengths up to 600 nm exhibit the typical slow waveform of a scotopic b-wave. At longer wavelengths, however, the shape of the response changes progressively with wavelength, indicating that most likely the cone system starts to contaminate the response. Finally, at 750 nm the response is dominated by a fast

187

waveform which resembles the photopic a and b wave of the cone system. At lower criteria the change in the dynamic characteristics shifts towards longer wavelengths. For example, at a criterion of 1 μV the scotopic dynamic characteristics could be obtained for wavelengts as long as 750 nm.

At first view, these data seem to imply that at the long wavelength side both rods and cones contribute to the criterion setting and, hence, that the spectral sensitivity curves would not reflect activity of a single pigment. Fourier transformation of the 'flash' responses results in the amplitude characteristics depicted in the centre of Fig. 3. For clarity the long and the short wavelengths are separated. They reveal that the contribution of the cones

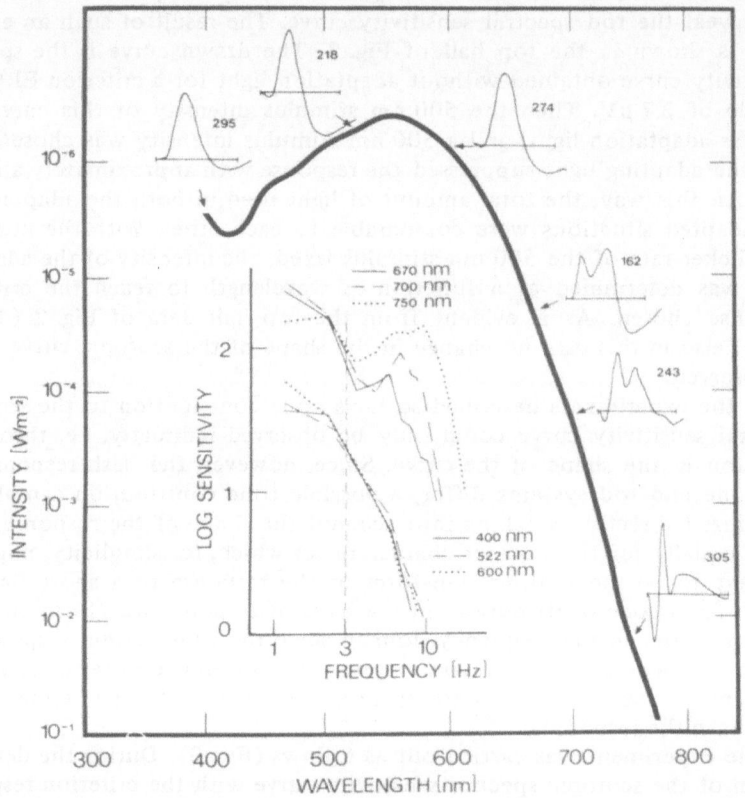

Fig. 3. The full line gives the scotopic spectral sensitivity curve determined in goldfish by the power that was needed to elicit an ERG amplitude of 5 μV. The monochromatic stimulus beam was sinusoidally modulated with a frequency of 3 Hz and a modulation depth of 35%. At the wavelenths indicated by arrows, the scanning monochromator was stopped and while maintaining the mean intensity the periodic modulation was changed into gaussian noise modulation with a bandwidth of 0 to 50 Hz, and a standard deviation of 35%. The cross-correlograms of input noise and output ERG obtained at the various wavelengths are depicted along the curve. To normalize these 'flash' responses, they have to be multiplied by the factors given to the right of the correlograms. Fourier analysis of the crosscorrelograms resulted in the amplitude characteristics that are presented as Bode plots in the center of the figure. The upper three plots are shifted upwards by about 1 log unit for clarity.

188

mainly elevates the sensitivity at high frequencies. At the frequency of 3 Hz used in the spectral measurements, the scotopic amplitude characteristic dominates. This follows immediately from the amplitude characteristics obtained at the short wavelength side of the spectrum. Therefore, although cones contribute to the response, they do not in the first instance, influence the long wavelength tail of the scotopic spectral sensitivity curve at low flicker rates. This is the reason why the shape of the spectral sensitvity curves of Fig. 1 remains invariant up till the highest criterion used. However, at this highest criterion (15 μV), and also at low stimulus frequencies, the cone contribution cannot be neglected. This results in a slightly broadened spectral sensitvity curve.

DISCUSSION

The visual process starts with the absorption of light quanta in a medium whose sensitivity, as a function of wavelength, is set by its spectral absorbance. This absorbance forms the basis for the spectral properties of the visual system. Determination of spectral sensitivity by e.g. electrophysiological measurements will, however, only reveal the absorbance of a single pigment if there is no contribution by other light sensitive media. To test for the absence of such contamination, a series of ERG experiments was designed. However, are the results presented conclusive on this point?

Let us assume for a moment that both the rod and cone systems contribute to the scotopic ERG in goldfish. From Fig. 1 we then have to decide that the 3 Hz response of both systems depends in the same way on intensity, since the shape of the scotopic spectral sensitvity curve is invariant over an intensity range of almost 3 log units. Following this line of thought, from Fig. 2 the conclusion must then be drawn that adaptive suppression takes place exclusively in those retinal units where the outputs from both rods and cones feed into, and that the adapting signal is generated in such summation pools. This, however, is an odd conclusion, since it is well established that at the receptor level, adaptation already plays an important role.

The 'flash' responses in Fig. 3 reveal that at progressively longer wavelengths another (cone) system becomes more important. In view of our working hypothesis that the scotopic curve reflects both cone and rod input, these observations would indicate that the spectral sensitivity of the combined (rod and cone) system drops faster at longer wavelengths than of the pure cone system. However, this interpretation is also unlikely, since at long wavelengths the rod sensitivity, according to the absorption data, is far below that of the red sensitive cones. To hold the initial assumption, it should, therefore, be concluded that cone activity dominates the scotopic spectral sensitivity. This, however, is in plain disagreement with the differing spectral sensitivity curves in the dark and the light adapted state (see Fig. 1).

We are thus inclined to conclude that the scotopic sensitivity curve, presented in this paper, originates solely from the rods.

In Fig. 4 the mean scotopic sensitivity curves of four goldfishes are gathered. The individual curves are so shifted with regard to each other that the long wavelength tails coincide, which leaves some scatter at the short wavelength side.

The dashed curve in Fig. 4 represents the absorption spectrum of porphyropsin brought in solution. This curve is corrected for screening
(WITKOWSKY, 1973). As is evident, the electrophysiological and absorption data differ. At the short wavelength side some of the difference in
spectral sensitivity can be attributed to the absorption in the eye media as
measured by BURKHARD (1966) which, at 400 nm, amounts to 0.4.
At the long wavelength side the effect of ocular absorption on the
slope of the spectral sensitivity curve can be neglected. Therefore,
even if the electrophysiological curves are corrected for ocular absorption on the basis of the data of BURKHARD (1966), it is clear that they
deviate systematically from the absorption curve of porphyropsin in solution.
Further study is needed to ascertain whether this difference will not be
present for *in situ* absorption measurements, or whether the ocular absorption has to be redetermined.*

SUMMARY

In man the psychophysical scotopic luminosity curve resembles the rhodopsin absorption curve only if the measurements are performed close to the
absolute threshold. At higher yet scotopic, criterion levels a broadening of
the scotopic curve occurs at the long wavelength side due to the activity of

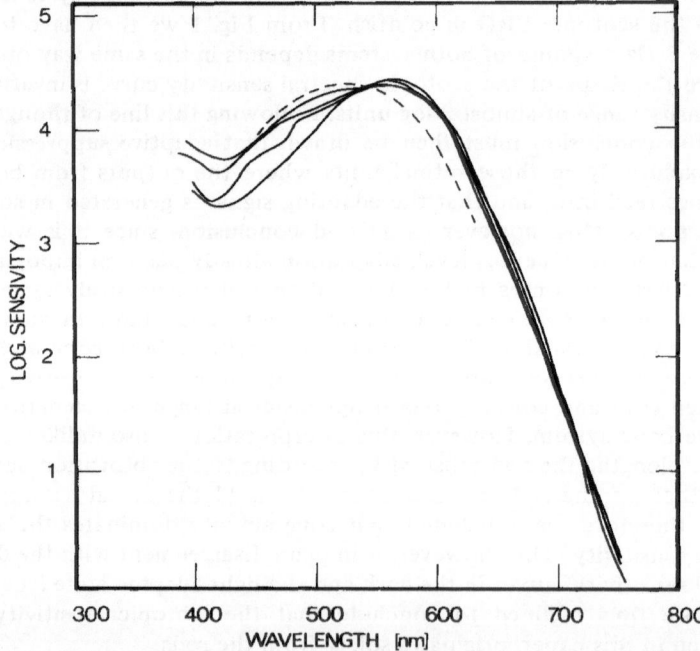

Fig. 4. Continuous curves represent the mean scotopic spectral sensitivity curves of
the 4 experimental animals of Fig. 1, 2 and 3. the dashed curve represents the absorption spectrum of porphyropsin in solution, corrected for screening. This curve is not
corrected for the absorption of the eye media, which amounts to about 0.1 log unit at
the leftmost point of the absorption curve.

the photopic system. It was, therefore, taken for granted that the deviation of the electrophysiologically determined scotopic spectral sensitivity curves in goldfish may also be attributed to cone contribution. In this paper experiments will be described to ascertain, whether this is, indeed, the case.

ACKNOWLEDGMENTS

This research was supported by a grant from the Netherlands Organization for the Advancement of Pure Research (ZWO).

REFERENCES

BURKHARD, D.A. The goldfish electroretinogram: relation between photopic spectral sensitivity functions and cone absorption spectra. *Vision Res.* 6, *517-532* (1966).

CRESCITELLI F. & DARTNALL, H.J.A. Human visual purple. *Nature (London)* 172, *195-196* (1953).

CRESCITELLI, F. & DARTNALL, H.J.A. A photosensitive pigment of the carp retina. *J. Physiol. (London)* 125, *607-627* (1954).

JAMESON, D. & HURVICH, L.M. Opponent-Response functions related to measured cone photopigments. *J. Opt. Soc. Am.* 58, *429-430* (1968).

MUNZ, F.W. & SCHWANZARA, S.A. A monogram for retinene$_2$ — based visual pigments. *Vision Res.* 7, *111-120* (1967).

PADMOS, P. & NORREN, D. VAN The vector voltmeter as a tool to measure electro-retinogram spectral sensitivity and dark adaptation. *Invest. Opthal.* 11, *783-788* (1972).

REYNAULD, J.P. Goldfish retina: sign of the rod input in opponent color ganglion cells. *Science* 177, *84-85* (1972).

SCHELLART, N.A.M.,SPEKREIJSE, H. & BERG, T.J.T.P. VAN DEN Influence of temperature on retinal ganglion cell response and ERG of goldfish. *J. Physiol.* 238, *251-267* (1974).

SPERLING, H.G. & HARWERTH, R.S. Red-green come interactions in the increment threshold spectral sensitivity of primates. *Science* 172, *180-184* (1971).

WALRAVEN, J. On the mechanisms of colour vision. University thesis, Utrecht (1962).

WITKOWSKY, P., NELSON, J. & RIPPS, H. Action spectra and adaptation properties of carp photoreceptors. *J. gen. Physiol.* 61, *401-423* (1973).

* Note added in proof: The latter proved to be sufficient to eliminate the difference between electrophysiological and absorption data.

CONTRIBUTION TO THE STUDY OF OCULAR INTERDEPENDENCE BY ELECTRO–OCULOGRAPHY

A. GARCIA-FRANCO & R. MTZ. DALMAU

(Madrid, Spain)

ABSTRACT

A relationship light peak (P) – dark trough (T) is established, $\dfrac{P-T}{T}$, and by means of it we observe how the performance from one eye is influenced by the other, being in the same state of adaptation or in darkness.

The illumination of the influencing eye decreases the $\dfrac{P-T}{T}$ ratio of the influenced one with respect to the value it would have in the condition of monocular illumination. This decrease is greater when the influencing eye has been illuminated in advance.

INTRODUCTION

Continuing the study of the interaction between both eyes, begun by us some time ago (GARCÍA-FRANCO & AGUILAR, 1970; GARCÍA-FRANCO, 1972), in this work the phenomena that are observed by another electrophysiological method, electro-oculography, are studied with the idea of giving a detailed account of the extension of same phenomena.

One could consider a different eye behavior with this work technique (EOG) than with ERG given that they manifest phenomena of a different origin: resting potential in the first case and reaction to a presented stimulus (action potential) in the ERG. However, in EOG the sensorial process is exhibited in the dark troughs and the light peaks, which are alterations of the resting potential produced by adaptation changes.

The difficulty of this technique is an extreme sensitivity at the moment of examination to previous adaptations, in other words, the difficulty of erasing from the slate, which is the retina, what has been written beforehand. Because of this, as has been confirmed by comparison, one needs to utilize preadaptation to a very high illumination (without reaching a glare level) or remaining more than 45 minutes in darkness, to obtain reliable results.

As a criterion for the quantitative evaluation of this process, the ratio, $\dfrac{\text{light peak} - \text{dark trough}}{\text{dark trough}}$ $\left(\dfrac{P-T}{T}\right)$, is adopted, given the property of the dark trough being the phenomenon least to be influenced by the different experimental conditions.

Five observers were used for the qualitative study of the phenomenon of ocular interaction by EOG, and one of them, well trained by other experiments, for the quantitative study of said phenomenon.

Taking as our base the ARDEN, BARRADA and KELSEY method (JAYLE, BOYER & SARACCO, 1965), we used a diffusing half sphere with two points of fixation at 39 ° either side of the median line to which points the observer alternatively looks at. This variation in the line of gaze gives rise to changes in the resting potential, which are the object of the present study.

The instrument used in this work is a Grass electroencephalograph, model 6, that was used in the following conditions:

Amplifier: with the 50 cycle filter on.

Sensitivity: 150 μV/cm. with a 2% precision.

Recording speed: 25 mm/s.

Base line in its normal mechanical position.

The connections to the observer are by cutaneous electrodes of silver, fixed to the skin, previously cleaned of grease and with an application of conducting paste, close to the nasal and temporal angles respectively. During these procedures, i.e. up to 5 minutes, an illumination is maintained of 1 cd/m^2 as a preadaptation.

The period of adaptation before beginning the session has been 10 minutes at 1500 cd/m^2 on observer 1 and 45 minutes at 1 cd/m^2 on observers 2, 3, 4 and 5.

During this time we perform the checking of the instrument, recording a known stimulus (rectangular wave of 1000 μV) with the same sensitivity to be used during the session (150 μV.).

Once the adaptation time is concluded, the session, properly speaking, begins. This is composed of a series of recordings effected every two minutes, which if they are performed in darkness we call 1st phase, or under illumination, 2nd and 3rd phase.

With observes 2, 3, 4 and 5, the sessions were performed with one eye occluded (one proceeds to the occlusion of this eye once the adaptation time is over) and these sessions consisted of two phases: the 1st phase (1ph) in darkness and the 2nd phase (2ph) at an illumination level of 555 cd/m^2. In observer 1, the study was performed:

A) With both eyes uncovered. Each session consisted of two phases:

— The 1st phase (1ph) in darkness during a period between 9 and 25 minutes.

— The 2nd phase (2ph) at an illumination level of 555 cd/m^2 for 15 minutes.

B) With one eye occluded. In this case, each session consisted of three phases:

— The 1st phase (1ph) was performed, likewise, in darkness, remaining this way for 9 minutes in some sessions and 15 minutes in others.

— In the 2nd phase (2ph) one examines with an illumination level of 555 cd/m^2 for 15 minutes (7500 cd/m^2 in a determined case)

— The 3rd phase (3ph) is recorded during the final 15 minutes of the session with the same illumination level as in the previous phase and is performed uncovering the eye that, up to this moment, had been occluded.

Several sessions were also carried out on observer 1 with the same adaptation and recording characteristics as in case A). In this new set of sessions we obtained the dark troughs and light peaks on the minutes 7, 9 and 11 of darkness and 7, 9 and 11 of illumination in two different conditions: a) with both eyes uncovered and b) occluding one eye instantly in the course of every recording.

Special care has been taken in each case, and we believe it fundamental that the occlusion does not exert any pressure, since pressure alters the results. So, the occlusion should be effective without putting pressure on the eye.

At the end of the sessions we proceeded to the compilation and evaluation of the data. Since the horizontal ocular movements give rise to deflections of opposite but of approximately the same value for each bipolar deviation, we measure — in mm. — the half of the total deflection, i.e. the value of the average amplitude of the resting potential.

Finally, the average values, previously transformed from mm to μV, of each series, are obtained. With these data the variation curves of the amplitude of the resting potential as a function of time are drawn for each observer and experience.

RESULTS AND DISCUSSION

On the curves obtained from observers 1, 2, 3, 4 and 5 (fig. 1 and 2) we see that each eye gives its characteristic response. One corresponding to an uncovered eye and the other one to an occluded eye, in such a way that

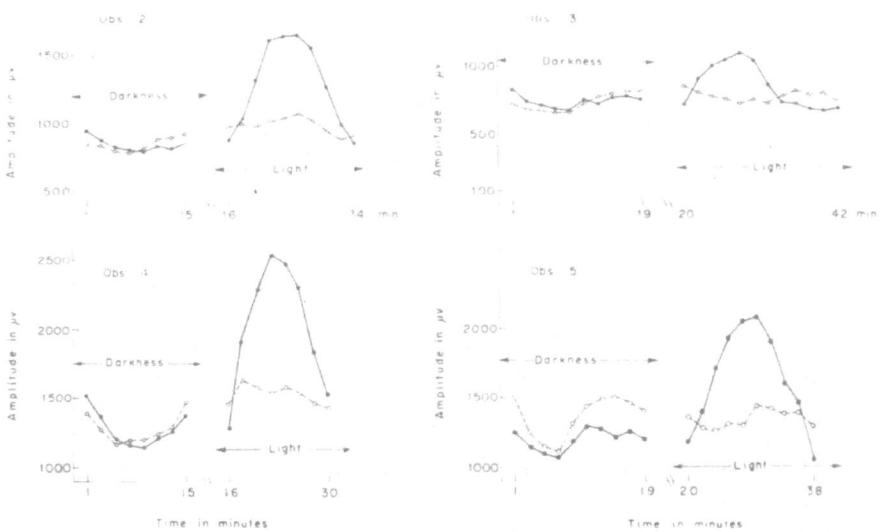

Fig. 1. Variation of amplitude of the resting potential with time. Preadaptation: 45 min at 1 cd/m² : ------- Covered eye; ——— Uncovered eye.

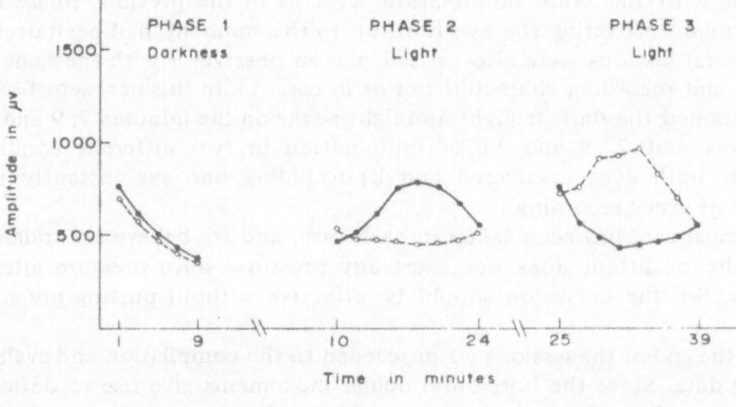

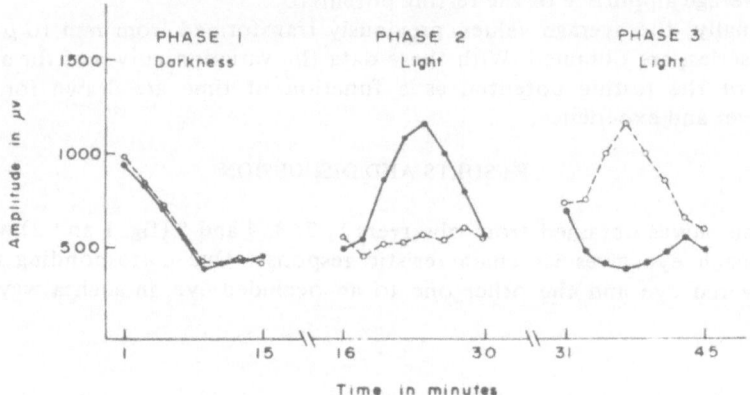

Fig. 2. Variation of amplitude of the resting potential with time. Observer: 1. Pre-adaptation: 10 min at 1500 cd/m^2 ;------ Covered eye in phase 1 and 2. Uncovered in phase 3. ———Uncovered eye in all phases.

while the first eye behaves with a normal amplitude/time variation (dark trough and light peak), although with variable amplitude, the second one does it with a variation corresponding to the lack of stimulus.

For a quantitative study of the interocular interaction, with the values obtained from observer 1, we have drawn figure 3. In it the values of the ratio $\dfrac{P-T}{T}$ are represented as a function of time.

This figure shows the curve of Permanent Binocular Illumination, AB, obtained from the sessions carried out with both eyes uncovered (simultaneous illumination) and from the ones in which the stay in darkness has been 9, 15 and 25 minutes, respectively, is observed that the ratio $\dfrac{P-T}{T}$

196

increases some 200%, approximately, on increasing the stay in darkness during the studied time.

Because of this, one can assert that the value of the ratio $\dfrac{P - T}{T}$ is related to the time of stay in darkness. ARDEN, BARRADA & KELSEY (JAYLE, BOYER & SARACCO, 1965) demonstrate that only the light peak is strictly linked to the state of adaptation to the light and that the amplitude of this peak varies, in a certain measure, with the time of the adaptation to the darkness and with the intensity of the adaptation light. In our experiments we have obtained similar results.

This relationship, $\dfrac{P - T}{T}$, established by us, is expressed in the curve AB, mentioned above, which we call the curve of Permanent Binocular Illumination (figure 3).

If we now study the experiments carried out with the occlusion of one eye (figure 3), curve CD, in which the observer stays 9 minutes (C) and 15 minutes (D) in darkness, one estimates that an increase of 50% and 25%, respectively, exist of the ratio $\dfrac{P - T}{T}$ with respect to values expressed in the Permanent Binocular Illumination curve.

In this same figure, curve EF represents the values of the ratio $\dfrac{P - T}{T}$ corresponding to the 3rd phase in which the illumination is already binocular. In this case, the values of the light peak considered are the ones corresponding to the eye that has remained occluded 25 minutes (E) and 31 minutes (F) while the contralateral eye has been exposed to the light since minutes 9 and 15, respectively.

Keeping in mind the stay in darkness of the occluded eye for a longer

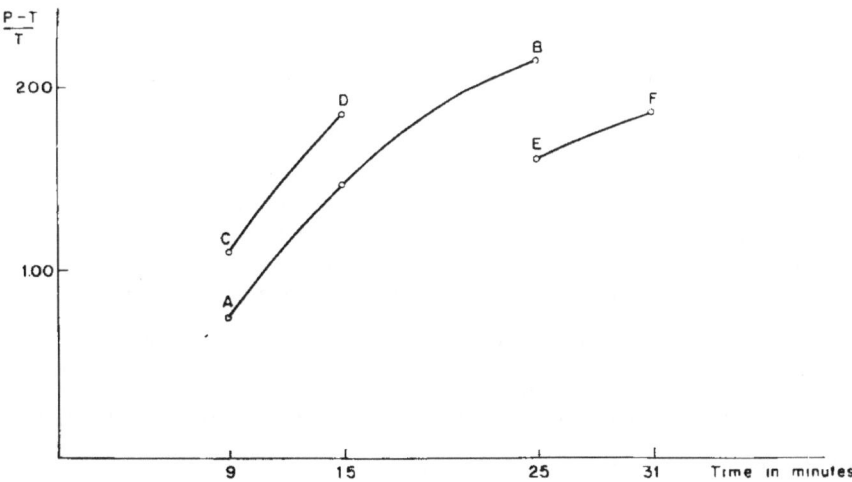

Fig. 3. (P − T)/T ratio as a function of the time that the influenced eye has been in darkness and of the state of adaptation of the influencing eye. AB: Permanent Binocular Illumination; CD: Monocular Illumation; EF: Delayed Binocular Illumination.

period, this curve EF, should have been a prolongation of the Permanent Binocular Illumination curve, AB. Nevertheless, it presents a decrease of the order of 25% with respect to the curve AB, from which one deduces that there has been an appreciable decrease, due to the contralateral eye's adaptation to the light.

The parallel between the three curves of figure 3, AB, CD and EF, is to be emphasized as a sign of the agreement in the results as much experimental as theoretical.

In the sessions carried out with an illumination of 7500 ca/m^2 in the 2nd phase ($\frac{P-T}{T} = 2.07$) and the 3rd phase ($\frac{P-T}{T} = 1.82$) the said influence is more clearly observed, due to the fact that the greater retinal illumination of the contralateral eye is more effective.

Finally, Table I summarizes the variation of the ration $\frac{P-T}{T}$ on passing rapidly from binocular illumination to monocular in six instances of the experiment: minutes 7, 9 and 11 of darkness (that correspond to the dark trough zone) and minutes 7, 9 and 11 of light (that correspond to the light peak zone). In it, a slight decrease of the ratio $\frac{P-T}{T}$ is observed when one eye is occluded. It is explainable by the confusion that this disparity of adaptations produces in the regulation systems and shows the necessity of the constancy in adaptation and not the instantaneous occlusion.

Time in minutes	$\frac{P-T}{T}$	
	One eye occluded	Both eyes uncovered
7	1.50	1.57
9	1.92	2.12
11	1.92	2.24

SUMMARY

As a summary, one arrives at the conclusion that be the electro-oculographic method, in the limits studied, a binocular interaction is observed, similar to that found by electroretinography.

The stay in darkness of the contralateral eye produces an increase of $\frac{P-T}{T}$ with respect to the value it would have if both eyes were maintained in the same adaptation conditions.

When the contralateral eye, adapted to darkness, is illuminated previous to the recording, it produces a decrease of $\frac{P-T}{T}$ with respect to the value that it would have if both eyes were maintained in the same adaptation conditions.

Also our conclusions can be expressed in other terms:

The illumination of the influential eye decreases the ratio $\dfrac{P-T}{T}$ of the influenced one (AB curve) with respect to the value it would have under conditions of monocular illumination (CD curve). This decrease is greater when the illumination of the influencing eye has been performed beforehand (EF curve).

ACKNOWLEDGEMENTS

We wish to express our gratitude to Drs. L . PLAZA for the helpful suggestions and R. VELASCO for the revision of the manuscript.

REFERENCES

A. GARCÍA-FRANCO & M. AGUILAR. – 'Estudio de la interdependencia ocular por Electrorretinografía'. Publication num. 31, Instituto de Optica. Madrid (1970).

A. GARCIA-FRANCO – Study of ocular interdependence by electroretinography. *Optica Pura y Aplicada*, 5, 16-21 (1972).

G.E. JAYLE, R.L. BOYER & J.B. SARACCO. – L'Electrorétinographie. Bases physiologiques et données cliniques. Masson & Cie Editeurs (1965) ³

CONTRALATERAL EFFECT IN THE ELECTRO–OCULOGRAM: EXPERIMENTAL VERIFICATION AND CLINICAL IMPLICATIONS

J.M. THIJSSEN & A. PINCKERS

(Nijmegen, The Netherlands)

INTRODUCTION

While studying the various types of what has been called the 'flat type' electrooculogram, we arrived at the conclusion that some of the results could be better understood if the EOG measured at one eye is partially determined by the standing potential of the contralateral eye. The literature revealed contradictory evidence for this phenomenon. For instance MILES (1938), ARDEN & KELSEY (1962a) and FRANCOIS et al. (1957) concluded that the EOG can be measured for both eyes independently. On the other hand, MILES (1939) reported results from patients with an enucleated eye displaying an EOG of reversed polarity at the artificial eye. Analogous results were given by IMAIZUMI (1966) and KELSEY (1967) for patients with unilateral diseases. Moreover, FRANCOIS et al. (1957) and ARDEN & KELSEY (1962b) observed EOG's displaying a light trough instead of a light peak in a case of a unilateral complete retinal detachment, and in a case of atrophia bulbi. This type of EOG curve has been called a 'paradoxical' EOG.

In our material (PINCKERS & THIJSSEN, 1974) we have found both the reversed polarity EOG and the paradoxical EOG. Additionally, a large group of patients displaying a unilateral subnormal EOG should be considered as well, since it may be expected that, the contralateral effect being present, the much larger standing potential of the healthy eye will diminish the potential measured at the impaired eye. This is due to the method of measuring the EOG. When the eye is simplified to a single dipole, then turning the eyes to the left means that the left temporal electrode will register a positive potential, whereas, the corresponding right nasal electrode, due to the contralateral effect, will record a negative potential. This potential will decrease the positive potential jump by the right eye itself.

We decided to investigate the presence and the magnitude of the contralateral effect by experiments with healthy subjects. Two types of experiment, viz. unilateral occlusion, and asymmetric fixation revealed a contralateral effect of the same order of magnitude as was found for patients with an artificial eye. Therefore, we have concluded that the contralateral effect does exist and that it can be described by a multiplicative constant: the contralateral effect factor. This factor represents the fraction of the measured EOG of the contralateral eye that spreads to the ipsilateral side. The magnitude of this factor appears to be 0.15.

In this paper we will present a calculation of the contralateral effect based on the electric dipole theory and also some representative patient data. The method for correcting the measured EOG curves and the light peak/dark trough ratio will also be given.

CALCULATION OF THE CONTRALATERAL EFFECT

In order to be able to calculate the contralateral effect, some simplifying assumptions have to be made. Firstly: that the eye is a part of a sphere covered with radially oriented electric dipoles, negative side outwards. Secondly: that the eye is embedded in an electrically homogeneous medium. Thirdly: that two measuring electrodes are located at 2 cm temporally of the center of the eyes at the line connecting both centers and the two nasal electrodes are placed at 2 cm nasally to the center of the eyes at the line connecting the center of the pupil after turning 20 degrees to the left or to the right (see Appendix, Fig. 8).

Electric dipole theory states that the potential resulting from a dipole covered surface equals the solid angle the surface is enclosing times the dipole moment per unit area. In the case of an almost closed surface (e.g. the eye minus the anterior chamber) this reduces to the solid angle comprising the border line (e.g. the limbus).* Moreover, the sign of the potential is reversed when the point of measurement is displaced from above to below this border area. The solid angle is proportional to the cosine of the angle between the normal at the surface and the line connecting the surface and the measuring point, and it is inversely proportional to the square of the length of this line.

Additionally, when both eyes are assumed to possess the same dipole moment, it will be clear that the absolute value of this moment can be neglected if only relative potential values are considered. The calculation is given in the appendix. The contralateral effect factor will be (see Apendix):

$$f = \frac{\Delta V_{LR}}{\Delta V_R} \times 100\% \approx 13.5\%$$

with ΔV_{LR} being the potential between the electrodes at the right, which is caused by the contralateral effect (viz. from the left eye) and ΔV_R being the potential at the same electrodes caused by the right eye. This means that the EOG measured at one eye is diminished by the contralateral spread of the potential of the other eye amounting to 13.5% of the EOG of the latter eye, and vice versa.

The calculation of the factor f as presented in the Appendix can be made more realistic by the incorporation of the limited dimensions of the medium surrounding the eye. At the corneal side this medium is totally absent, so the electric field is distorted. This distortion can be simulated by hypo-

---

*   The eye is thought to be closed by the missing part of it, and this part is electrically rebalanced by a flat dipole covered disc coinciding with the limbus. The potential from a closed surface being zero, the potential can be calculated by taking into account the disc only.

thetically extending the medium to infinity and placing a dipole disc before the cornea. The positive side of this disc faces the cornea and it possesses a dipole momentum equal to that of the eye. Since the solid angle covered by this hypothetical disc will be approximately equal to the solid angle covered by the limbus of the eye, it may be concluded that the above mentioned value of f will be sufficiently accurate.

In a recent paper we presented a mathematical derivation of the formulas for calculating the correction factor from particular experimental results and for correcting the measured light peak and dark trough values. (THIJSSEN & PINCKERS, 1974). The formulas are

$$dt_L = \frac{DT_L + f.\,DT_R}{1 - f^2} \tag{1}$$

$$lp_L = \frac{LP_L + f.\,LP_R}{1 - f^2} \tag{2}$$

and $$r_L = \frac{LP_L + f.\,LP_R}{DT_L + f.\,DT_R} \tag{3}$$

where dt, DT = dark trough
  1p, LP = light peak
  r = light peak/dark trough ratio
  L, R = left, and right eye respectively

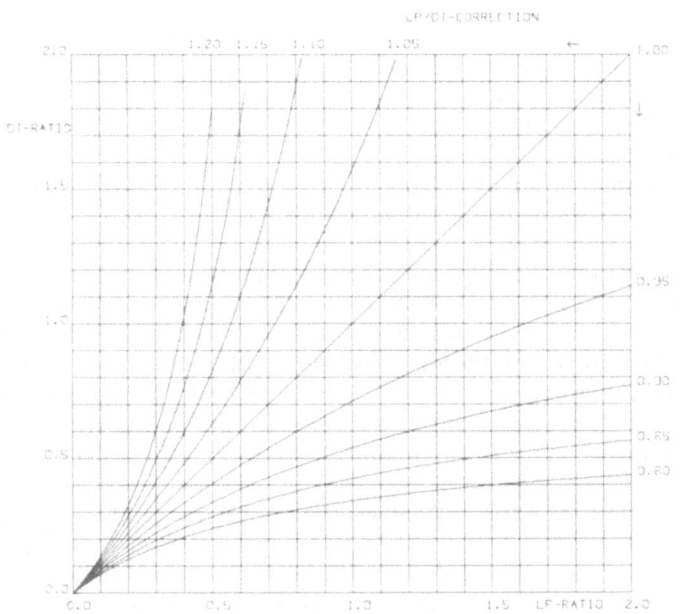

Fig. 1. Correction of the light peak/dark trough ratio; contralateral effect (c.e.) factor f = 15%.

The symbols in lower case (dt, etc.) represent the 'real' values, and the symbols in capitals (DT, etc.) the measured values.

Analogous formulas are valid for the right eye. Since, LP_L/DT_L equals the measured ratio R_L, equation (3) can be rewritten:

$$r_L = R_L \cdot \frac{1 + f.\ LP_R/LP_L}{1 + f.\ DT_R/DT_L} \qquad (4)$$

It follows from this equation, that the correction factor at the right part of equation (4) is dependent on the light peak ratio LP_R/LP_L and on the dark trough ratio DT_R/DT_L. This is illustrated in Figure 1. As can be seen from this figure the correction will be necessary only in the case of either a non-unity light ratio, or a non-unity dark trough ratio.

The value of the contralateral effect factor f has been determined recently (THIJSSEN & PINCKERS 1974). The data are obtained from two kinds of experiments, viz. unilateral occlusion and , symmetric fixation and from clinical measurements, viz. the EOG aft enucleation. The data of 18 healthy subjects and 12 patients ar.   ayed in Figure 2. The overall average being 15%, which value appears to be close to the value that has been calculated above.

CLINICAL RESULTS

The first group of patients that is illustrative of the applicability of the correction method is the group with uniocular severe impairment (e.g. a complete retinal detachment), or an enucleated eye. The EOG that is shown in Figure 3 was obtained from such a patient. The right eye has been removed, but, nevertheless, the EOG seems to react to the light stimulation. However, the potentials are negative. This type of EOG has been called a 'reversed polarity' EOG (PINCKERS & THIJSSEN, 1974). Recalculation of the EOG by using the factor f = 0.12 results in a completely flat and zero EOG at the right eye.

The second group of patients is characterized by a so-called 'paradoxical' EOG curve. Although the potentials are positive, a light trough instead of a light peak is observed (OS, Figure 4), which yields a light peak/dark trough ratio smaller than one. After correction (equation 1 or 2) the curve becomes almost flat, which corresponds to a light peak/dark trough ratio of 0.94 instead 0.68. It may be concluded that this type of EOG is caused by a severe impairment of the eye resulting in the absence of a light reaction, although a standing potential is present. The healthy right eye of the patient in Fig. 4 is corrected also, but now all the data points are shifted upwards by an approximately fixed amount. Therefore, a slight decrease in the ratio results.

The third type of EOG that will be considered is illustrated in Figure 5, i.e. the 'subnormal' EOG. This type is characterized by a mainly normal dark trough value, but a subnormal light peak. Hence, the light peak ratio in equation 4 will be larger than one, and consequently, the corrected ratio will be larger than the measured ratio. Moreover, the corrected ratio of the normal eye will be lower than the measured one. The data from 25 patients

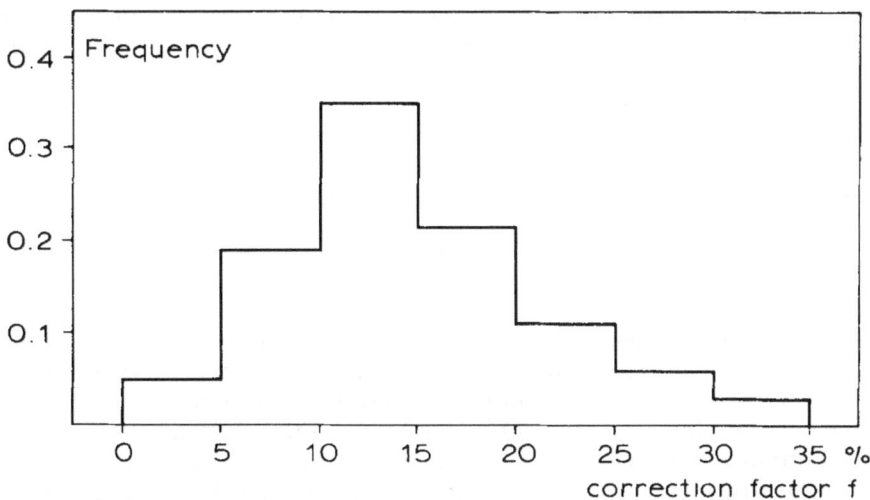

Fig. 2. Histogram of c.e. factor values obtained from 12 patients and 18 healthy subjects. Mean value 15%.

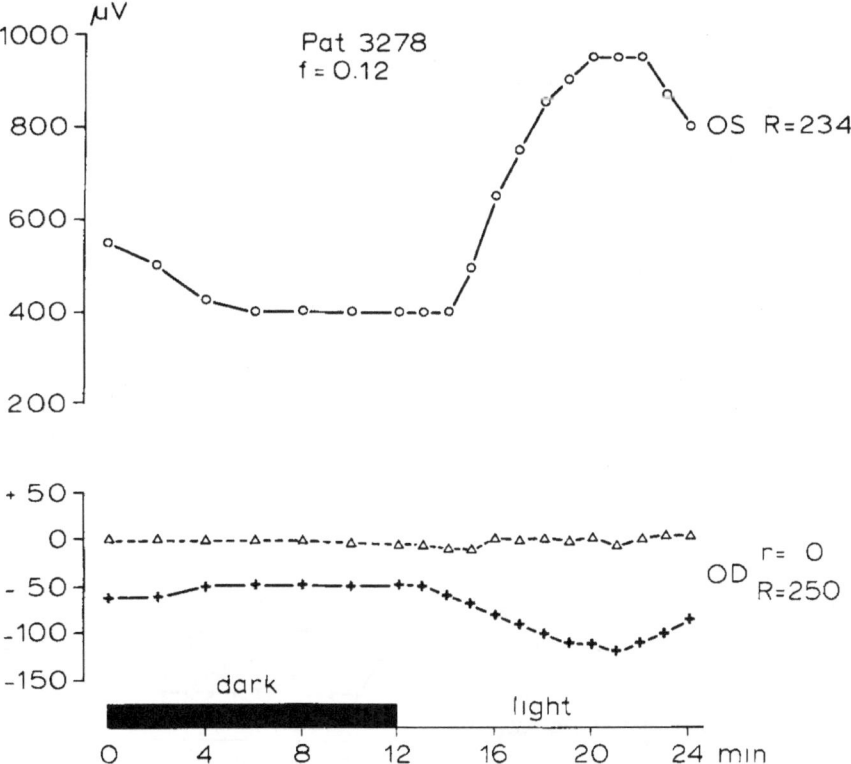

Fig. 3. EOG curves from a patient with an artificial eye. Light adaptation 2500 Lux. (o) healthy eye, (x) artificial eye, (Δ) artificial eye after correction, R = light peak/dark trough ratio before, and r = ratio after correction.

205

with a unilateral subnormal EOG are shown in Fig. 6. The solid lines of this cumulative frequency curves are the original data, the dotted lines are the corrected data. As can be seen the subnormal ratio values are shifted to the right, 4% of the data even becomes normal (larger than 180%). The ratio values of the normal eye display a steepening of the frequency curve, which means a decrease in the spread of the data. This latter result will be important for the separation of normal and subnormal ratio values.

DISCUSSION

In this and in previous papers we have shown that the contralateral effect does exist. It has been demonstrated by experiments and by EOG measurements in patients with a prosthetic eye. The order of the effect appears to be 15%; theoretical considerations yield a figure of the same order of magnitude. The usefulness of the correction based on the above mentioned figure is illustrated by the group of patients with a unilateral subnormal EOG (R ≤ 180%). After the correction has been applied it is possible to distinguish a really flat EOG, i.e. no light reaction at all, from a small reaction. The

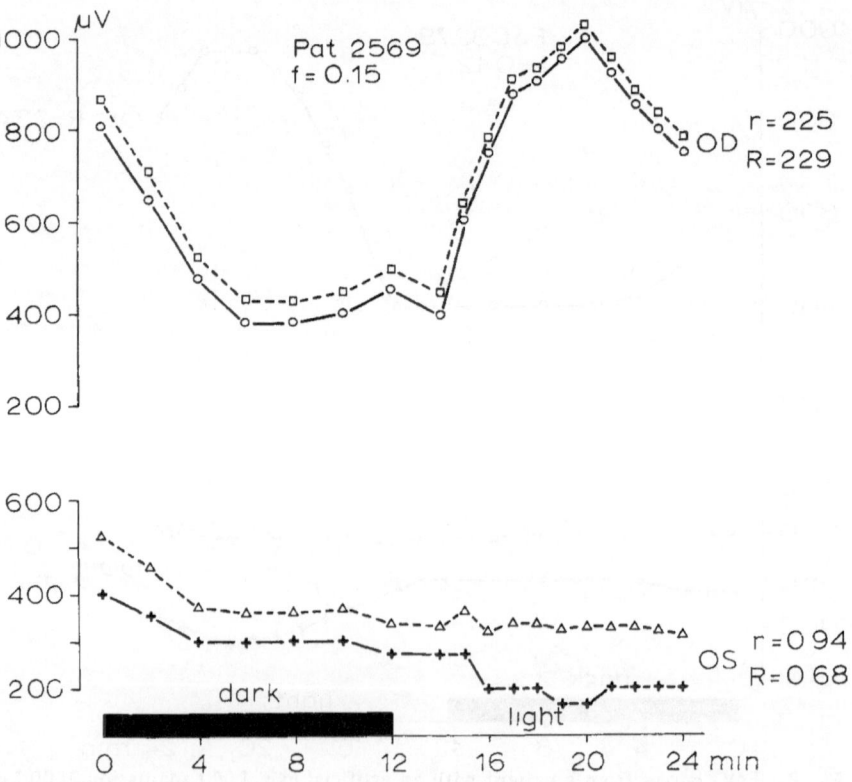

Fig. 4. EOG curves from a patient with a 'paradoxical' type of curve at the left eye. The solid curves are measured, the dashed curves are obtained after correction.

206

second argument is derived from the observations on the healthy eye of this group of patients: the inter-individual spread in the ratio values decreases on application of the correction. Therefore, it will be possible to make a sharper distinction between normal and subnormal EOG's. It should be stressed that the correction is necessary in cases of unilateral impairment yielding a non-unity light peak ratio or dark trough ratio. Since it is very easy to construct a device to carry out the correction, we have decided to build it into our equipment. The design of the device is shown in Fig. 7. The principle is to substract one seventh of the potential measured at one eye from the potential measured at the other eye. Since, the contralateral potential has a reversed polarity this substraction will result in an increase of the ipsilateral EOG.

APPENDIX

The relative potential values will be obtained from the distances of the electrodes to the center of the pupil in both positions of the eye (20 ° to the left and to the right, just as in a real EOG measurement), and from the

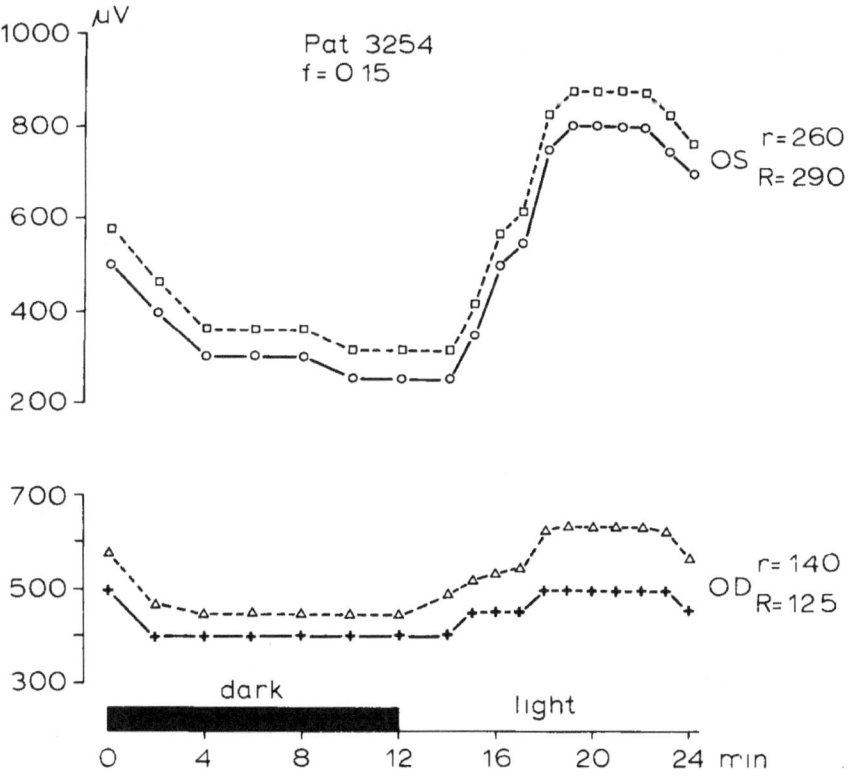

Fig. 5. EOG curves of a patient with a subnormal type of curve at the right eye. The solid curves are measured, the dashed curves are obtained after correction.

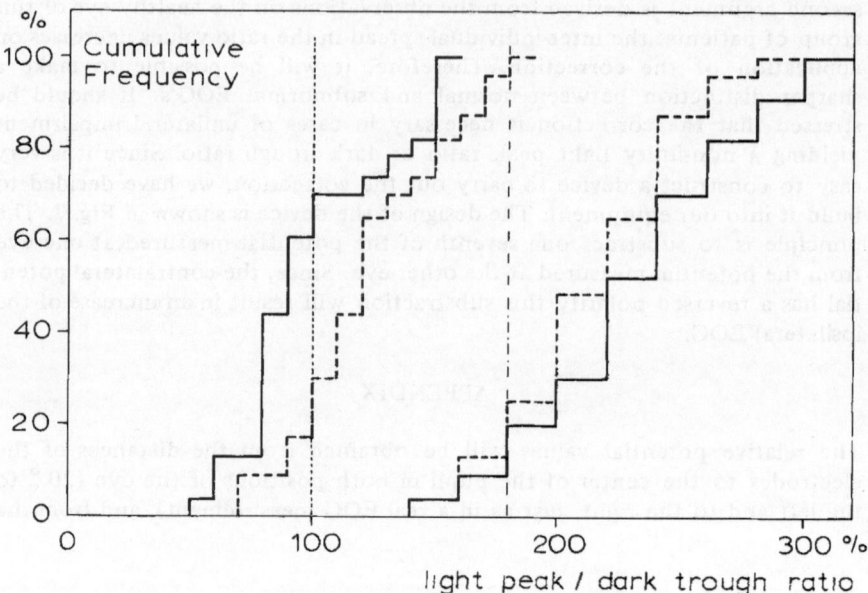

Fig. 6. Cumulative histogram of 25 patients with a unilateral subnormal EOG. Solid lines are measured data, dashed lines are corrected values.

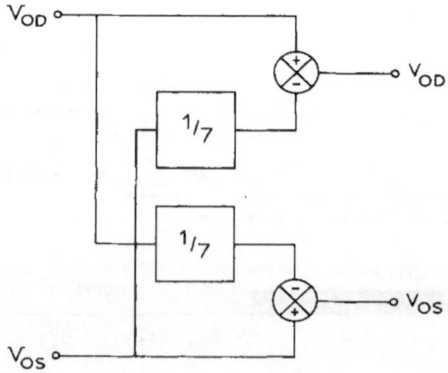

Fig. 7. Scheme of a device to correct automatically the measured EOG potentials.

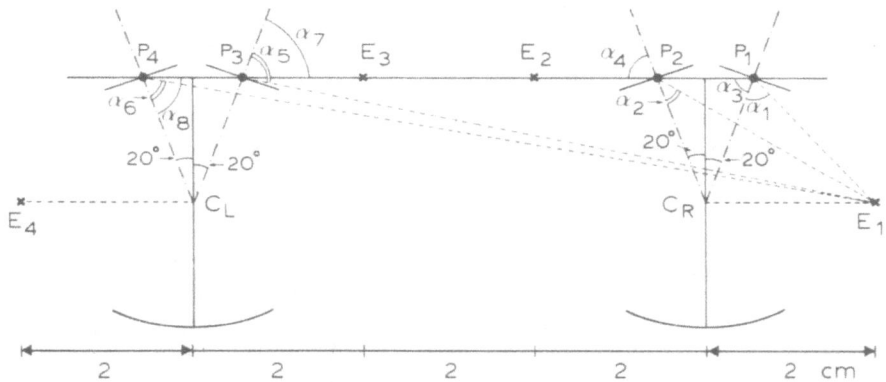

LEFT EYE   RIGHT EYE

Fig. 8. Scheme of the calculation of the contralateral effect: E_1 to E_4 electrodes, P_1 to P_4 extreme positions of the eyes during the measurement of the EOG, C_R and C_L centers of the eyes. The radius of the eye (e.g. $C_R P_1$) equals one centimeter.

cosine of the angles between the normal at the center of the pupil and the line connecting this center to the electrodes (see also Fig. 8). The radius of the eyes being 1 cm, it follows that:

$$\overline{E_1 P_1} = \{(\cos 20)^2 + (2 - \sin 20)^2\}^{\frac{1}{2}} = 1.90$$

$$\overline{E_1 P_2} = \{(\cos 20)^2 + (2 + \sin 20)^2\}^{\frac{1}{2}} = 2.51$$

$$\alpha_1 = \{20 + \arc\sin(\frac{2 - \sin 20}{\overline{E_1 P_1}})\} = 80°\,46'$$

$$\alpha_2 = \{\arc\sin(\frac{2 + \sin 20}{\overline{E_1 P_2}}) - 20\} = 48°\,55'$$

So $V_{11}\;(:) - \dfrac{\cos \alpha_1}{(\overline{E_1 P_1})^2} = -0.045$

and $V_{12}\;(:) - \dfrac{\cos \alpha_2}{(\overline{E_1 P_2})^2} = -0.104$

The potentials measured at the nasal electrode (2) are determined as follows:

$$\overline{E_2 P_1} = 2 + \sin 20 = 2.342$$

$$\overline{E_2 P_2} = 2 - \sin 20 = 1.658$$

$$\alpha_3 = 70°$$

$$\alpha_4 = 70°$$

209

So, $\quad V_{21} (:) - \dfrac{\cos \alpha_3}{(E_2 P_1)^2} \quad = -0.062$

$\qquad V_{22} (:) + \dfrac{\cos \alpha_4}{(E_2 P_4)^2} \quad = +0.124$

The potentials resulting from the left eye at electrode (1):

$$\overline{E_1 P_3} \quad = \quad \{(8 - \sin 20)^2 + (\cos 20)^2\}^{\frac{1}{2}} \quad = \quad 7.7$$

$$\overline{E_1 P_4} \quad = \quad \{(8 + \sin 20)^2 + (\cos 20)^2\}^{\frac{1}{2}} \quad = \quad 8.4$$

$$\alpha_5 \quad = \quad \{180 - 20 - \text{arc sin} \left(\dfrac{8 - \sin 20}{E_1 P_3} \right) \} = \quad 76°$$

$$\alpha_6 \quad = \quad \{\text{arc sin} \left(\dfrac{8 + \sin 20}{E_1 P_4} \right) - 20\} \qquad = \quad 63° \, 16'$$

So, $\quad V_{13} (:) \dfrac{\cos \alpha_5}{(E_1 P_3)^2} \qquad = 0.004$

$\qquad V_{14} (:) - \dfrac{\cos \alpha_6}{(E_1 P_4)^2} \qquad = -0.007$

And at electrode 2 the left eye will produce:

$$\overline{E_2 P_3} \quad = \quad (4 - \sin 20) \quad = \quad 3.658$$

$$\overline{E_2 P_4} \quad = \quad (4 + \sin 20) \quad = \quad 4.342$$

$$\alpha_7 \quad = \quad 70°$$

$$\alpha_8 \quad = \quad 70°$$

So, $\quad V_{23} (:) \quad \dfrac{\cos \alpha_5}{(E_2 P_3)^2} \qquad = \qquad 0.026$

$\qquad V_{24} (:) - \dfrac{\cos \alpha_6}{(E_2 P_2)^2} \qquad = -0.018$

The potential difference between electrodes 1 and 2 due to the movements of the right eye will be:

$$\Delta V_R \quad = \quad (V_{11} - V_{21}) - (V_{12} - V_{22})$$

$$= \quad (-0.045 + 0.062) - (-0.104 - 0.124)$$

$$= \quad +0.017 + 0.228 = +0.245$$

Whereas the potential difference due to the movement of the left eye (the contralateral effect) will be:

$$\Delta V_{LR} = (V_{13} - V_{23}) - (V_{14} - V_{24})$$
$$= (0.004 - 0.026) - (-0.007 + 0.018)$$
$$= 0.022 - 0.011 = -0.033$$

SUMMARY

The influence of the standing potentials from one eye to the other is present while measuring the Electro-oculogram (EOG). The experimental results of the so-called contralateral effect factor (c.e.f.) from a previous paper are reviewed. The applicability of a method to correct the EOG measurements is demonstrated, and a device is outlined that makes the correction by fractional subtraction of the EOG potentials. The calculation of the contralateral effect from electric field theory is presented in the Appendix. The result of it agrees fairly well with the experimental c.e.f. of 0.15.

REFERENCES

ARDEN G.B. & J.H. KELSEY Changes produced by light in the standing potential of the eye. *J. Physiol.* 161, *189-204* (1962a).

ARDEN G.B. & J.H. KELSEY Some observations on the relationship between the standing potential of the human eye and the bleaching and regeneration of visual purple. *J. Physiol.* 161, *205-226* (1962b).

FRANCOIS J., G. VERRIEST & A. DE ROUCK L'Electro-oculographie en tant qu'examen fonctionnel de la rétine. Progrès en Ophthalmologie Vol. VII, pp. *1-67* (1957).

IMAIZUMI K. The clinical application of electro-oculography. Proc. IIId ISCERG Symposium pp. *311-326*. Ed. H.M. BURIAN & J.H. JACOBSON, Pergamon, New York (1966).

KELSEY J.H. The combined use of the EOG and ERG as a routine clinical procedure. Proc. VIth ISCERG Symposium, pp. *19-28*. Ed. E. SCHMÖGER, G. THIEME, Leipzig (1967).

MILES W.R. The polarity potential of the human eye. *Science* 90, *437* (1938).

MILES W.R.: The steady potential of the human eye in subjects with unilateral enucleation. *Proc. Nat. Acad. Sci.*, 25, *349-358* (1939).

PINCKERS A. & J.M. THIJSSEN. Flat type electro-oculogram (EOG) *Acta Ophthalmologica* 52, *429-440* (1974).

THIJSSEN J.M. & A. PINCKERS. Contralateral effects in the electro-oculogram. *Acta Ophthalmologica* 52, *441-454* (1974).

RECENT DATA ON TWO PUTATIVE INHIBITORY TRANSMITTERS IN THE RETINA: TOURINE AND GABA

N. BONAVENTURE, N. WIOLAND & M. BEZAUT

(Strasbourg, France)

It is commonly accepted that a substance has to fulfil six main criteria, if it is to be recognized as a neurotransmitter; it must
1. be localized in nerve endings
2. be synthetized *in situ*
3. be removed from postsynaptic sites through a specific mechanism
4. be released on stimulation
5. be identical in effect to natural synaptic activation
6. be antagonized by specific substances.

Several amino acids are thought to be involved in inhibitory mechanisms in the nervous system. In the retina, there are a number of experimental facts which point to the possible role of amino acids, in particular of taurine and γ aminobutyric acid (GABA), as inhibitory transmitters. The aim of this paper is to summarize and to discuss some of the evidence concerning mainly physiological processes i.e. points 5 and 6.

1. Taurine is present at high concentrations in the retina of several species (KUBICEK & DOLENK, 1968). PASANTES-MORALES et al. (1972) showed that taurine accounts for 41 p. cent of the total amount of free aminoacids in the chicken retina while GABA accounts for 13 p.cent. Both aminoacids were found at high concentrations in the amacrine cells (GRAHAM, 1972; EHINGER, 1970). But an uptake by MÜLLER cells was observed for GABA (IVERSEN & NEAL; 1972) and for taurine (EHINGER, 1973).

In a previous work, PASANTES-MORALES et al. (1973) measured, following intravitreal injection of labelled taurine, the distribution of this aminoacid in the different retinal layers isolated according to the technique of LOWRY (1953). One hour after injection, at the time of maximal inhibitory effect on the ERG, radioactivity was concentrated in the inner plexiform layer and in the innermost part of the inner nuclear layer. Fourteen hours after injection of taurine, when the ERG had recovered, the radioactivity was more diffusely distributed.

2. The biosynthesis of GABA is catalysed by an enzyme, glutamic acid decarboxylase (GAD). In the frog retina, GRAHAM (1972) has shown that GAD activity is predominantly localized in the inner synaptic layer and to a lesser degree in the outer plexiform layer. He also showed that GABA content among the retinal layers is parallel to that of GAD. KLETHI et al. (1974) showed that biosynthesis of taurine is catalyzed by the cysteine

sulfinate decarboxylase in the chicken retina, as it is in the brain; they observed that the level of this enzyme follows that of taurine during onto-genesis.

3. Two possible mechanisms of inactivation of taurine were described in the retina. In the rat retina (STARR & VOADEN, 1972) and in the chicken retina (PASANTES-MORALES et al., 1972) a specific uptake process was found which might be responsible for active removal of released taurine from its site of action. In the chicken retina, KLETHI et al. (1974) showed the existence of another mechanism by which taurine may be inactived, as they isolated in the incubation medium isethionic acid which is a product of taurine catabolism. A mechanism of active uptake of GABA has been demonstrated in the isolated frog retina by VOADEN et al. (1974) and in the goldfish retina by LAM & STEINMAN (1971). In the latter case, the uptake by horizontal cells was increased by light stimulation.

4. The release of GABA and taurine from the retina in response to photic or electrical stimulation has been demonstrated by PASANTES-MORALES et al. (1974). Radioactivity was measured in the efflux of per-

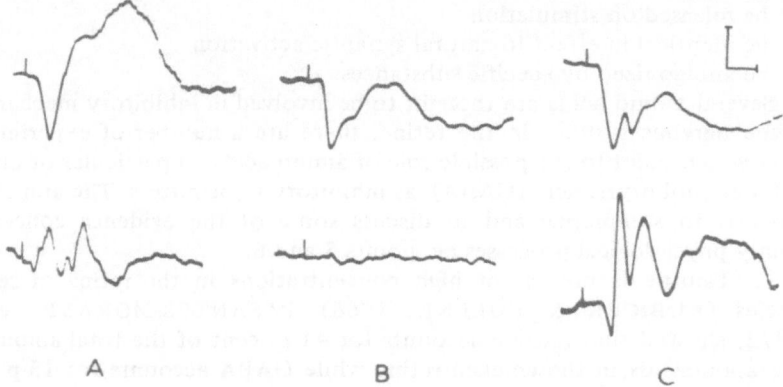

Fig. 1. ERG (upper traces) and T.E.R. (lower traces) before (A) 1 hour and 3 hours (B and C) after intravitreal injection of taurine. The calibration lines indicate 25 ms and 100 μV.

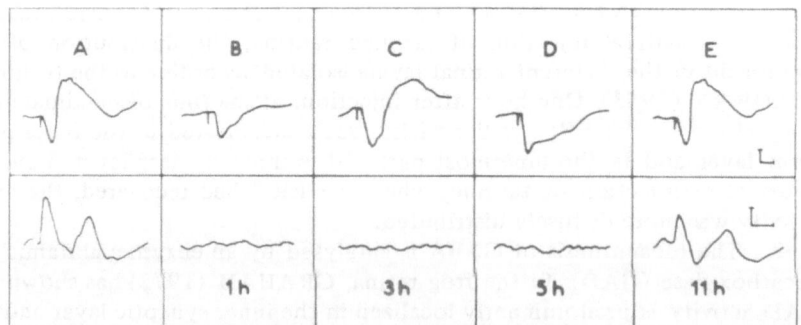

Fig. 2. ERG (upper traces) and T.E.R. (lower traces) before (A), 1 hour (B), 3 hours (C), 5 hours (D) and 11 hours (E) after intravitreal injection of GABA. The calibration lines indicate 25 ms and 100 μV.

fused chicken retina which had been preloaded with various labelled amino-acids. A single flash induced a marked increase in the efflux of radioactive taurine. An increase in the efflux of GABA was only seen with the successive application of 15 flashes. The same effect was obtained with electrical stimulation applied to the perfused retina and it was also more important for taurine than for GABA. This increase in the efflux was closely related to the intensity of photic or electric stimulation. These effects were not observed when calcium was absent from the perfusion medium. It is well known that the release of transmitter agents from nervous tissues is a calcium dependant mechanism. These two points, i.e. calcium-dependence and relation to stimulus intensity, bring further support to the assumption that taurine and GABA act as neurotransmitters in the retina.

5.   The effects of intravitreal injection of taurine or GABA on the ERG have been published in detail elsewhere (PASANTES-MORALES et al., 1973). But a few major points may be briefly recalled. The injection of taurine or GABA provokes a progressive reduction in the b-wave amplitude, whereas the a-wave amplitude remains unchanged (Fig. 1, Fig. 2). Once the b-wave has entirely disappeared, GABA (but not taurine) has a further effect of its own: it induces an increase in the a-wave amplitude and the appearance of a positive component of long latency (ROBERTS et al., 1968; PASANTES-MORALES et al., 1973). The effect of either aminoacids is maximal 5 to 7 hours following injection; the b-wave recovers its initial amplitude about 6 hours later. Furthermore, it was shown that the depressant effect of these aminoacids increases with increasing intensity of photic stimulation.

Intravitreal injection of taurine or GABA produces a progressive decrease and a total disappearance of the tectal evoked responses (T.E.R.), with the same time-course as the decrease of the b-wave of the ERG. But two hours after injection of taurine (this time-span varies according to the concentration of the injected aminoacid), the T.E.R. reappear although the b-wave of the ERG is still maximally depressed (Fig. 1). On the contrary, the T.E.R. remain totally depressed after GABA injection, as long as the b-wave itself remains depressed (Fig. 2). The double-phased action of taurine on the T.E.R. is similar to that found by TRUBATCH et al. (1973) following intravitreal injection of glutamate. It clearly points to a rather complex action of taurine, which must intervene at more than one synaptic site in the retina.

6.   If GABA and taurine act as neurotransmitters in the retina, they must be antagonized by specific substances. In a study of spinal cord motoneurones, ECCLES et al. (1963) showed that various aminoacids are involved in two types of synaptic inhibition with different pharmacological characteristics and different sites of action. 'GABA-like' aminoacids can be antagonized by picrotoxin or bicuculline and they are responsible for a presynaptic inhibition. 'Glycine-like' aminoacids can be antagonized by strychnine and they are responsible for post-synaptic inhibition. Taurine is considered as a 'glycine-like' aminoacid (ECCLES et al., 1963).

These two types of inhibitory transmission were observed by various authors on many other central nervous structures: spinal cord motoneurones and Renshaw cells (CURTIS et al., 1968, a, b, and 1969; PIERCEY et al., 1973); brain stem (HAAS & HÖSLI, 1973 a); medulla oblongata (HAAS & HÖSLI, 1973 b): cuneate nucleus (DAVIDSON & SOUTHWICK, 1970, 1971; DAVIDSON & REISINE, 1971; GALINDO, 1969); nucleus interpositus neurones (KAWAGUCHI & ONO, 1973). and thalamus (CURTIS & TEBECIS, 1972). The question was raised as to whether the model derived from the spinal cord might also be applied to the retina. In other words, our purpose was to investigate the mechanisms of action of taurine and GABA, and more specifically to uncover any antagonism between taurine and strychnine on one hand, GABA and picrotoxin (or bicuculline) on the other. We first showed that strychnine and picrotoxin have no effects by themselves on ERG and T.E.R. with the concentrations used (strychnine: 0.05 M; picrotoxin: 0.001 M). But with higher concentrations the amplitudes of both a-wave and b-wave decrease and T.E.R. amplitude is enhanced. Furthermore, pitrotoxin changes the morphology of the T.E.R. and increases their latency.

Intravitreal injection of taurine entailed a rapid decrease in the b-wave amplitude, without affecting the a-wave. If 50 μl of strychnine 0.05 M were injected at a time when the b-wave was maximally depressed, it rapidly reversed this depressant effect and the b-wave recovered its initial amplitude in less than 40 minutes. If strychnine was injected a few minutes before taurine, the inhibitory effect of taurine on b-wave amplitude was considerably reduced, and was even totally absent in some cases (Fig. 3).

Similar experiments were made following intravitreal injection of GABA. Strychnine has no antagonistic effect on the inhibitory action of GABA, and it did not prevent the decrease in b-wave amplitude at any concentration used. Intravitreal injection of picrotoxin did not prevent the decrease in b-wave amplitude due to a previous injection of taurine. But, it antagonized

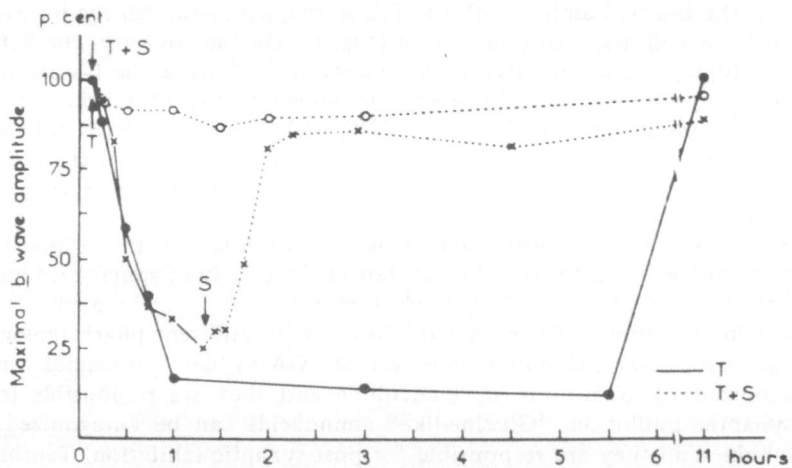

Fig. 3. Time-course of ERG b-wave amplitude after intravitreal injection of taurine (0.3 M). Solid line _____ effect of taurine alone; dotted line — 0 — effect of simultaneous injections of taurine and strychnine; — x — effect of an injection of strychnine when the effect of taurine is maximal.

216

the inhibitory action of GABA. The latter antagonistic action is only partial and the b-wave never reaches its initial value. Furthermore, the action is transient and it never exceeds 45 minutes. Fig. 4 shows that the increase in b-wave amplitude always goes with increase in a-wave amplitude of very short duration.

Preliminary data obtained with bicuculline indicate that this compound might have the same antagonistic action as picrotoxin: it seems to antagonize the action of GABA, but not that of taurine, on the ERG. So, in the chicken ERG, strychnine was shown to antagonize the inhibitory action of taurine, but not that of GABA; on the other hand, picrotoxin antagonizes the inhibitory action of GABA, but not that of taurine. These results are in agreement with those obtained by CURTIS et al. (1968) on the motoneurones of the spinal cord, and with those obtained by a number of authors on various central nervous structures. In the retina α and β aminoacids like glycine and taurine which are specifically antagonized by strychnine through a competitive mechanism at a synaptic site, may be responsible for post-synaptic inhibitions. On the other hand, aminoacids like GABA which are antagonized by picrotoxin and not by strychnine, may be responsible for a presynaptic inhibition.

Thus, there is good evidence indicating that GABA and taurine may act as inhibitory neurotransmitters in the retina, but with different modes and sites of action.

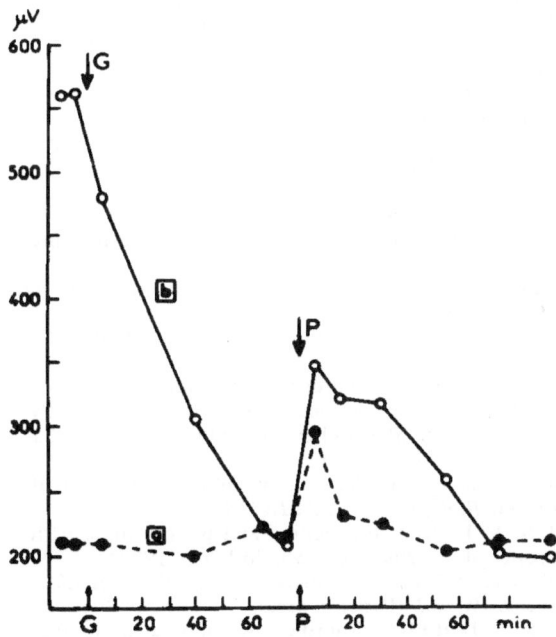

Fig. 4. Time course of ERG a-wave (dotted line) and b-wave (solid line) amplitudes after intravitreal injection of GABA (G) and of picrotoxin (P). Picrotoxin is injected when b-wave is maximally depressed.

SUMMARY

Strychnine and picrotoxin were tested as possible antagonists of two putative inhibitory transmitters in the retina: taurine and GABA, Strychnine was shown to antagonize the depressive action of taurine on the ERG b-wave, but it did not affect the depressive action of GABA. Conversely, picrotoxin had no effect on the depressive action of taurine on the ERG b-wave, but it antagonizes to some extent the depressive effect of GABA.

These data, as well as those obtained through recording tectal evoked responses, lead to the conclusion that taurine and GABA do not act in the same way in retinal inhibitory synaptic transmission.

REFERENCES

CURTIS, D.R., A.W. DUGGAN & G.A.R. JOHNSTON. Glycine, strychnine, picrotoxine and spinal inhibition. *Brain Res.* 14, *759-762* (1969).

CURTIS, D.R., L. HÖSLI & G.A.R. JOHNSTON. A pharmacological study of the depression of spinal neurones by glycine and related aminoacids. *Exp. Brain Res.* 6, *1-18* (1968 a).

CURTIS, D.R., L.HÖSLI, G.A.R. JOHNSTON & I.H. JOHNSTON. The hyperpolarization of spinal motoneurones by glycine and related aminoacids. *Exp. Brain Res.* 5, *235-258* (1968 b).

CURTIS, D.R. & A.K. TEBECIS. Bicuculline and thalamic inhibition. *Exp. Brain Res.* 16, *210-218* (1972).

DAVIDSON, N. & H. REISINE. Presynaptic inhibition in cuneate blocked by GABA antagonists. *Nature New Biology* 234, *223-224* (1971).

DAVIDSON, N. & C.A.P. SOUTHWICK. The effect of topically applied aminoacids on primary afferent terminal excitability in the rat cuneate nucleus. *J. Physiol.* 210, *172p-173p* (1970).

DAVIDSON N. & C.A.P. SOUTHWICK. Aminoacids and presynaptic inhibition in the rat cuneate nucleus. *J. Physiol.* 219, *689-708* (1971).

ECCLES, J.C., R. SCHMIDT & W.D. WILLIS. Pharmacological studies on presynaptic inhibition. *J. Physiol.* 168, *500-530* (1963).

EHINGER, B. Autoradiographic identification of rabbit retinal neurons that take up GABA. *Experientia* 26, *1063-1064* (1970).

EHINGER, B. Glial uptake of taurine in the rabbit retina. *Brain Res.* 60, *512-516* (1973).

GALINDO, A. GABA-picrotoxin interaction in the mammalian central nervous system. *Brain Res.* 14, *763-767* (1969).

GRAHAM, L.T. Intraretinal distribution of GABA content and G.A.D. activity. *Brain Res.* 36, *476-479* (1972).

HAAS, H.L. & L. HÖSLI. The depression of brain stem neurones by taurine and its interaction with strychnine and bicuculline. *Brain Res.* 52, *399-402* (1973 a).

HAAS, H.L. & L. HÖSLI. Strychnine and inhibition of bulbar reticular neurones. *Experientia* 29, *542-544* (1973 b).

IVERSEN, L.L. & M.J. NEAL. Autoradiographic localization of ^{3}H-GABA in rat retina. *Nature New Biology* 235, *217-218* (1972).

KAWAGUCHI, S. & T. ONO. Bicuculline and picrotoxin sensitive inhibition in interpositus neurones of cat. *Brain Res.* 58, *260-265* (1973).

KLETHI, J., P. MALLORGA & P. MANDEL. Synthèse et dégradation de la taurine dans la rétine. *J. Physiol.* (Paris) in press.

KUBICEK, R. & A. DOLENK. Taurine and aminoacids in the retina of animals. *J. Chromatogr.* 1, *266-268* (1958).

LAM, D.M.K. & L. STEINMAN. The uptake of GABA (γ [3]Haminobutyric acid) in goldfish retina. *Proc. Nat. Acad. Sci. U.S.A.*, 68, *2777-2781* (1971).

218

LOWRY, H.O., The quantitative histochemistry of the brain. *J. Histochem. Cytochem.* 1, *420-428* (1953).

PASANTES-MORALES, H., J. KLETHI, M. LEDIG & P. MANDEL. Free aminoacids of chicken and rat retina. *Brain Res.* 41, *494-497* (1972).

PASANTES-MORALES, H., N. BONAVENTURE, N. WIOLAND & P. MANDEL. Effect of intravitreal injections of taurine and GABA on chicken electroretinogram. *Int. J. Neurosciences*, 5, *235-241* (1973)

PASANTES-MORALES, H., J. KLETHI, P.F. URBAN & P. MANDEL. The physiological role of taurine in retina uptake and effect on electroretinogram (ERG). *Physiol. Chem. et Physics.* 4, *339-347* (1972).

PASANTES-MORALES, H., J. KLETHI, P.F. URBAN & P. MANDEL. The effects of electrical stimulation, light and glutamic acid on the efflux of 35$_S$-taurine from retina of the domestic fowl. *Exp. Brain Res.* 19, *131-141* (1974).

PIERCEY, M.F., J. GOLDFARB & R.W. RYALL. Effects of picrotoxin and bicuculline on the excitation and inhibition of Renshaw cells. *Neuropharmacol.* 12, *975-982* (1973).

ROBERTS, E. & K. KURIYAMA. Some correlations in studies of the GABA system. *Brain Res.* 8, *1-35* (1968).

STARR, M.S. & M.J. VOADEN. The uptake, metabolism and release of ^{14}C Taurine by rat retina in vitro. *Vision Res.* 12, *1261-1270* (1972).

TRUBATCH, J., F.C. VERHULST & A. VAN HARREVELD. Glutamate as a transmitter; comparison between the crustacean neuromuscular junction and the chicken retina. *Comp. Biochem. and Physiol.* 45, *183-194* (1973).

INCREASED SIZE OF B–WAVE IN THE RABBIT AFTER INTRAVENOUS DIPHENYLHYDANTOIN

G. CAVALLACCI, G. TOTA & A. WIRTH

(Pisa, Italy)

During the past years our laboratory has been mainly engaged in studies of the effect of ionic changes on the electroretinogram (ERG) in the intact eye. A number of substances were tried and the results are summarized in Table I.

Diphenylhydantoin, a well known anticonvulsivant, is routinely used as sodium salt and it is administered *per os*: the drug is metabolized by the kidney. Diphenylhydantoin (DPH) is a drug of choice for the symptomatic therapy of epilepsy, having no sedative-hypnotic effects, but it is also employed in heart diseases. In ophthalmology it has been recently tried in glaucoma therapy, for it seems to improve the visual field (BECKER et al. 1972).

Of particular interest is the fact that DPH has a marked ability to influence the excitability of the cell membrane: JENSEN & KATZUNG (1970) have shown that it reduces the action potentials of isolated heart atria of the frog at a concentration $2 - 4 \times 10^{-5}$ M, whereas at a concentration 4×10^{-6} it has the reverse effect, viz. a voltage increase. Other authors (ESPLIN, 1957; TUTTLE & PRESTON, 1963) have reported that DPH stimulates both the segmentary and suprasegmentary fibres of the spinal cord because of its depressing effect on the synaptic interneurones of the inhibitory type.

As far as changes of the ERG are concerned, HONDA et al. (1973 a) found that DPH diminishes both P_{II} and P_{III} components at concentration 10^{-3} M, whereas it increases the amplitude of both at concentration 10^{-4} - 10^{-5} M within 60-90 minutes. At concentration 10^{-6} M no effect was observed. Further experiments (HONDA et al. 1973 b) showed that DPH protects the retinal activity from hypoxia and that it increases the size of P_{II} when the potassium concentration in the extracellular fluid is 3-6mM, but has no effect whatsoever at higher concentration (6-10, 1mM).

The experiments so far reported were performed *in vitro*: we have, therefore, considered it to be of interest to test the effect, if any, of the DPH in the intact eye of the rabbit by conventional electroretinography.

METHODS AND RESULTS

The experiments were carried out on 15 pigmented rabbits of both sexes, weighting 1500-2000 gr. and of 3-4 months age. After anesthesia with

Table 1. See the text for explanation.

Substances	Dosage (mg/Kg)	Effect on b-wave (%)	Peak Time (minutes)
Aldosterone	0,25	+39	32
Furosemide	10	+45	44
Dichlorophenamide	30	+55	10
Triamterene	25	+44	20
Ethacrinic Acid	25	−24	30

Nembutal (20 mg/kg) we first recorded the basal ERG in full dark adaptation. Then sodium DPH was given intravenously at a dose of 40 mg/kg; the course of the ERG was followed for at least 1 hour. The recording technique was that employed routinely in our laboratory: a special ring electrode mounted in a Plexiglas blepharostat served as the active electrode, the indifferent one being inserted in the ear skin. Leads were taken to a condenser-coupled amplifier of 1 sec. time-constant. The sweep of the oscilloscope was synchronized with the light stimulus by means of a photodiode. The stimulus was provided by a gas discharge lamp of 1 Joule instantaneous energy placed at 30 cm from the eye of the animal. The tracings were photographed on stationary film.

The results are reported in Figure 1: it can be seen that DPH, at the dose mentioned above (40 mg/kg) produces a large increase of the b-wave, the maximum increament of 58% being reached after 35 minutes (median value). In Figure 2 changes of the mean b-wave size are plotted as a function of time. Statistical treatment of the results (Student t) showed a highly significant difference (P 0,01).

DISCUSSION

The mechanism of action of DPH on the ERG is not clear, but it seems justified to suggest that the reduction of intracellular sodium (WOODBURY, 1955) may be responsible for the changes in retinal photocurrent. The increase of the b-wave could depend upon a hyperpolarization of the cell membrane in those structures which contribute to its origin. The variations induced on the ERG by DPH have been interpreted in two ways. According to some authors (see LEWIN & BLECK, 1971), DPH facilitates the passage of sodium from the intracellular to the extracellular compartment stimulating the membrane enzyme ATPase. However, this hypothesis, suggestive from the theoretical point of view insofar as it explains the reduction of intracellular sodium in the cortex and the higher uptake of labeled Na, seems to be contradicted by some recent investigations, which showed (see PINCUS et al. 1970) that DPH inhibits the ATPase Na-K dependent and increases the inhibition of this enzyme produced by ouabain. These effects are a function not only of the DPH concentration but also of Na and K concentration as well, for it exhibits the activity in a rather constant way, when the ratio varies from 3:1 to 1:2. At different concentrations, far indeed from physiological, viz. 30-50:1, the ATPase is on the contrary stimulated (FELSTOFF & APPEL, 1968). According to recent work (PIN-

222

CUS et al. 1970) DPH decreases the intracellular sodium without activating either the ATPase or any other energy mechanism related to the sodium-potassium pump. Its rôle seems simply to be that of limiting the passage of sodium from the extracellular to intracellular compartment with a mechanism similar to that of tetrodotoxin (TTX). As it is known TTX may enter the sodium channels (KAO, 1966) in the excitable membrane and may form some bonds with certain membrane structures to close off these channels

N. of RABBITS	VOLTAGE OF b WAVE IN μV (MEAN ± s.d.)		
	BEFORE	AFTER 35'	Δ + %
15	374 ± 89	593 ± 105	58
DPH 40 mg/kg			

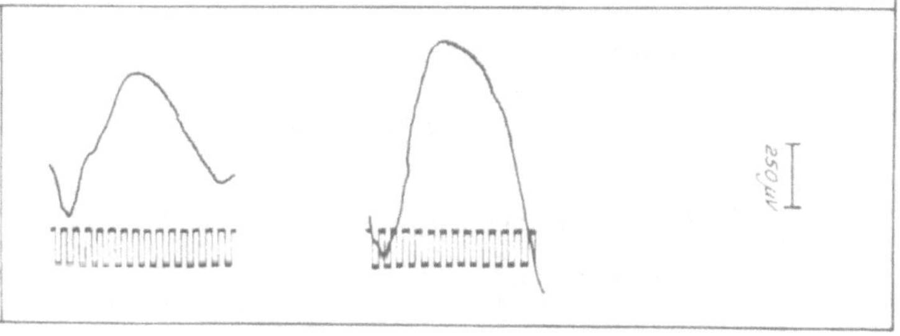

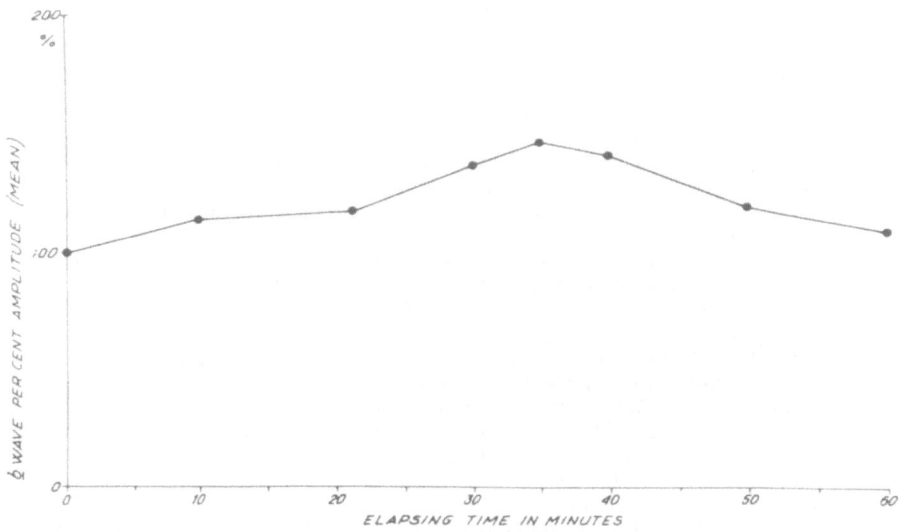

Fig. 1. Results reported, see the text for experimental details.

Fig. 2. Changes of the mean b-wave size plotted as function of time.

for sodium movement. A mechanism of this kind has been suggested by WALD (1973) to explain excitation in vertebrate photoreceptors. However, since the b-wave is considered a side phenomenon not necessarily concerned with excitation (see: WIRTH & PONTE, 1964; FRANÇOIS et al. 1973) it appears likely that the point of action of DPH could be in the Müller cells (glial cells) as it it actually does in the CNS.

SUMMARY

DPH at the dose mentioned (40 mg/Kg) produces a large increase of the b-wave in the rabbit, the maximum increament of 58% being reached after 35 minutes (median value). The mechanism of action of DPH on the ERG is not clear, but it seems justified to suggest that the reduction of intracellular sodium may be responsible for the changes in retinal photocurrent. According to recent advances DPH decreases the intracellular sodium without activating the ATPase of the sodium-potassium pump. Its rôle seems to that of limiting the passage of sodium from the extracellular to intracellular compartment with a mechanism similar to that of tetrodotoxin (TTX). The point of action of DPH could be in the Müller cells.

REFERENCES

BECKER, B., STAMPER, R.L. & ASSEFF, C. Effect of diphenylhydantoin in glaucomatous field loss: A preliminary report. *Trans. amer. Acad. Ophthal. Otolaryng.* 76, *412*, 1972.

ESPLIN, D.W. Effects of diphenylhydantoin on synaptic transmission in cat spinal cord and stellate ganglion. *J. Pharm. exp. Ther.* 120, *301*, 1957.

FESTOFF, B.X. & APPEL, S.H. Effect of diphenylhydantoin on synaptosome sodium-potassium ATPase. *J. clin. Invest.* 47, *2752*, 1968.

FRANÇOIS, J., DE ROUCK, A., CAMBIE, E. & ZANEN, A. 'L'electrodiagnostic des affections retiniennes' *Bull. Soc. belge Ophtal.* 166/1, 1974.

HONDA, Y. PODOS, S.M. & BECKER, B. The effect of diphenylhydantoin on the electroretinogram of rabbits. I. Effect of concentration. *Invest. Ophthalmol.* 12, *566*, 1973a.

HONDA, Y., PODOS, S.M. & BECKER, B. The effect of diphenylhydantoin on the electroretinogram of rabbits. II. Effects of hypoxia and potassium. *Invest. Ophthalmol.* 12, *573*, 1973b.

JENSEN, R.A. & KATZUNG, B.G. Electrophysiological actions of diphenylhydantoin on rabbit atria. *Circulat. Res.* 26, *17*, 1970.

KAO, C.Y. Tetrodotoxin, Saxitoxin and their significance in the study of excitation phenomena. *Pharmacol. Rev.* 18, *998*, 1966.

LEWIN, E. & BLECK, V. The effect of diphenylhydantoin administration on sodium-potassium-activated ATPase in cortex. *Neurology* 21, *647*, 1971.

PINCUS, J.H., GROVE, I., MARINO, B.B. & GLASER, G.E. Studies on the mechanism of action of diphenylhydantoin. *Arch. Neurol.* 22, *566*, 1970.

TUTTLE, R.S. & PRESTON, J.B. The effects of diphenylhydantoin (Dilantin) on segmental and suprasegmental facilitation and inhibition of segmental motoneurones in the cat. *J. Pharm. exp. Ther.* 141, *84*, 1963.

WALD, G. Visual pigments and photoreceptor physiology. in 'Biochemistry and physiology of visual pigments'. ed. H. Langer, 1973.

WIRTH, A. & PONTE, F. 'Fisiopatologia e clinica dell'elettroretinogramma' Industria Grafica Nazionale, Palermo 1964.

WOODBURY, D.M. Effect of diphenylhydantoin on electrolytes and sodium turnover in brain and other tissues of normal, hyopnatremic and potictal rats. *J. Pharm. exp. Ther.* 115, *74*, 1955.

PRESERVATION OF ERG IN THE ISOLATED PERFUSING EYE BY FLUOROCARBON AS THE ERYTHROCYTE SUBSTITUTE

KITETSU IMAIZUMI, YUTAKA TAZAWA, TADAHIRO OTSUKA &
HIROO IMAIZUMI

(Morioka, Japan)

INTRODUCTION

Since a method of recording the electroretinogram (ERG) from an isolated bovine eye under perfusion was reported in 1969 by TAZAWA & SEAMAN (1969, 1972), the technique has been employed as an excellent experimental procedure in the electrophysiological study of the retina of warm-blooded animals (IMAIZUMI, et al., 1972; MERA, 1972; OTSUKA, 1973; TAZAWA, 1973).

It is difficult in this preparation, nevertheless, to perform studies under experimental conditions beyond the physiological limits of bovine blood used as perfusate, although the isolated eye can be maintained in a state closer to the physiological condition than in the case of perfusion with Eagle's minimum essential medium (MEM) described by GOURAS & HOFF (1970) and NIEMEYER & GOURAS (1973 a, b).

With a view to improving the experimental technique in this respect, a study was attempted to find a suitable substitute for erythrocytes to deliver sufficient amount of oxygen to the retina.

The present investigation was performed in an attempt to determine the optimal composition of the emulsified fluorocarbon (FC) as a erythrocyte substitute for perfusion to maintain normal ERG waves from the isolated bovine eye, by altering concentrations or kind of solvents in the emulsion, and the flow rate of the perfusion.

METHODS

1. Emulsification of FC

From among several varieties of FC preparations with different oxygen solubilities, i.e. FC-43, FC-75, FC-80, etc. (Minnesota Mining Mfg. Inc., USA), FC-43 was chosen in this investigation.

Liquid fluorocarbon, a solvent and a surface active agent were combined in the specified proportions and the resulting mixture was emulsified by ultrasonic treatment (20 KHz) for 2 to 3 hours, using several platinum needles, 1 mm in diameter and 15 mm in length, as vibratory rods to cause efficient cavitation.

Used as solvents were Krebs' solution, physiological saline, MEM (EAGLE, 1959) and bovine plasma. A non-ionic surfactant (Plonon; Nippon Oils & Fats Co., Ltd.) was made up as solution in physiologic saline at a concentration of 10^{-4} mol/l and was added 10 volume per cent to the FC-solvent mixture, for emulsification.

Prepared FC emulsions, containing homogeneously distributed concavo-concave discoid FC particles, 2 to 3 microns in diameter, were used as perfusates after equilibrated with pure oxygen at the atmospheric pressure.

2. *Perfusion of an isolated whole bovine eye*

Perfusion of an isolated whole bovine eye was performed in accordance with the procedure described by TAZAWA & SEAMAN (1969; 1972). Namely, a bovine eye isolated immediately after slaughter was perfused with oxygenated heparinized bovine blood at a pressure of 800 mmH$_2$0 via the cannulated ciliary artery. The perfusion was maintained consistently at a flow rate of approximately 2 ml per minute at 32°C.

3. *ERG recording*

ERGs of the isolated eye were recorded, according to the methods described by TAZAWA & SEAMAN (1969; 1972), MERA (1972) and OTSUKA (1973), by stroboscopic lighting (xenon lamp with an intensity of 20 joule; 1,730 candela) under dark adaptation by a cathode-ray oscilloscope via a differential amplifier, with a time constant of 0.3 sec.

After stabilization of the ERG wave under perfusion with bovine blood (being taken as control), the perfusate was exchanged to various FC emulsion and ERGs were recorded at 30-second intervals to observe changes in amplitude of a- and b-waves.

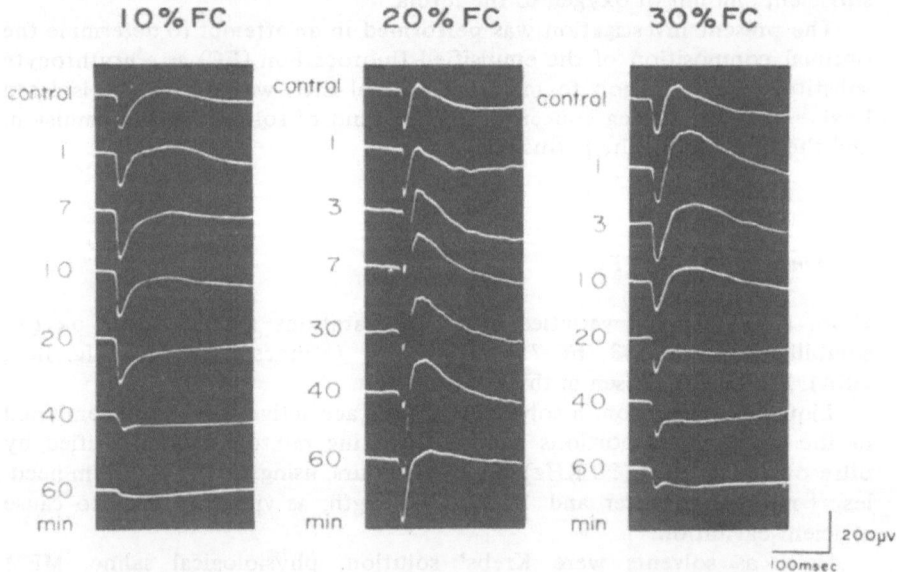

Fig. 1. ERG waves recorded from the isolated bovine eyes perfused with different concentrations of 10, 20 or 30 per cent fluorocarbon emulsion in Krebs' solution.

1. Optimal concentration of FC

With a view to determining the optimum concentration of FC in the emulsion for the best maintenance of a- and b-waves of ERG of the perfused bovine eye, ERGs were recorded to compare changes of these waves due to different concentration of FC; i.e. 10, 20, or 30 volume per cent FC in Krebs' solution (referred her eafter as 10, 20, or 30% FC-K respectively).

The ERGs recorded under these conditions are exemplified in Figures 1 and 2. ERGs from the eye being perfused with 20% FC-K showed a- and b-waves with increased amplitudes by more than 200 per cent over the control level at 7 minutes after initiation of perfusion and these waves continued to exhibit increased amplitudes over the ensuing 60 minutes. ERGs from the eye under perfusion with 10 or 30% FC-K, by contrast, failed to maintain the control level for more than 10 minutes (Figures 1 and 2).

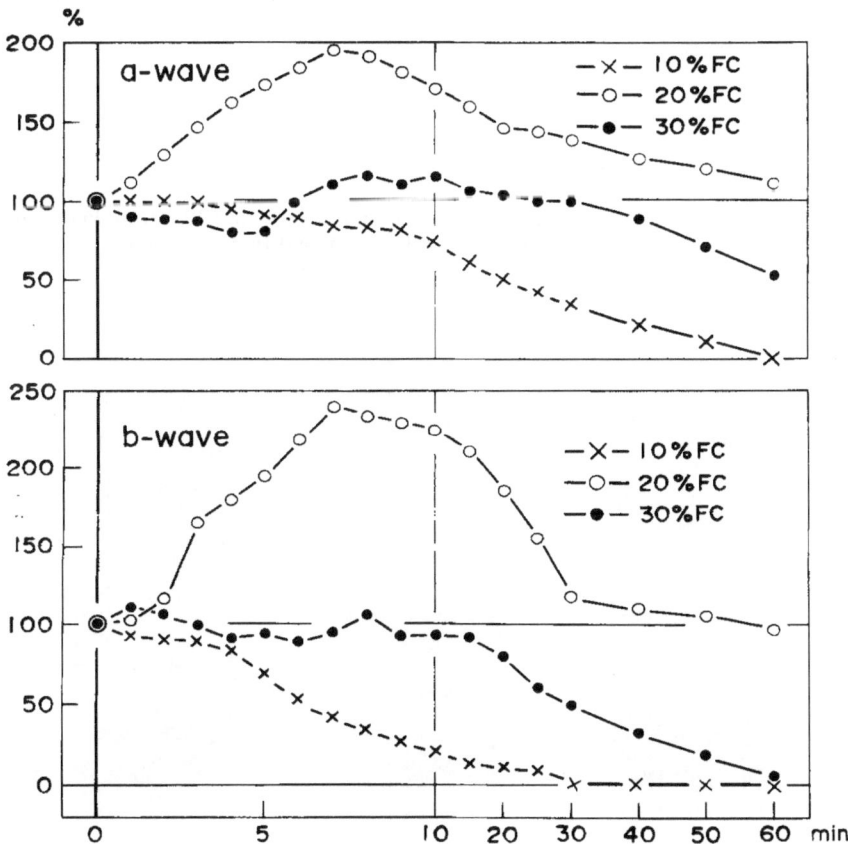

Fig. 2. Variations in relative amplitudes of a- and b-waves of ERGs recorded from the isolated bovine eyes perfused with different concentrations of 10, 20 or 30 per cent fluorocarbon emulsion in Krebs' solution.

227

2. Alternate perfusion with oxygenated blood and 20% FC-K

Figure 3 illustrates the ERG waves obtained under perfusion alternately with normal blood and 20% FC-K. The increase in amplitudes of a- and b-waves perfused with 20% FC-K was noted to be sognificantly reproducible (Figure 3).

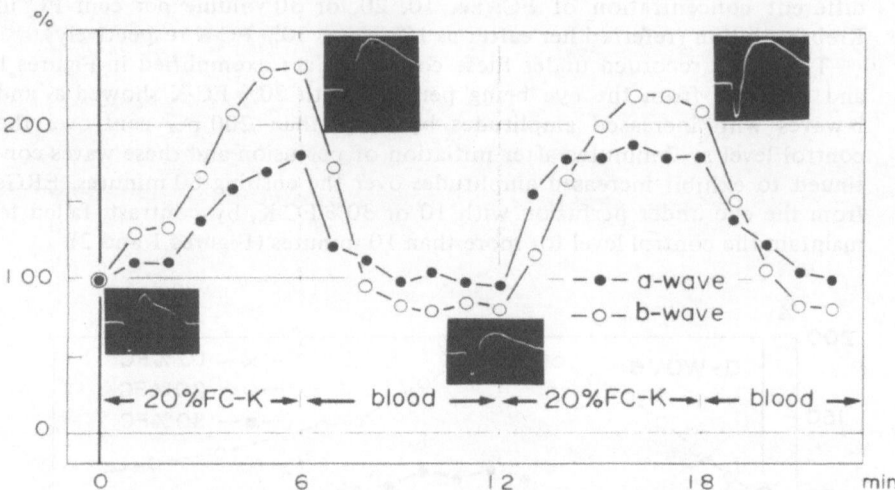

Fig. 3. Variations in relative amplitudes of a- and b-waves of ERGs recorded from an isolated bovine eye perfused alternately with 20 per cent fluorocarbon-Krebs' solution and the normal bovine blood.

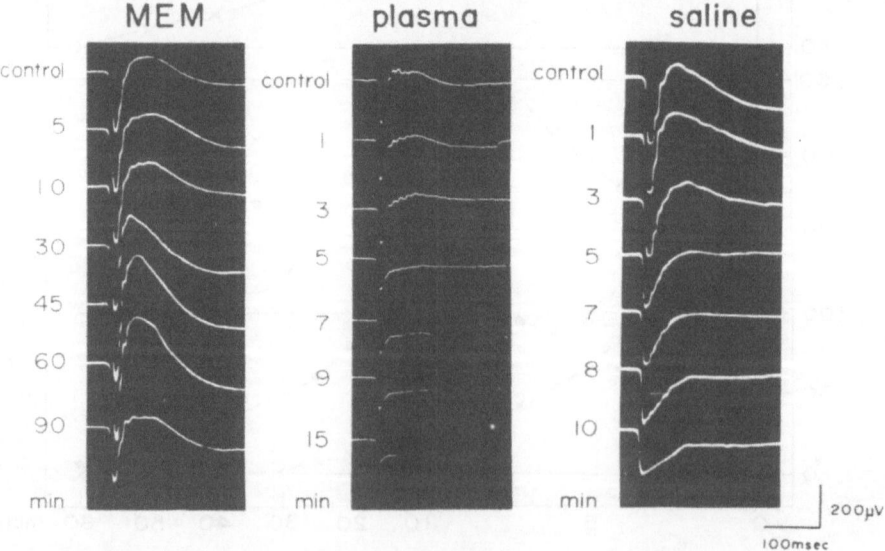

Fig. 4. ERG waves recorded from the isolated bovine eyes perfused with fluorocarbon emulsions in different solvents such as physiological saline, MEM or the bovine plasma.

228

3. Effects of solvents

Emulsion of 20 per cent FC using various other solvents such as physiological saline (20% FC-saline), MEM (20% FC-MEM) or bovine plasma (20% FC-plasma) were assessed as perfusates for the isolated eye. As shown in Figures 4 and 5, perfusion with 20% FC-MEM has proven to effect increased amplitudes of a- and b-waves over 90 minutes, whereas 20% FC-saline and plasma failed to facilitate sustained increase in amplitude for more than 5 minutes (Figures 4 and 5).

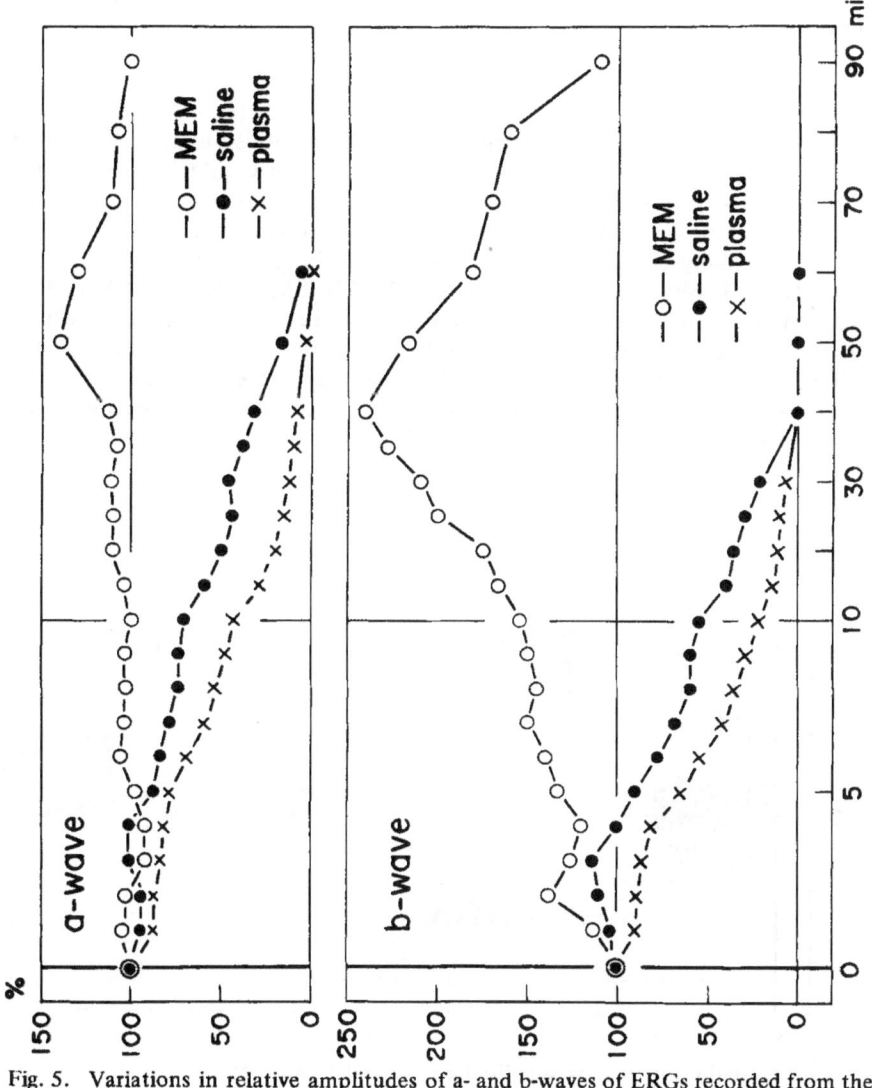

Fig. 5. Variations in relative amplitudes of a- and b-waves of ERGs recorded from the isolated bovine eyes perfused with fluorocarbon emulsions in different solvents such as physiological saline, MEM or the bovine plasma.

229

4. *Effect of flow rate*

When the FC emulsion was allowed to flow at the same perfusion pressure as in the case of the normal blood perfusion, 800 mmH$_2$O, the flow rate of emulsion was approximately three times as high as that of blood because of lower viscosity. In view of the possibility that the increased amplitude of a- and b-waves under perfusion with 20% FC-K might be attributable, at least in part, to the increased flow rate, an attempt was made to determine the lower limit of perfusion pressure to obtain a sustained ERG wave closest to the control, by gradually lowering the perfusion pressure. Perfusion with 20% FC-K at 500 mmH$_2$O was found to be suitable for the said condition (Figure 6).

DISCUSSION

The principal problem which arises in the electrophysiological study of the retina using an isolated whole eye under perfusion would be the means of adequate oxygen supply to the retina. The methods that have been described may be classified grossly into two: (a) perfusion with the whole blood by taking the advantage of hemoglobin in erythrocytes (TAZAWA & SEAMAN, 1969; IMAIZUMI, et al., 1972; MERA, 1972; OSTUKA, 1973; TAZAWA, in press) and (b) the use of perfusates other than blood where a high concentration of oxygen is supplied continuously (GOURAS & HOFF, 1970; NIEMEYER & GOURAS, 1973). In the former, the disadvantage is that, as described above, it is impracticable to conduct any experimentation under the condition beyond the physiological limits of erythrocytes. The disadvantage that the non-blood perfusate should be flowed at an aphysio-

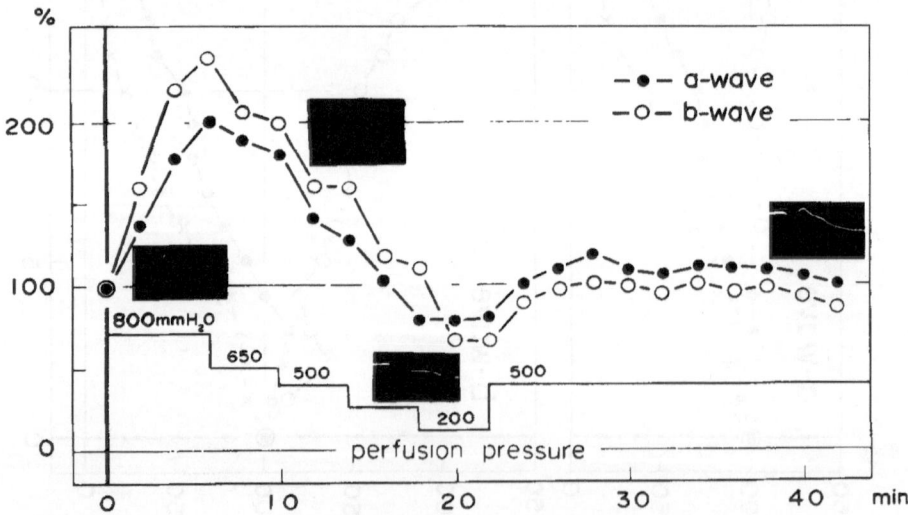

Fig. 6. Variations of relative amplitudes of a- and b-waves of ERGs recorded from an isolated bovine eye perfused with 20 per cent fluorocarbon-Krebs' solution due to changes of the perfusion pressure.

230

logically high rate or under elevated oxygen pressure, is inherent in the letter inasmuch as the amount of oxygen dissolved in the perfusate under atmospheric pressure is physically limited.

In order to remove these limitations of the existing experimental procedures and eventually widen the application of experimental techniques of this sort, we thought it reasonable to explore the possible usefulness of FC with proven high oxygen solubility as a substitute for erythrocytes in perfusion of an isolated eye.

Fluorocarbon, with the empirical formula $(C_4F_9)_3N$ and a specific gravity of $1,87 \, g/cm^3$, is a colorless transparent liquid insoluble in various solvents. It shows high solubilities for various gasses; 34 ml of oxygen or 123 ml of carbon dioxide can dissolve in 100 ml of FC at 32 °C (Flourinert 3M Co., 1965).

In the present study, the concentration of 20 per cent has proven to be most adequate in the perfusate emulsion in that a- and b-waves of the isolated eye were best maintained. HUSTSON et al. (1968) reported the optimal concentration of FC to be 15 per cent for the isolated canine heart perfusion, while 33 per cent was determined for total blood exchange in rats by GEYER et al. (1968). The state of emulsion was noted to be unstable at over 30 per cent FC concentration prepared by the procedure herein reported, causing fusion of FC particles in a short period of time to yield greater particles more than 7 microns in diameter and hence giving rise to circulatory disturbances, as previously reported by one of the present authors (OTSUKA, 1973).

With an emulsion containing 10 per cent FC, it is evident that the amount of oxygen conveyed to the retina does not suffice for satisfactory maintenance of the ERG in that both a- and b-waves diminished progressively.

Under alternate perfusion with the bovine blood and 20% FC-K emulsion, the ERGs exhibited characteristic patterns corresponding to the respective perfusates, alternately. This seems to imply that FC, at least for this period of time, was of little harm to the retina, and suggests a highly advantageous property of FC emulsion as a substitute for blood in the present ocular perfusion study.

As for effects on ERG waves of various solvents for the FC emulsion, 20% FC-saline caused a marked decrease in the amplitude of a- and b-waves, as a natural consequence of the electrolytes contained in the solvent being sodium and chlorine alone. The finding, moreover, that the use of MEM facilitated prolonged maintenance of favorable ERG waves, as compared with Krebs' solution, may well be construed as ascribable to the constituents of the former solvent being more adequate for the retinal metabolism.

The use of FC emulsions in bovine plasma failed to produce any favorable result. The cause of the failure might be sought in the fact that the technique employed for emulsification could not prevent precipitation of FC particles in the plasma.

It is yet to be determined, whether the marked enhancement in amplitudes might be due to greater amounts of oxygen supply to the retina by the FC than by the blood or, otherwise, due to some other mechanism. In order to meet the initial purpose of finding a perfusate with the ability of oxygen transport as a substitute for blood, it was important to find such a perfusate which would permit ERGs with well sustained amplitudes of a- and b-waves almost comparable to those in the case of perfusion with blood. An experiment carried out with 20% FC-K, from this view point, by gradually reducing the perfusion pressure, disclosed that ERG comparable to the control could be accomplished by perfusion at 500 mmH$_2$O.

In previous studies undertaken to determine the level of oxygen in the perfusate for maintenance of normal ERG, we investigated the ERG changes under hypoxia induced (a) by dilution of the perfusion blood or (b) by reducing the flow rate of the blood perfusion (IMAIZUMI, et al., 1974, in press). These previous studies demonstrated that a virtually constant amount of oxygen per unit time is required for maintenance of normal ERGs. The results of the present investigation seem to indicate oxygen deficiency from the low FC concentration in 10% FC-K, and the excessively high flow rate of 20% FC-K. Thus, a particular interrelationship was found to exist between the concentration of FC and the flow rate of perfusion. Thus, evidence has been obtained that potential usefulness of emulsified FC as an efficient erythrocyte substitute for perfusion will be provided if a relationship between concentration of FC and flow rate would be established as a relationship comparable to that of the oxygen transporting capacity of erythrocytes and blood flow rate.

SUMMARY

To explore the possibility of the use of fluorocarbon emulsion as erythrocyte substitute to deliver oxygen to an isolated perfused bovine eye, experiments were carried out to assess the effect of various concentrations of fluorocarbon, solvents for emulsion, and perfusion pressure with simultaneous ERG recordings to monitor the physiological activity of the eye. The results were as follows.

1. Emulsion containing 10 or 20 per cent of FC show homogeneous particles which remain in uniform size of 2 to 3 micron in diameter and satisfactorily stable for 3 to 4 hours.

2. Perfusion with 20 per cent FC emulsion was noted to be most appropriate to facilitate well maintained a- and b-waves of ERG of an isolated eye.

3. The a- and b-waves were best maintained (for 90 minutes) under perfusion with FC emulsion in MEM, followed in order, by emulsion in Krebs' solution (60 minutes) and in physiological saline (10 minutes). Bovine plasma proved to be unsuitable as solvent for fluorocarbon emulsion as it failed to maintain the emulsive state.

4. With 20 per cent FC emulsion in Krebs' solution, the amplitudes of b-wave were best maintained at the control level when the perfusion was carried out at pressure of 500 mmH$_2$O. With the perfusion pressure raised to 800 mmH$_2$O, however, the amplitudes of b-wave increased over the control level, whilst the amplitudes decreased progressively with in decrease in perfusion pressure below 500 mmH$_2$O.

5. Evidence has been obtained for adequate capacity of emulsified FC as an efficient erythrocyte substitute in the perfusate to deliver oxygen to an isolated bovine eye as to permit maintenance of a- and b-waves of ERG.

232

BIBLIOGRAPHY

EAGLE, H. *Science*, 130: *432* (1959).

'Fluorinert' Brand Electronic Liquids 3M Campany 1965.

GEYER, D.G., et al. Organ Perfusion and Preservation, pp. *85*, Appleton-Century-Crofts, New York. 1968.

GOURAS, P. & HOFF, M. *Invest. Ophth.*, 9: *388*. 1970.

HUSTSON, D.G., et al. Organ Perfusion and Preservation, pp. *77*, Appleton-Century-Crofts, New York. 1968.

IMAIZUMI, K., et al. The 5th Afro-Asian Congress of Ophthalmology, Tokyo, (in press). 1972.

IMAIZUMI, K., et al. *Jap. J. Ophthalm.* 18: *177*. 1974.

MERA, H. *Acta Soc. Opthalm. Jap.* 76: *921*. 1972

NIEMEYER, G. & GOURAS, P. *Vision Res.* 13: *1603*. 1973 a.

NIEMEYER, G. & GOURAS, P. *Vision Res.* 13: *1613*. 1973 b.

OTSUKA, T. *Acta Soc. Ophthalm.* Jap. 77: *1102*. 1973.

TAZAWA, Y. & SEAMAN, A.J. *Invest. Ophth.* (Abst.), 8: *238*: 1969.

TAZAWA Y. & SEAMAN, A.J. *Invest. Ophth.* 11: *691*. 1972.

TAZAWA, Y., et al. *F. Opthal. Jap.* 24: *1134*. 1973.

THE EFFECTS OF GLYCINE ON THE RABBIT RETINA
AVERAGED ERG AND MICROSCOPIC ANATOMY*

S. KOROL, J.J. MEYER & P.M. LEUENBERGER

(Geneva, Switzerland)

There is evidence that glycine can act as an inhibitory neurotransmitter in the central nervous system (CURTIS, HÖSLI, JOHNSTON & JOHNSTON 1968, CURTIS & WATKINS 1965, HÖSLI & HAAS 1972, MATUS & DENNISON 1971, NEAL & PICKLES 1969, WERMAN , DAVIDOFF & APRISON 1968). This action was originally suggested by APRISON & WERMAN (1965).

The criteria for evaluating a substance as a synaptic transmitter is based on its presence, storage, release, postsynaptic action and inactivation. COHEN (COHEN, MCDANIEL & ORR 1973) showed in mice, a large concentration of glycine, gaba and taurine in the inner retina. These amino acids in the retina tend to match or exceed the highest local values reported in the central nervous system.

The retina uptake of glycine, storage and retention mechanism were demonstrated by BRUUN & EHINGER (1972), EHINGER (1970, 1972) and EHINGER & FALCK (1971). This studies demonstrated an active uptake mechanism for glycine into the rabbit retina. Certain retinal neurons, mainly the amacrine cells, dispose of a specific uptake mechanism for glycine (EHINGER 1970, EHINGER & FALCK 1971, EHINGER 1972).

Glycine has been found to have inhibitory actions on the retina by AMES (AMES & POLLEN 1969) 'in vitro', and by KOROL (1973) 'in vivo'. In that previous paper we have shown the effects of glycine in the rabbit retina (averaged ERG and averaged VER), characterized by a loss of the oscillatory potentials during the effect of glycine, with a partial blocking of the AVER's early components. Maximal inhibitions takes place between 3 to 10 hours with recovery by 20 to 24 hours.

This present paper is a morphological and quantitative analysis of the b-wave and OPs of the rabbit AERG in different conditions of stimulation before and during the effect of glycine. Light and electron-microscopic examinations were carried out in different stages of glycine's action. Autoradiography was used to show the cellular location of the uptake of glycine.

* Partly supported by SNSF grant No 3. 1150.73.

Experiments were carried out on both eyes of 18 unanaesthetised rabbits (i.e. 36 eyes).

Group I: Flicker AERGs were recorded before and after injection of 0.003 gr of glycine (ρH 6.58) in the vitreous body to determine the time of onset, maximal effect, and of recovery (18 eyes). A quantitative analysis of the b-wave and OPs was performed on 12 eyes from this group.

Group II: 8 rabbit eyes were injected with glycine for light and electron-microscopic examination of the retina. Autography was performed in 4 rabbit eyes after injection of 3×10^{-4} M $2H^3$ Glycine (1.35 Ci per milli-mole). 6 rabbit eyes were used as normal or technical controls for micro-scopic anatomy.

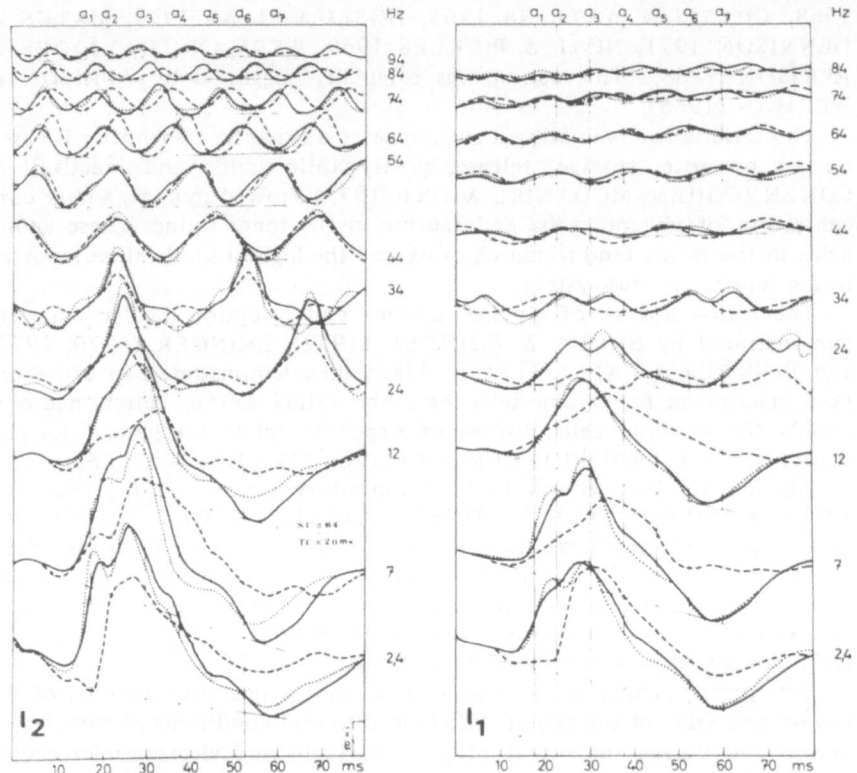

Fig. 1. Rabbit 178 (right eye)
Averaged flicker ERG: ....: normal control;
- - - - - : 4 hours after glycine injection;
_____: 24 hours after glycine injection.
I_1 and I_2 : two different stimulation intensities.
Abscissa: time in msec., ordinate: stimulation frequency in Hz. a 1 to a 7: the latencies in which the amplitude of the b-wave was measured. SC = sweep count; TC = time constant.

The light source was a Ahrend-van Gogh n.v. (si-lc) stimulator in an indirectly illuminated wall 30 cm in front of the subject. The pupil was dilated with Mydriaticum Roche (1%) and a corneal needle was used for electrical pickup. After light adaptation for 3 minutes with a bright light (2000 lux), the flicker AERG was recorded for a set of frequencies from one Hz to 80 Hz. The intensity was provided with a constant background (100 lux) for

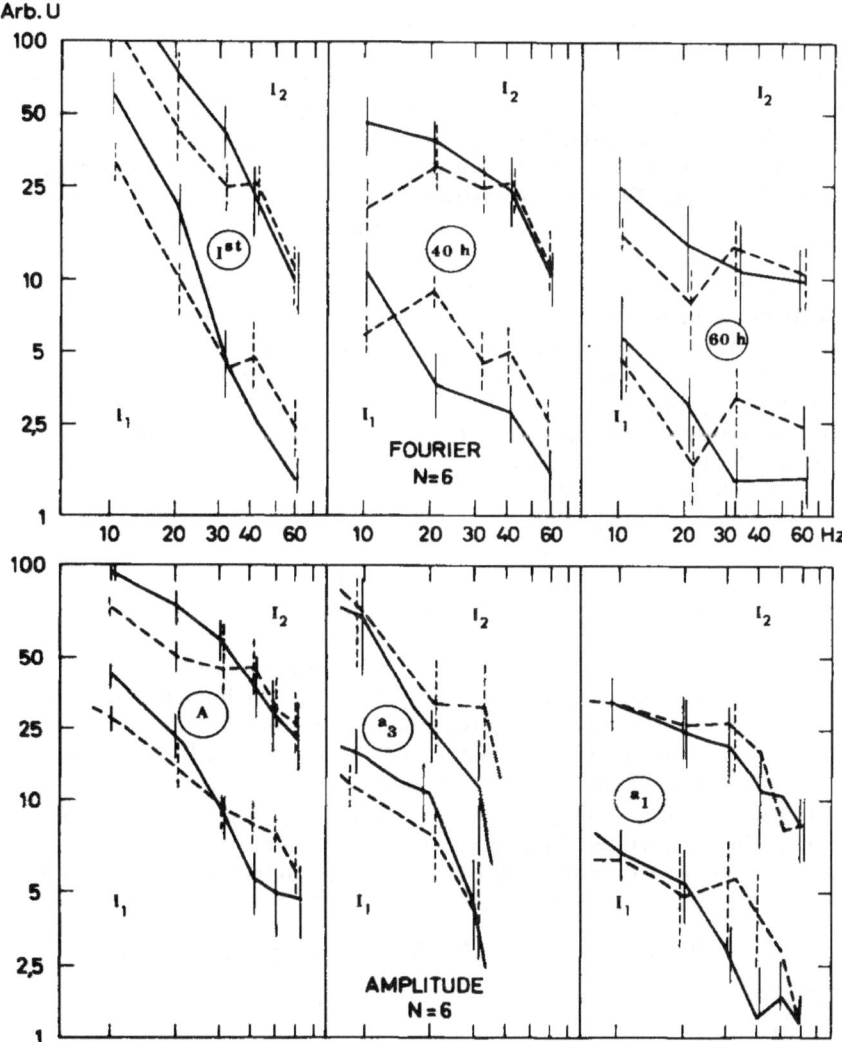

Fig. 2. Mean values and standard deviation for normal ERG ———— and after 4 hrs. glycine injection - - - - -. *Bottom*: amplitudes for two different stimulation conditions. A: maximal b-wave amplitude; a 1: amplitude of the b-wave at 17 msec. and a 3: amplitude of the b-wave at 30 msec. *Top*: Fourier analysis for different stimulation frequencies (see text).

two stimulus conditions (I_1 and I_2). The ERG responses were amplified with a AC Tektronix preamplifier type FM 122 with low and high frequency cut off at 0.8 and 250 Hz, and displayed on a dual beam Tektronix oscilloscope type A502; 64 responses were averaged with a Biomac 1000 averaged (Data Lbo).

Flicker AERG results

We have used two methods of analysis:

Method I: To quantify the form and latency variations of the flicker AERG, we measured the amplitude of the b-wave at different latencies from a base line joining the negative waves (Fig. 1). Three values are measured for two different stimulation conditions (I_1 and I_2) and for each frequency: A = maximal b-wave amplitude; a_1 and a_3 = the latencies in which the amplitude of the b-wave was also measured (a_1 at 17 msec., a_3 at 30 msec.).

Method II: The ERG was transformed into digital values for Fournier analysis. The computed values of Fourier components, for the different stimuli and frequencies, the first harmonic, one harmonic corresponding to 40 Hz and an other to 60Hz oscillations were plotted as arbitrary values versus frequency on a double logarithmic scale (Fig. 2).

Mean values and standard deviation were compared before (normal values) and after 4 hours of glycine injection. Our findings for 12 eyes are illustrated by Fig. 2:

a) The b-wave amplitude shows the same amplitude behaviour as the amplitude of the Fourier 1st harmonic.

b) The whole glycine ERG curves are outside the normal regions.

c) The b-wave curve (A) and the first harmonic amplitude curve (I) are abnormal in the glycine group.

d) The other components, amplitude at different latencies (a_1, a_3) and the other harmonics (40 Hz, 60 Hz) also lie outside the corresponding reference values.

In general, the A and I curves are of the same type: decreasing amplitude for lower frequencies, and increasing amplitude for higher frequencies. On the other hand, this effect is more evident with weaker stimulation.

A classical morphological analysis of the ERG (Fig. 1) at one Hz shows that during the maximum effect of glycine there is a loss of the oscillatory potentials of the b-wave with relative increase of a-wave and b-wave peak-times. The recuperated ERG does not have an identical shape to the initial normal ERG of the same rabbit before glycine injection, but the amplitude and the OPs become normal again after 20 to 24 hours.

MICROSCOPIC ANATOMY RESULTS (Fig. 3 and Fig. 4)

Light microscopy

1.15 hs. after glycine injection, certain cells in the innermost layers of the inner nuclear layer show edematous changes of the cytoplasm. The clear cell-processes within the inner plexiform layer presumably belong to the same cells. On the basis of their cytological and topographical characteristics, we have identified these cells as being amacrine cells.

Electron microscopy

The cytoplasm appears almost devoid of organelles; chromatin is partially clumped, and partially released through disrupted nuclear envelopes into the cytoplasm. Karyorrhexis is frequently observed. The swollen cell processes show an almost complete loss of the neurotubules (Fig. 4).

AUTORADIOGRAPHY

Autoradiography demonstrates that 30 after injection there is a rather uniform distribution of radioactive labelled material through all retinal layers, whereas at 1.10 h. ever and more marked at 4.30 hrs. after the injection the bulk of labelled material is concentrated around and over the amacrine cells showing edematous alterations.

RETINA 10 HRS. AFTER GLYCINE

Light microscopy

The edematous changes are in regression.

Electron microscopy

Cell organelles are again discernible. ER cisternae are distended, and neurotubules are frequently observed in the neuropil. Synaptic contacts between amacrine cell processes and bipolar (axons) display the ultrastructural components of a normal synapse.

RETINA 24 HRS. AFTER GLYCINE

Light microscopy

The inner nuclear layer appears normal.

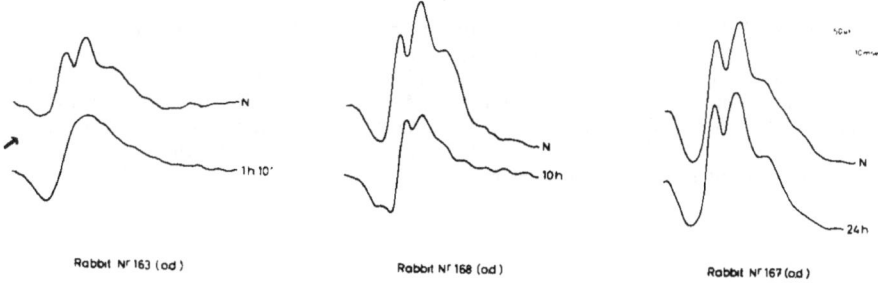

Rabbit Nr 163 (od)   Rabbit Nr 168 (od)   Rabbit Nr 167 (od)

Rabbit's averaged ERG before and after Glycine

Fig. 3.   Averaged ERG normal (N) and 1,10, 10 and 24 hours after glycine injection. Arrow: rabbit ERG corresponding to the micrography of the Fig. 4.

239

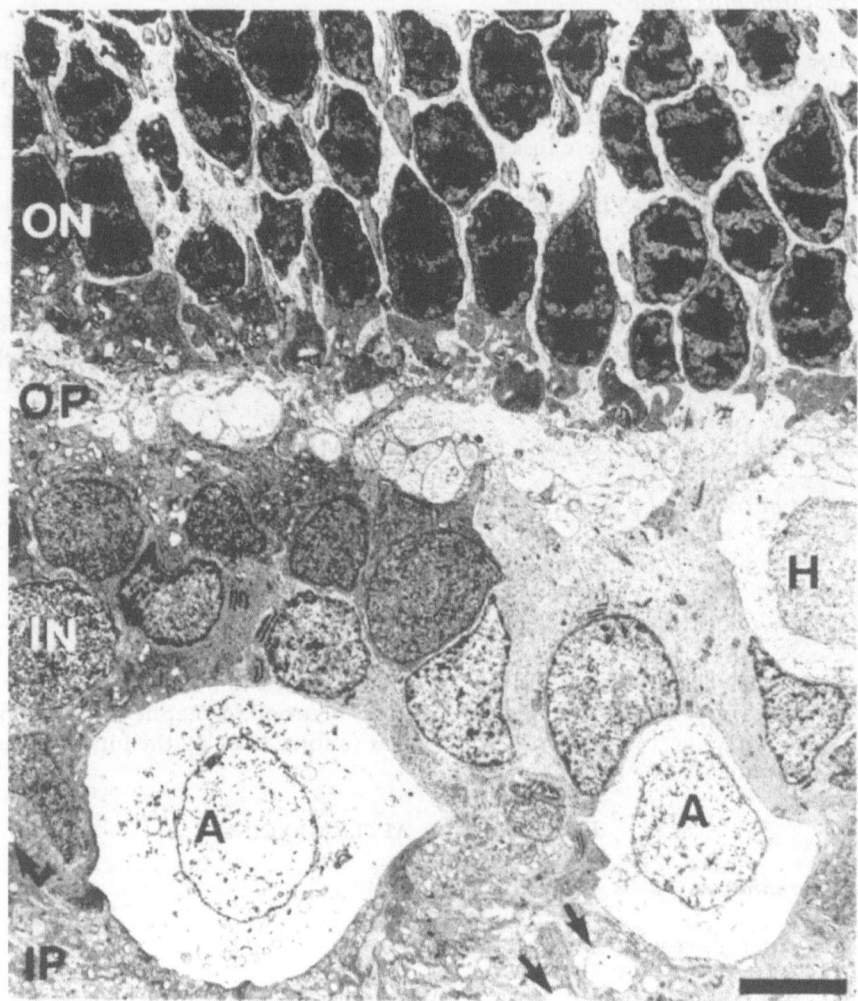

Fig. 4 Rabbit 163. Low power electron micrography of a rabbit retina _____5 μm
1.15 hrs after intravitreal injection of glycine.
ON = outer nuclear layer; OP = outer plexiform layer; IN = inner nuclear layer; IP =
inner plexiform layer; H = horizontal cells; A = amacrine cells; amacrine cell processes
(arrows) (see text). The cytoplasm of the amacrine cells is almost devoid or organelles,
chromatin is released through disrupted nuclear envelopes into the cytoplasm. The
arrows show the swollen cell processes.

Electron microscopy

Some amacrine cells show pyknotic nuclei, characterizing marked cellular
degeneration. In others we observed a conspicuous increase of neurotubules
indicating regenerative processes.

240

CONCLUSIONS

Glycine has reversible inhibitory effects on the rabbit retina *in vivo*. During the maximal effect of glycine, the ERG shows a loss of the oscillatory potentials and a statistically significant reduction of amplitudes (attenuation amplitude curves and Fourier analysis). Recovery takes place 10 to 24 hours after glycine injection.

Light and electron-microscopic pictures show changes of the amacrine cells and their processes during the maximal electrophysiological effect of glycine. These changes were partially reversible. Autoradiography shows glycine-labelled material surrounding the amacrine cells during the maximal inhibition, which is probably related to the cellular location of glycine.

DISCUSSION

Our electrophysiological and morphological results support the assumption (AMES & POLLEN 1969, BRUUN & EHINGER 1972, EHINGER 1970, EHINGER & FALCK 1971, EHINGER 1972) that glycine may be an neurotransmitter inhibitor related to certain nervous cells and their synaptic contacts in the inner plexiform layer of the rabbit retina. Perhaps these synaptic amacrine contacts have a function related to the origin of the fast oscillatory components of the b-wave (OPs).

In another paper we describe how the effects of glycine on the rabbit ERG can be antagonized specifically by an appropriate concentration of strychnine.* The inhibitory action of glycine is specifically antagonized by strychnine in other regions of the central nervous system (HOSLI & HAAS 1972).

The presence of glycine in the inner nuclear layers (COHEN, MCDANIEL & ORR 1973), its experimental active uptake and storage in the amacrine cells (BRUUN & EHINGER 1972, EHINGER 1970, 1972, EHINGER & FALCK 1971) and its inhibitory action on the living retina relates it to the group of the amino acids such as gaba and taurine with probable neurotransmitter function in the retina (PASANTES MORALES, BONAVENTURE, WIDLAND MANDEL 1973).

SUMMARY

Experiments were carried out on both eyes of 18 unanaesthetised rabbits (i.e. 36 eyes). AERG was recorded before and after injection of 0,003 g of glycine into the vitreous body (1 to 24 hours).

Light- and electron microscopic examinations of the retina at intervals after glycine injections revealed cytoplasmic lesions at the level of the amacrine cells. These lesions were only partly reversible.

Our results are quite compatible with the assumption that glycine may be an inhibitory neurotransmitter in certain nervous cells of the inner nuclear layer, whose functions are probably related with the origin of the oscillatory potentials.

* KOROL, S. & OWENS, G. Glycine, strychnine and retinal inhibition. *Experientia* (Basel) 30, *1161-1162*, 1974.

REFERENCES

AMES, A. POLLEN, D.A. – Neurotransmission in central nervous tissue; a study of isolated rabbit retina. *J. Neurophysiol.* 32, *424-442*, 1969.

APRISON, M.H. & WERMAN R. – The distribution of glycine in cat spinal cord. *Life Sci.*, 4, *2075-2083*, 1965.

BROWN, K.T. – The electroretinogram: its components and their origings. *Vision Res.*, 8, *633-677*, 1968.

BRUUN, A. & EHINGER, B. – Uptake of the putative neurotransmitter, glycine, into the rabbit retina. *Invest. Opthal.*, 11, *191-198*, 1972.

COHEN, A.I., MCDANIEL, M. & ORR, H. – Absolute levels of some free amino acids in normal and biologically fractionated retinas. *Invest. Ophthal.* 12, *686-693*, 1973.

CURTIS, D.R., HÖSLI L., JOHNSTON, G.A.R. & JOHNSTON, I.H. – The hyperpolarization of spinal motoneurones by glycine and related amino acids. *Exp. Brain Res.*, 5, *235-258*, 1968.

CURTIS, D.R. & WATKINS, J.C. – The pharmacology of amino acids related to gamma amino butyric acid. *Pharmacol. Rev.*, 17, *347-391*, 1965.

DOWLING, J.E. – Organization of vertebrate retinas. *Invest. Ophthal.*, 9, *655-680*, 1970.

DOWLING, J.E. & BOYCOTT B.B. – Organization of the primate retina: electron microscopy. *Proc. roy. Soc. B.*, 166, *80-111*, 1966.

EHINGER, B. – Cellular location of uptake of same amino acids into the rabbit retina. *Brain Res.* 46, *297-311*, 1972.

EHINGER, B. & FALCK, B. – Autoradiography of some suspected neurotransmitter substances: GABA, glycine, aspartic acid, glutamic acid, histamine, dopamine, and L-dopa. *Brain Res.*, 33, *157-172*, 1971.

EHINGER, B. – Autoradiography identification of rabbit retinal neurons that take up GABA. *Experientia (Basel)*, 26, *1063-1064*, 1970.

HÖSLI, L. & HAAS, H.L. – The hyperpolarization of neurons of medulla oblongata by glycine. *Experientia (Basel)*, 28, *1057-1058*, 1972.

KOROL, S. – The effects of glycine on the rabbit retina: averaged ERG and averaged visual evoked responses. *Experientia (Basel)*, 29, *984-985*, 1973.

MATUS, A.I. & DENNISON, M.E. – Autographic localization of tritiated glycine at 'flat vesicle' synapses in spinal cord. *Brain Res.*, 32, *195-197*, 1971.

NEAL, M.J. & PICKLES, H.G. – Uptake of ^{14}C-glycine by spinal cord. *Nature (Lond.)*, 222, *679-680*, 1969.

PASANTES MORALES, H., BONAVENTURE, N., WIOLAND, N. & MANDEL, P. – Effect of intravitreal injections of taurine and GABA on chicken electroretinogram. *Intern. J. Neurosciences*, 5, *235-241*, 1973

VÖRKEL, W. & HANITZSCH, R. – Effect of strychnine on the electroretinogram of the isolated rabbit retina. *Experientia*, 27, *296-297*, 1971.

WERMAN, R., DAVIDOFF, R.A. & APEISON, M.H. – Inhibitory action of glycine on spinal neurons in the cat. *J. Neurophysiol.*, 31, *81-95*, 1968.

AZIDE POISONING: ITS EFFECTS ON P III RESTING POTENTIAL OF THE ISOLATED RETINA

L. WÜNDSCH, J.H. REUTER* & A. v. LÜTZOW

(Vienna, Austria)

The properties of azide as a retinal poison were first described by NOELL (1952). Noell showed that low dosages of azide produce a rise of the resting potential of the eye and enhance the c-wave of the ERG. Both affected potentials have been shown to be closely related to the pigment epithelium (NOELL 1952, STEINBERG 1970). However, there is some evidence for retinal factors being involved in the azide response as well:

1) The isolated pigment epithelium does not give an azide response (NOELL 1952).

2) Small azide responses could be evoked from iodate poisoned eyes with histologically verified major destructions in the pigment epithelium (NOELL 1952).

3) In isolated retinae of frog (SICKEL 1965, HÖHNE 1971) and of rabbit (WÜNDSCH et al. 1974) an azide response could be recorded.

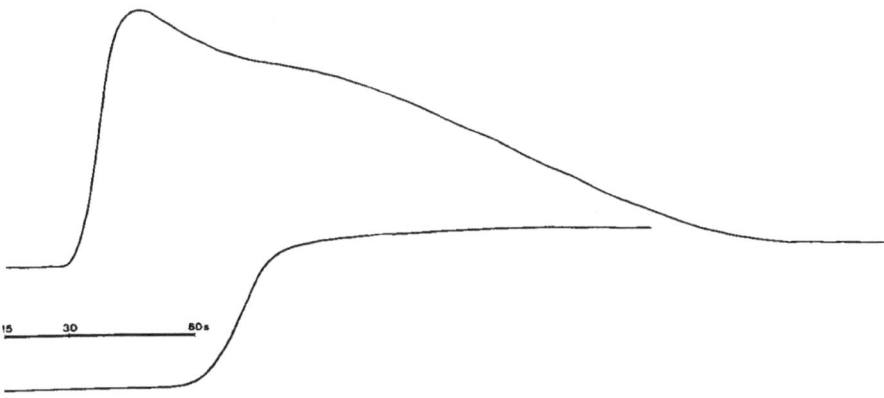

Fig. 1. Recordings of the azide effect on the standing potential of the isolated rabbit retina. Injection of 20 mg azide into the tubing transporting the media to the retina (upper recording). The high concentration gradient causes a steep rise of the potential 30 s after injection. Final azide concentration 3 mM/1, amplitude of potential 0,6 mV. Lower recording: 3 mM/1 of azide were dissolved in the total perfusion medium. Onset of the potential rise immediately after arrival of the substance at the retina.

* J.H. REUTER received a grant from the Netherlands organization for the advancement of pure research (Z.W.O.).

Consequently, one can assume that it is not merely the pigment epithelium but also the neural retina and/or the functional connection between the neural retina and pigment epitheliun which are affected by azide. Therefore, azide can be expected to influence the ERG, as has actually been shown by TOMITA (1963) who reported that azide concentrations of 0,1% affected the local ERG in the frog, abolishing P II and part of P III.

It was the purpose of the present investigation to elucidate in mammals the role of the receptors in the ERG changes following azide poisoning. However, the toxicity of the drug prevents systematic investigations with higher dosages *in situ* and, furthermore, the presence of the pigment epithe-

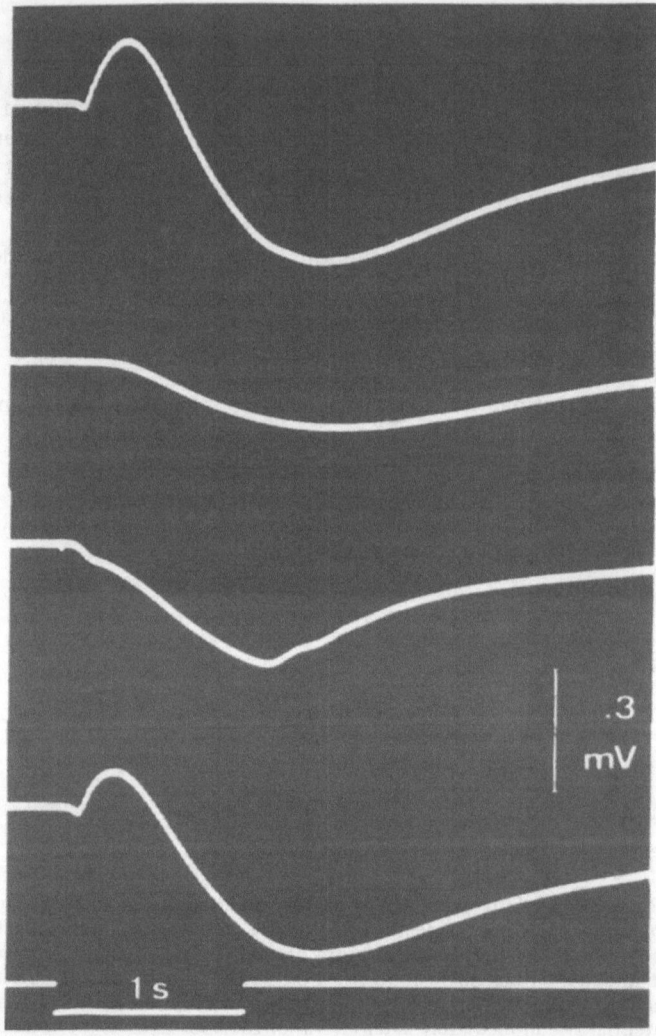

Fig. 2. ERG if isolated rabbit retina. Recordings from above: 1) before 2) 6 min after application of 5 mM/1 of azide 3) 2 min 4) 30 min after switching back to azide free media, light stimulus: 1 mlx, 1 s.

lium in this case would impede exact identification of the site of action of the drug. Therefore, azide was applied to the isolated rabbit retina, the pigment epithelium of which had been carefully removed.

From this preparation an azide response can be evoked (Fig. 1), the amplitude of which depends on the concentration gradient. In the case of the upper curve, azide was injected in a single dosage of 20 mg into the tubing containing the perfusion fluid. The steep rise of the potential (up to 1 mV) is followed by a slow decrease, indicating the drug being washed out. If azide was homogeneously dissolved in the total perfusion medium, no potential drop would follow the initial rise.

Fig. 2 demonstrates the effect of 5 mM/1 azide on the ERG of the isolated retina. Six min. after azide application the b-wave is abolished, the remaining response consisting merely of a small P III. Two min. of azide free perfusion thereafter, a small hump following the onset of the enhanced P III indicates the starting regeneration of the P II. Partial regeneration is completed within 30 minutes.

Since ERGs containing a b-wave cannot supply sufficient information about the receptors, the b-wave was eliminated prior to the azide application in a further series of experiments (Fig. 3).

In the upper row P III evoked by two different light intensities is shown in azide free media, in the lower row 15 min after administration of 3 mM azide. The considerable decrease in the amplitude of the potential is obvious.

Amplitude diminution of P III depends on the azide concentration (Fig. 4). There is no significant effect of the light intensity. With 10 mM azide only a small P III was left. The lower graph (4b) shows the potential drop with time following azide application. The major portion of the amplitude reduction is achieved after 2 min. No systematic differences could be found between different light intensities. However, P III diminution by azide

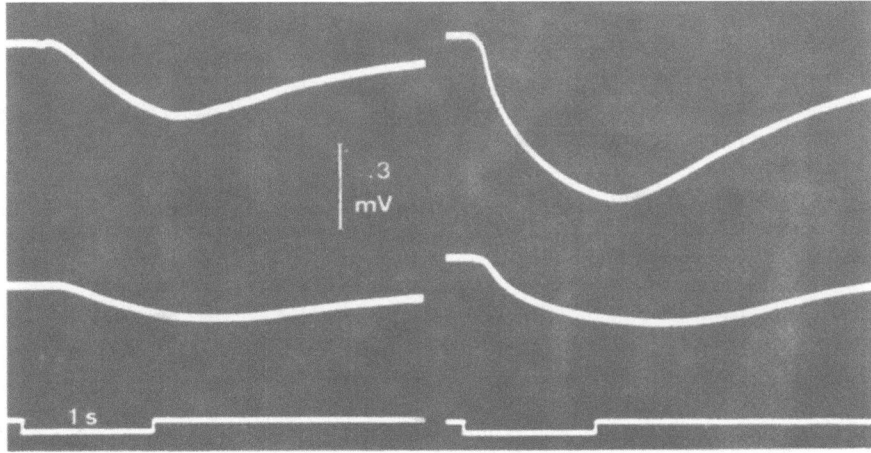

Fig. 3. Isolated P III before (upper recordings) and 14 min after application of 3 mM/1 of azide, light intensities: 4 mlx (left curves), 63 mlx (right curves).

does not necessarily mean that it is the receptors that are affected. In 1966 MURAKAMI & KANEKO showed P III to be composed of two parts. For warmblooded animals similar results were obtained by HANITZSCH (1973), who suggested even 3 parts of P III. Little doubt remains that the earliest of the components originates within the receptors. From what was stated above concerning the receptor- pigment epithelium connection, azide would be expected to affect this first component. In order to investigate this, high speed recordings were made to show clearly the onset of the potential (Fig. 5). With brighter lights (upper curves), as well as with dim lights (lower curves), considerable delays of the P III onset could be observed after azide application. In these cases, only low dosages of azide were applied to avoid major amplitude reductions which would necessarily result in slope changes.

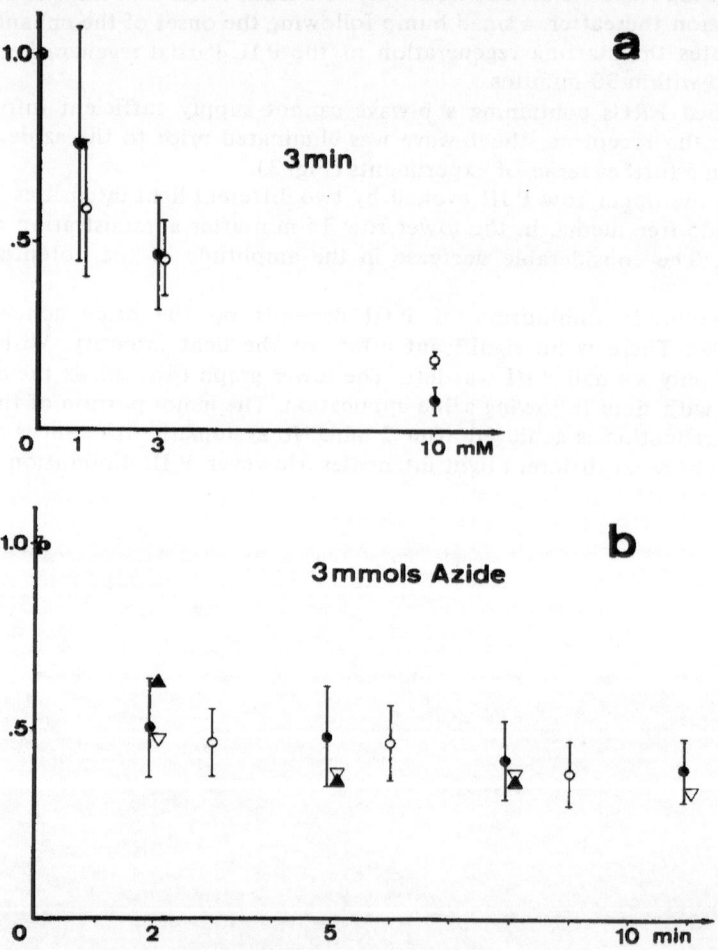

Fig. 4. Normalized amplitudes of P III, a) as function of azide concentration 3 min after application of the drug. Mean values and standard deviations (1 and 3 mM...n = 8, 10 mM...n = 2) light intensity ● 4 mlx, ○ 63 mlx, b) as function of time following application of 3 mM of azide. Different light intensities: ▽ 1 lx, ▲ 0,25 lx.

246

These results demonstrate a direct toxic effect of azide on the receptors. It cannot be excluded, however, that proximal P III may also contribute to the amplitude reduction of P III. In addition to the effects described above, azide produced in some cases changes in the off-response of the retina (Fig. 6). Especially at medium light intensities a small positive hump could be observed at 'off'. This hump was increased by low azide dosages, despite the amplitude decreases of the P III. With light intensities increased tenfold

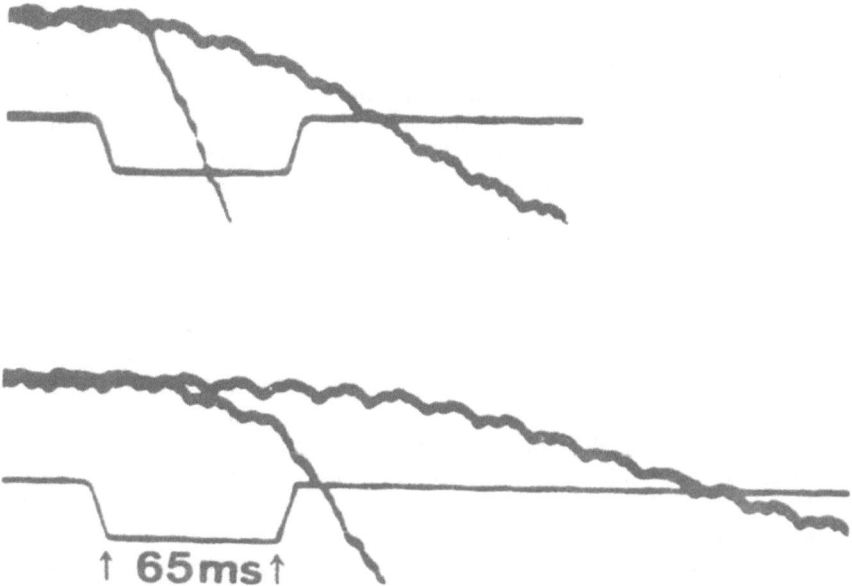

Fig. 5. Onset of P III before (faster decaying curves) and after 3 min of application of 3 mM of azide (delayed decaying curves), light intensities: 63 mlx (upper curves), 4 mlx (lower curves).

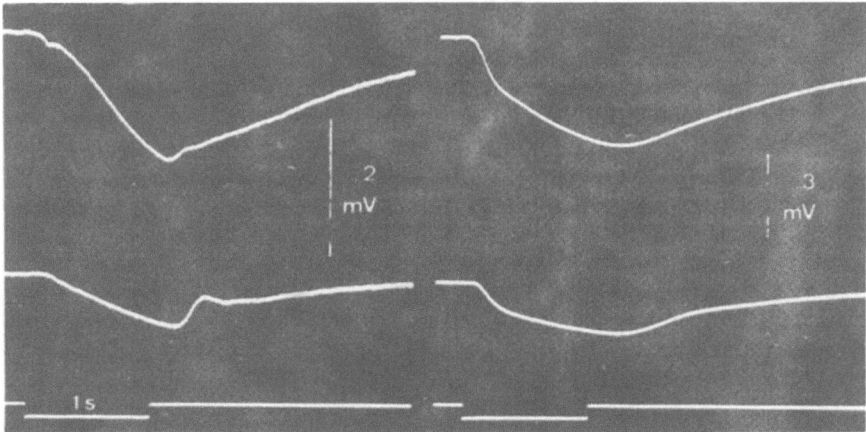

Fig. 6. Isolated P III before (upper recordings) and 10 min after 3 mM of azide (lower recordings), light stimuli: 1 s, 4 mlx (left curves), 63 mlx (rights curves).

the curves failed to reveal such an effect (right hand side). Occasionally at 'off', instead of the single hump, a sequence of humps resembling a dampened oscillation appeared. The amplitudes of these humps were also enhanced by low azide dosages. The interpretation of this effect remains unclear since the generation mechanism of this kind of off-response is not yet known.

The effect of azide on the onset of P III strongly suggests that the receptors are involved, as had been assumed on the basis of the earlier data on the azide response. As the site of action of azide is the carbohydrate metabolism, it is not surprising that, in addition to the pigment epithelium and receptors, proximal layers of the retina are also involved in the response as indicated by the simultaneous abolishment of the b-wave of the ERG. Nevertheless, the relative fraction of receptor participation is considerably higher than with other drugs which also affect the b-wave of the ERG, but which are not known to have a similarly striking effect on the resting potential of the eye.

SUMMARY

The retinal toxicity of azide has been known since the investigations of NOELL (1952). In the present study sodium azide was applied to the isolated rabbit retina by adding concentrations from 0,5 − 10 mMol to the perfusion media. Azide produces a rise of the resting potential which amounts up to 1 mV depending on the azide gradient. The b-wave of the ERG is abolished by low concentrations of azide and the amplitude of the remaining P III diminished. The P III latency is distinctly prolonged, indicating damage of the receptors. The decay of the negative potential at light 'off' was also in the off-effect which resembled a dampened oscillation. Higher concentrations resulted in slowing down the potential decay.

REFERENCES

HANITZSCH, R. *Vis. Res.* 13, *2093* (1973).
HÖHNE, W. *Acta biol. med. germ.* 27, *307* (1971).
MURAKAMI, M. and KANEKO, A. *Vis. Res.* 6, *627* (1966).
NOELL, W.K. *Amer. J. Physiol.* 170, *217* (1952).
SICKEL, W. *Science* 148, *648* (1965).
STEINBERG, R.H. SCHMIDT, R. and BROWN, K.T. *Science* 227, *728* (1970).
TOMITA, T. *J. Opt. Soc. Amer.* 53, *49* (1963).
WÜNDSCH, L. et al., *Experientia* 30, *627* (1974).

C–WAVE AMPLITUDE OSCILLATIONS IN THE SHEEP ERG

B. CALISSENDORFF, B. KNAVE & H.E. PERSSON

(Stockholm, Sweden)

The *c*-wave component ERG has been analysed with different experimental approaches. In 1933 GRANIT selectively abolished the *c*-wave by use of light ether anaesthesia. About 20 years later NOELL found that sodium iodate selectively eliminated the *c*-wave and at the same time destroyed the pigment epithelium cells. These observations indicated the pigment epithelium layer as the origin of the *c*-wave, a finding which was later confirmed and extended in intracellular recordings (STEINBERG et al. 1970). The characteristics of the *c*-wave as a function of factors such as state of adaption, spectral sensitivity, stimulus intensity and duration has been investigated by several authors (see review, CALISSENDORFF et al. 1974). To our knowledge, however, no study has been published on the long-term variations of the *c*-wave amplitude. In the present paper a report is given on some experiments in sheep in which were found that the *c*-wave amplitude changed as a function of time and stimulus frequency.

The method has been described in detail in a previous work (KNAVE, MØLLER & PERSSON 1972); the technique allows us to record d.c. responses from the intact eye in long-term studies during constant experimental conditions.

Fig. 1 shows the results from an experiment in which the *a*-, *b*- and *c*-wave amplitudes were studied for 300 min. During a period of about 12 hours before the actual experiment the sheep was kept in darkness. The operative preparations were performed in dim light and care was taken not to throw light upon the eye. After application of the electrodes the sheep was kept in darkness for another 2-3 hours before testing. With this procedure the *b*-wave amplitude obtained with stimulus intervals more than 30 sec was constant which was taken as evidence of full dark adaptation. In the experiments the stimulus intensity was 5 log units above the *b*-wave threshold of the dark adapted eye, the stimulus duration 1 sec and the stimulus interval 2 min. The *c*-wave amplitudes were found to change in an oscillatory way with a slow frequency of about 0.3 per hour. The *a*- and *b*-wave amplitudes remained unchanged during the whole experiment. In the *c*-wave amplitudes there is also an indication of a faster oscillation, with a

This work was supported by grants from the Swedish Medical Research Council, the Magn. Bergvall Foundation for Scientific Research, the Hierta Foundation for Ophthalmological Research and Karolinska Institutet.

249

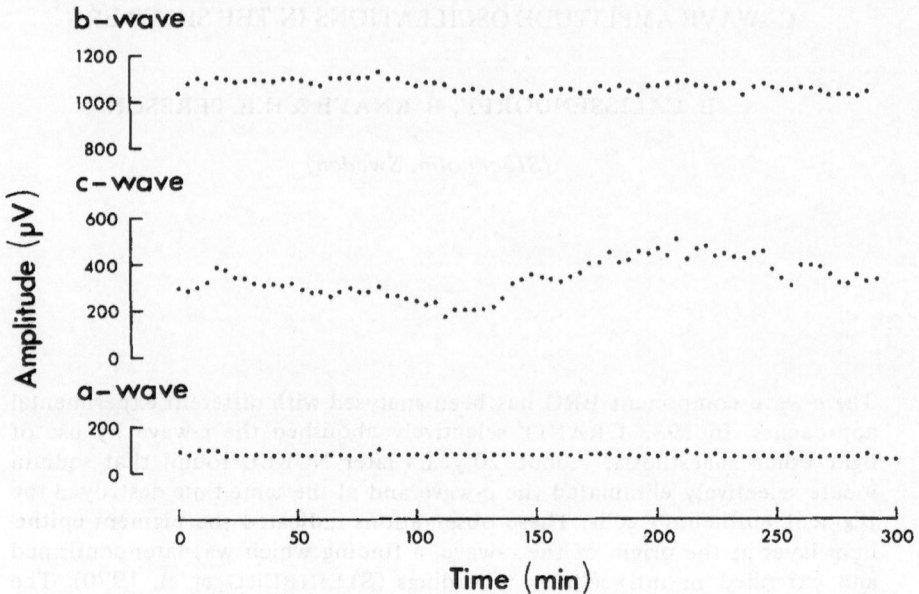

Fig. 1. Amplitudes of the *a*-, *b*- and *c*-waves of the ERG as a function of time. Stimulus interval: 2 min. Stimulus duration: 1 sec. Stimulus intensity: 5.0 log units above *b*-wave threshold.

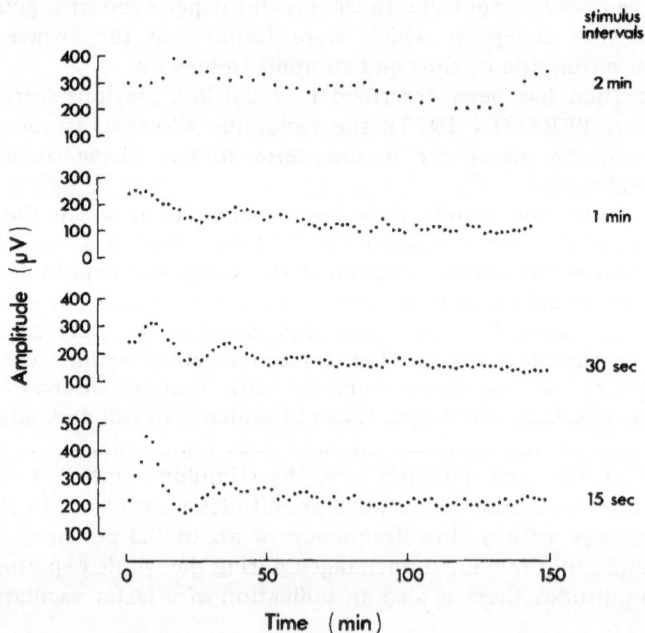

Fig. 2. Amplitudes of the *c*-waves of the ERG as a function of time. Stimulus intervals: 2 min, 1 min, 30 sec and 15 sec. Stimulus duration: 1 sec. Stimulus intensities: 5.0-5.3 log units above *b*-wave threshold.

frequency of 2 per hour, superimposed upon the slow one. This is more clearly seen in Fig. 2 in which the results from 4 different experiments are shown. The ERG was studied with stimulus intervals of 2 min (top record), 1 min, 30 sec, and 15 sec (bottom record).

With stimulus intervals of 1 min or less the c-wave amplitude can be seen to oscillate with a frequency of about 2 per hour. With a stimulus frequency of 1 per min or more the oscillations at first were of large amplitudes, diminished with time and after about 70-100 min a constant level was reached.

The a- and b-wave amplitudes were constant throughout the experiments with stimulus intervals of 2 min, 1 min and 30 sec. This was not the case, however, when using a stimulus interval of 15 sec. Fig. 3 shows the a-, b- and c-wave amplitudes from such an experiment. The a-wave diminished during the first 5 min, whereupon a constant level was reached. A similar initial decrease was noted in the b-wave amplitude. After the initial drop also a slow decrease of the amplitude was observed, probably representing an adaptation effect of the tightly spaced stimulus flashes.

As mentioned in the introduction the c-wave is known to be generated in the pigment epithelium cells. The activity of these cells is also reflected in the standing potential of the eye. From studies on the human electro-oculogram (EOG), used in clinical practice as an expression for the standing potential of the eye, damped oscillations with a frequency of just 2 per hour

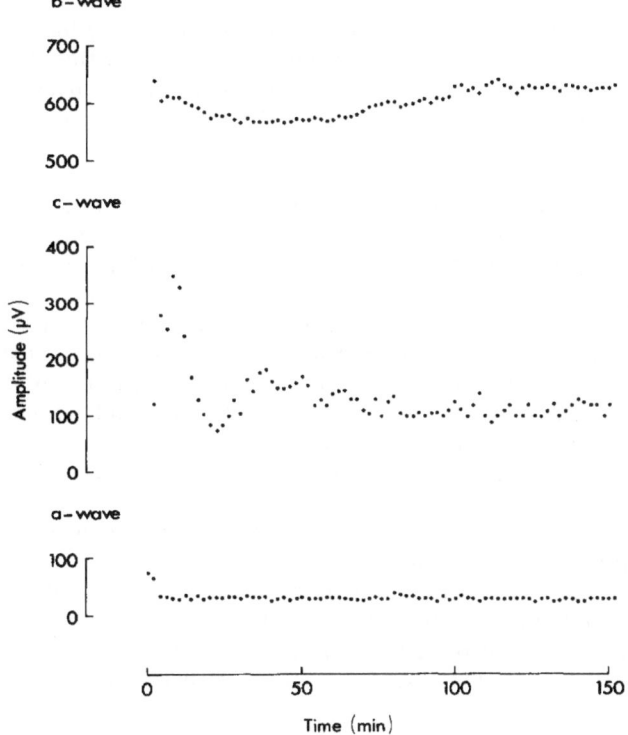

Fig. 3. Amplitudes of the a-, b- and c-waves of the ERG as a function of time. Stimulus interval: 15 sec. Stimulus duration: 1 sec. Stimulus intensity: 5.3 log units above b-wave threshold.

251

have been found (KRIS 1958, KOLDER 1959). Furthermore, long-term cyclic variations of the EOG potential have also been described (KRIS 1960, DAVIS & SHACKEL 1960).

The exact origin and mechanism of these cyclic variations are not known. ARDEN & KELSEY (1962) provided evidence from observarions on diseased eyes that the cyclic variations of the standing potential was related to the activity of the pigment epithelium cells and presumably due to the bleaching and biochemistry of rhodopsin. In our experiments with the stimulus intensity used, only 0.03 per cent of the available rhodopsin was bleached. Due to this fact, it seems less likely that the oscillations of the c-wave and the standing potential are induced by retinal and retinol molecules released from bleached rhodopsin. Since the sensitivity of the rods has been shown to be affected also by relatively small bleachings (e.g. DONNER & REUTER 1968), the possibility cannot be excluded that the oscillations may be due to changes in rod sensitivity. Finally, it seems relevant to suppose a relationship with changes in retinal metabolism, since the c-wave has been found to be closely related to redox process in the retina (SICKEL 1972).

SUMMARY

The c-wave component of the electroretinogram (ERG) has been analysed with different experimental approaches. The characteristics of the c-wave as a function of factors such as state of adaptation, spectral sensitivity, stimulus intensity, and stimulus duration have been previously investigated, but to our knowledge, no study has been published on the longterm variation of the c-wave amplitude.

The c-wave of the sheep electroretinogram was studied in the present investigation during long-term experiments. It was found that its amplitude changed as a function of time and that these alterations were dependent on the intervals of the stimulus flashes. A slow oscillation (frequency about 0.3-0.5 per hour) was observed with long flash intervals (2 min) when using one sec light stimuli. Shorter flash intervals gave rise to oscillations with a frequency of about 2 per hour. These fast oscillations initially were of relatively large amplitudes but decreased with time and reached a constant level after about 100 min. Shortening of stimulus duration (0.1 sec) resulted in c-waves of less amplitude, but the cyclic variation pattern described above did not change.

The c-wave is known to be generated in the pigment epithelium cells. The activity of these cells is also reflected in the standing potential of the eye (SP). In this connection it is relevant to refer to findings obtained in studies on the human electrooculogram (EOG) used in clinical practice as an expression for the SP of the eye. From these studies it is known that the EOG potential oscillates with frequencies similar to those obtained in the present study.

REFERENCES

ARDEN G.B. & KELSEY J.H. Some observations on the relationship between the standing potential of the human eye and the bleaching and regeneration of visual purple. *J. Physiol., Lond.* 161, *205-226* (1962 b).

CALISSENDORFF B., KNAVE B. & PERSSON H.E. Cyclic variations in the *c*-wave amplitude of the sheep ERG. *Vision Res.* 14, *1141-1145* (1974).

DAVIS J.R. & SHACKEL B. Changes in the electrooculogram potential level. *Brit. J. Ophthal.* 44, *606-618* (1960).

DONNER K.O. & REUTER T. Visual adaptation of the rhodopsin rods in the frog's retina. *J. Physiol.* 199, *59-87* (1968).

GRANIT R. The components of the retinal action potential in mammals and their relation to the discharge in the optic nerve. *J. Physiol. Lond.* 77, *207-239* (1933).

KNAVE B., MØLLER A. & PERSSON H.E. A component analysis of the electroretinogram. *Vision Res.* 12, *1669-1684* (1972).

KOLDER H. Spontane und experimentelle Änderungen des Bestandspotentials des menschlichen Auges. *Arch. ges. Physiol.* 268, *258-272* (1959).

KRIS C. Corneo-fundal potential variations during light and dark adaptation. *Nature, Lond.* 182, *1027-1028* (1958).

KRIS C. *Medical Physics* (edited by Glaser O.), Vol. 3 p. *692.* Year Book Publishers, Chicago. (1960).

NOELL W.K. Studies on the electrophysiology and metabolism of the retina. *USAF School of Aviation Medicine, Project* No. 21-1201-0004. Report No. I. (1953).

NOELL W.K. The origin of the electroretinogram. *Am. J. Ophthal.* 38, *78-90.* (1954).

SICKEL W. *Handbook of Sensory Physiology* (edited by Fuortes M.G.F.), Vol. VII:2, *667-727.* Springer Verlag, Berlin (1972).

STEINBERG R.H., SCHMIDT R. & BROWN K.T. Intracellular responses to light from cat pigment epithelium: Origin of the electroretinogram *c*-wave. *Nature, Lond.* 227, *728-730.* (1970).

INTENSITY – AMPLITUDE RELATIONSHIP AND CYCLIC VARIATIONS OF THE C–WAVE OF THE HUMAN D.C. REGISTERED ERG

SVEN ERIK G. NILSSON & KLAS-OLAV SKOOG

(Linköping, Sweden)

ABSTRACT

The c-wave of the human ERG was studied with a new method, using d.c. amplification and averaging technique. A linear relationship between log stimulus intensity and the c-wave amplitude was found within the investigated range of intensities (2 log units). In long-term experiments the c-wave amplitude showed cyclic changes, in most cases damped, with a frequency of 2/hour. These results should be of importance for the development of a routine clinical method.

A new method for d.c. registration of the human ERG at low and conventional stimulus intensities has recently been described by KNAVE, NILSSON & LUNT (1973). It has been further developed by SKOOG & NILSSON (1974 a) and now gives recordings which are stable and reproducible enough for the quantitative study of the human c-wave, even for experiments of long duration. It should be of interest to develop it into a routine clinical procedure.

It has been rather easy to record the c-wave of animals, as the eyes can be immobilized in different ways etc. GOTCH (1903) recorded the first complete ERG with the initial, comparatively fast a- and b-waves, the slow, positive c-wave and the off-effect, the d-wave. Early ERG work has been reviewed by BRÜCKE & GARTEN (1907) and KOHLRAUSCH (1931). In Granit's component analysis of the ERG (1933) the c-wave is mainly built up by PI, although its form may be modified by PII and PIII. Granit proposed that PI is a rod-dependent process, which disappears at light adaptation and is not directly related to the firing of impulses in the optic nerve (1947). Later authors (NOELL 1954, BROWN & WIESEL 1961, STEINBERG, SCHMIDT & BROWN 1970) have suggested, that the c-wave originates in the pigment epithelium. Intracellular recordings from pigment epithelial cells in the cat showed slow, light-evoked responses, which were 'identified positively as the origin of the c-wave' (STEINBERG et al. 1970). Similar responses from the pigment epithelium were obtained by NIEMEYER (1973). Other authors have published results which suggest that other structures than the pigment epithelium may contribute to the c-wave potential. When the central retinal artery was occluded in the monkey (GOURAS & CARR 1965) the c-wave amplitude diminished. SICKEL (1972) and HÖHNE (1971, 1972, 1973) claim to have recorded c-waves

This investigation was supported by a grant from the Swedish Medical Research Council (Project No 12X-734).

255

from isolated frog retinas. However, YAMASHITA (1959) could not demonstrate a c-wave from the isolated toad retina. DOWLING & RIPPS (1972) obtained a c-wave from the intact aspartate treated skate retina in situ but failed to do so from the isolated aspartate treated retina. RODIECK (1972) considers the c-wave as the result of an interaction between a large, negative receptor potential and a large, positive potential from the pigment epithelium. In their analysis of the low-intensity sheep ERG KNAVE, MØLLER & PERSSON (1972) suggest as ERG components a rod and a cone receptor potential, a positive and a negative d.c. response and a slow, late, positive potential corresponding to the c-wave at higher stimulus intensities.

The c-wave requires very stable recording conditions because of its slowness. This has been very difficult to achieve in experiments with human volunteers and only very little has been written about the human c-wave component. Apparently with great difficulties and with unstable and varying results KAHN & LÖWENSTEIN (1924), HARTLINE (1925), SACHS (1928 and 1931), COOPER, CREED & GRANIT (1933), BERNHARD (1941), WIRTH (1951) and DODT (1951) and a few others obtained human electroretinograms with c-waves. The earlier authors do not state whether mydriatic drugs were used to eliminate iris potentials, which may simulate c-waves, a fact which was pointed out by BRÜCKE and GARTEN already in 1907. DODT (1951) separated the secondary rise into a retinal component (the c-wave) and a pupillary component. Furthermore, he could record the c-wave only after the first flash in a series of recordings. HANITZSCH, HOMMER & BORNSCHEIN (1966) made a few measurements in patients during general anesthesia prior to surgery. Our present method for the first time allows stable and reproducible recordings of the human c-wave without the aid of general anaesthesia.

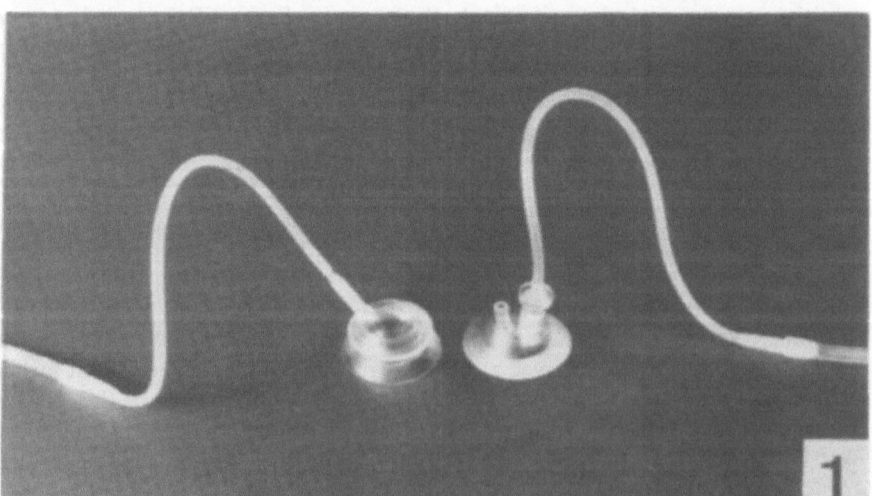

Fig. 1. The scleral contact lens to the left and the plastic chamber for the forehead to the right. The electrode tips are inserted in their holders. (From SKOOG & NILSSON 1974 a).

The present paper presents an analysis of the relationship between stimulus intensity and c-wave amplitude in the human as well as an investigation of the c-wave oscillations with time. More detailed reports are being published elsewhere (SKOOG & NILSSON 1974 a, 1974 b).

METHODS

The recording technique has been described in detail elsewhere (KNAVE, NILSSON & LUNT 1973, SKOOG & NILSSON 1974 a, 1974 b). Seven healthy volunteers, females between 20 and 30 years old, were chosen. They were not under the influence of drugs or stimulants. Three of the volunteers were used in the study of the c-wave amplitude at varying stimulus intensities, and all seven were included in the study of the long-term variations in the c-wave amplitude. Both pupils were dilated to 8 mm more with 0,5% tropicamide and 10% metaoxedrine given topically. After 30 minutes of dark-adaptation a scleral contact lens (Fig. 1.) was applied to one of the eyes (Fig. 3). After cleaning the skin with alcohol, the tip of the reference electrode was placed on the forehead by means of a plastic chamber (Figs. 1 and 3). Both this chamber and the contact lens were filled with Methocel^R. One of the arms was grounded. The illumination of the eyes during this procedure did not exceed 5 Lux. If necessary, a correcting lens corresponding to the volunteer's refraction was placed in front of the free eye, which

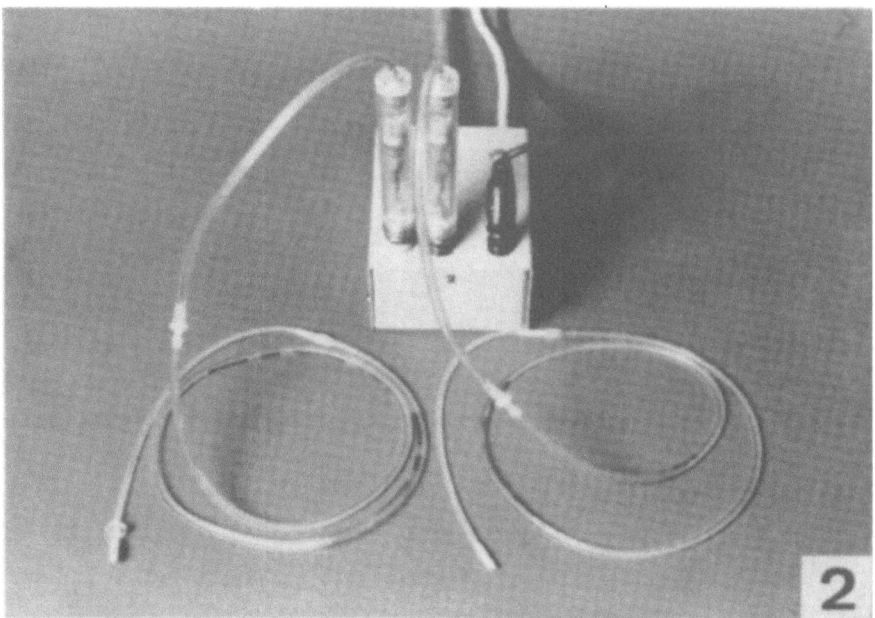

Fig. 2. The matched calomel half-cells used as recording and reference electrodes. Between the half-cells and the electrode tips are saline bridges in agar-filled polyethylene tubes. (From SKOOG & NILSSON 1974 a).

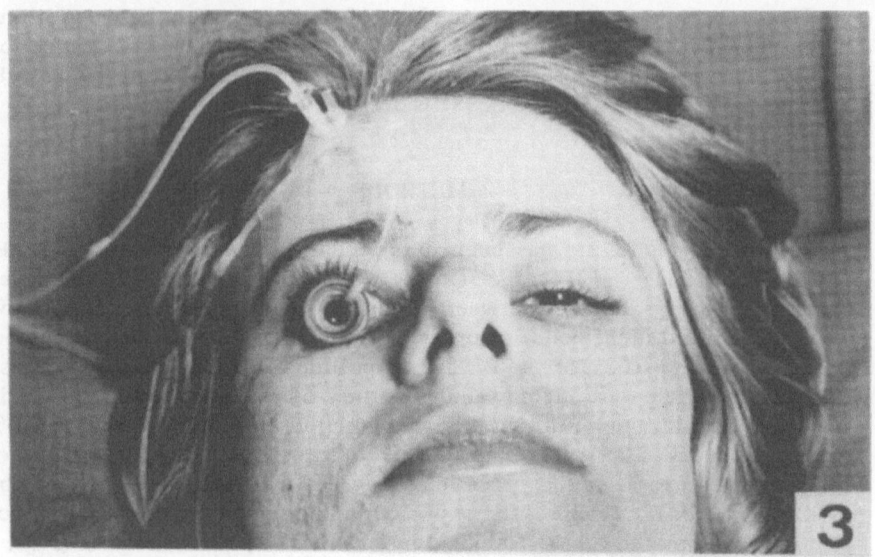

Fig. 3. The contact lens and the plastic chamber applied. (From SKOOG & NILSSON 1974 a).

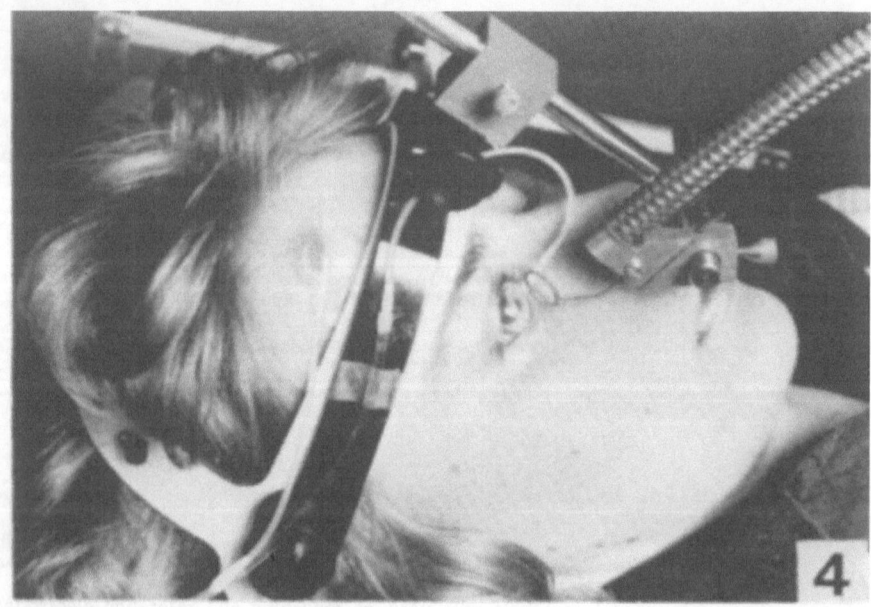

Fig. 4. The fiber optics and its holder attached to the patient. (From SKOOG & NILSSON 1974 a).

258

was used to fix upon a very weak deep red light in the ceiling. A grounded wire-net cage was lowered over the volunteer and the electrode system to exclude artefacts from alternating current etc. After the application of the contact lens etc. the volunteer was kept in darkness for 20 minutes.

The scleral contact lens and the plastic chamber on the forehead were connected to matched calomel half-cells by means of saline bridges in agar-filled polyethylene tubes (Figs. 2 and 3). The calomel cells served as recording and reference electrodes. The signal from the electrodes was fed into the differential inputs of a low-drift d.c. amplifier. It was lowpass-filtered (220 Hz cut off 18 dB/octavc) before it reached a Hewlett-Packard signal analyzer 5480 S either directly or after being displayed in a digital buffer connected to an oscilloscope. The noise level of the electrode system was 5-10 μV and the d.c. drift 10-15 μV/h.

The stimulus light came from a 150 Watt ozone-free Osram XBO xenon lamp with an approximately flat spectral emission curve within the visible

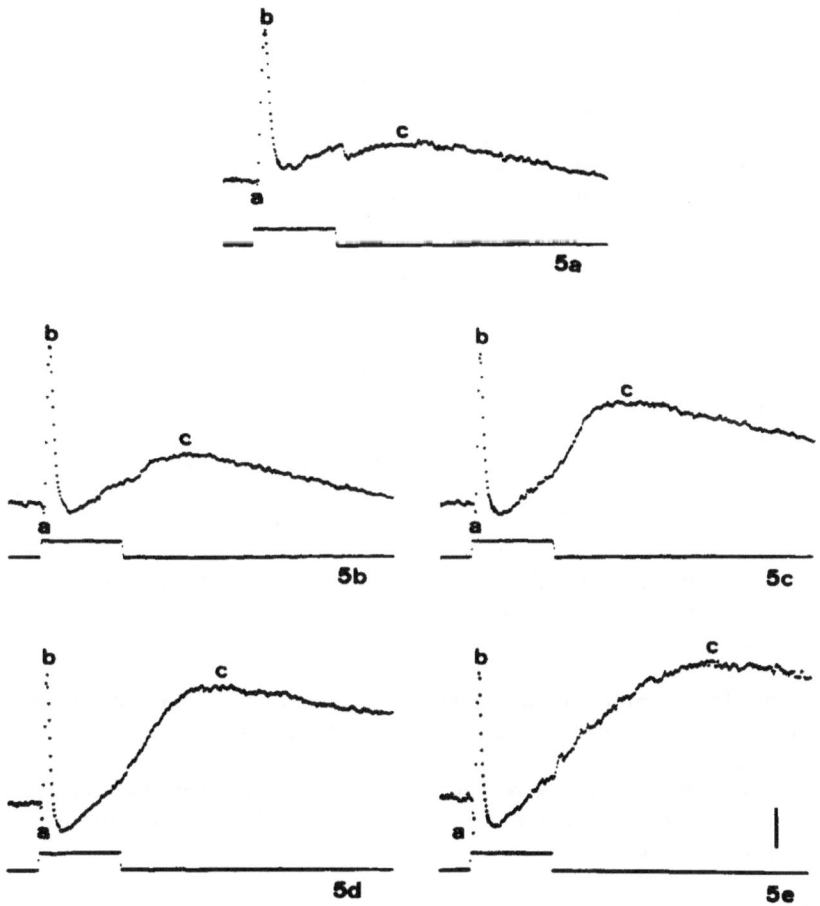

Fig. 5. The d.c. recorded human ERG in response to stimulus intensities of a. 3.5, b. 4.0, c. 4.5, d.5.0 and e. 5.5 rel. log units above the b-wave threshold. Stimulus duration 1.0 sec., indicated on lower line. Amplitude calibration 100 μV.

259

part of the spectrum. It passed heat reflection and heat absorbing filters (Zeiss) as well as neutral density filters (Balzer), which were used to change the light intensity. The lowest intensity eliciting a single flash b-wave (threshold at 30-40 μV) is referred to as log relative intensity 0. The light was led to the eye through a quartz fiber optics (Schott), which was held in front of the eye by an adjustable helmet (Fig. 4). Stimulus duration was varied with the aid of an electromagnetic shutter (Zeiss).

In the amplitude-intensity study a stimulus duration of 1 sec. was used. Relative stimulus intensities of 3.5, 4, 4.5, 5 and 5.5 log units above the b-wave threshold were used. The flash interval was 15 sec. at log rel. intens. 3.5 and 4 and 30 sec. at log rel. intens. 4.5 and 5. Four responses were averaged at log rel. intens. 3.5 and 4. Two responses were averaged at log rel. intens. 4.5 and 5. Single recordings were used at log rel. intens. 5.5. A total of 15 series of measurements (4-6 per volunteer), each consisting of responses with stimulus intensities from 3.5 to 5.5 relative log units, were carried out. A series of measurements lasted 5 minutes. The interval between the series was 2-3 min.

In the study of the long-term variations of the c-wave the stimulus duration was 1 sec. The stimulus interval was either 30 sec. or 2 min. A stimulus intensity of 4.5 rel. log units was used. With the short and long stimulus interval four and two responses were averaged respectively. Every measurement lasted at least 5 sec., thus always allowing the peak of the c-wave to be measured. 20 experiments were carried out.

RESULTS

Fig. 5 demonstrates a series of recordings with rel. stimulus intensities from 3.5 to 5.5 log. units above the b-wave threshold. The relationship between the c-wave amplitude and the logarithm of the stimulus intensity was linear within the range studied. Fig. 6 shows this relationship when the c-wave amplitude is measured from the base-line and Fig. 7 when it is measured from the bottom of the preceding trough. The means of 15 experiments with 95% confidence limits of the mean are plotted.

Fig. 8 shows the long-term variation of the c-wave amplitude on repetitive stimulations with a stimulus interval of 30 sec. The c-wave is measured from the base-line. The change in c-wave amplitude resembles a damped oscillation with a frequency of about 2/hour. The oscillation is quite small after one hour.

The slow stimulus frequency (0.5/min) resulted in similar 2/hour oscillations, which were less pronounced than with the shorter stimulus frequency, however.

A much slower change was also evident in many recordings, regardless of the stimulus interval. The experiments were not long enough to reveal whether this slower change was cyclic or not.

The relationship between stimulus intensity and the size of ERG components has been noted by many authors. DEWAR & MCKENDRICK (1876) found a linear relationship between the amplitude of their recordings, presumably corresponding to the b-wave, and the logarithm of stimulus light intensity within a range of two log units. BROSSA & KOHLRAUSCH (1913) state that all ERG components increase with increasing stimulus light. HARTLINE (1925) showed that the curve which describes the relationship between the sum of the a- and b-wave amplitudes (ordinate) and log stimulus light intensity (abscissa) is more or less S-shaped, tending to go horizontally at low and at high intensities with a linear relationship in between. Similar findings have been reported by WIRTH & ZETTERSTRÖM (1954), MÜLLER-LIMMROTH (1953, 1959), ASHER (1959) and others. According to MÜLLER-LIMMROTH (1953) an S-shaped curve is obtained when the c-wave amplitude (frog) is plotted against log stimulus intensity. In animal experiments many other workers have noted, that the c-wave disappears at light adaptation but increases with rising stimulus intensities at dark adaptation (EINTHOVEN & JOLLY 1908, BROSSA & KOHLRAUSCH 1913, GRANIT 1933, 1947, BROWN & WIESEL 1961, WÜNDSCH & BORNSCHEIN 1972, BROWN 1968, KNAVE, MØLLER & PERSSON 1972 and others). This has been noted to some extent also in

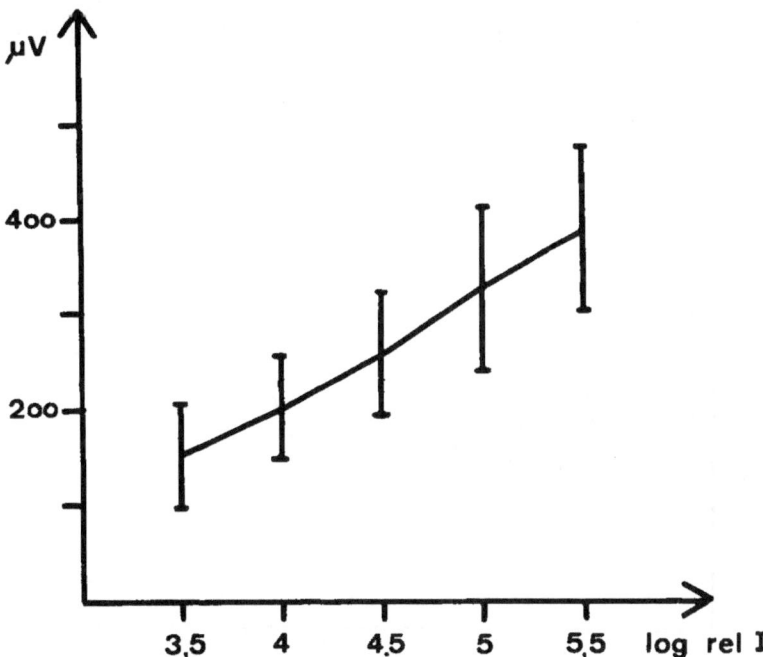

Fig. 6. The relationship between the amplitude of the c-wave, measured from the base-line, and log rel. stimulus intensity. Mean and 95% confidence limits. (From SKOOG & NILSSON 1974 a).

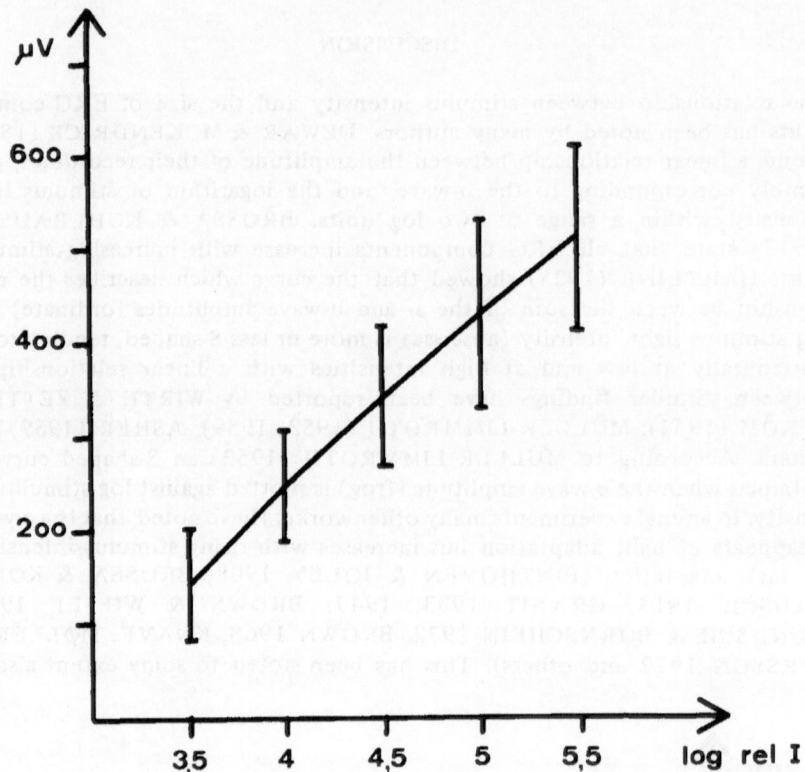

Fig. 7. The relationship between the amplitude of the c-wave, measured from the bottom of the preceding trough, and log rel. stimulus intensity. Mean and 95% confidence limits. Stimulus duration 1.0 sec., indicated on lower line. (From SKOOG & NILSSON 1974 a).

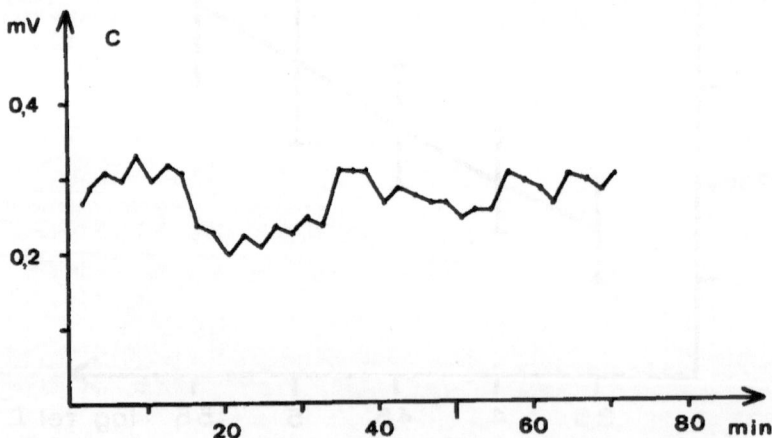

Fig. 8. The cyclic change of the c-wave amplitude on repetitive stimulations. Light intensity 4.5 rel. log units. Flash duration 1.0 sec. Stimulus interval 30 sec. Four responses averaged. (From SKOOG & NILSSON 1974 b).

262

recordings on humans (WIRTH 1951, DODT 1951, HANITZSCH, HOM-MER & BORNSCHEIN 1966). Due to technical difficulties or for other reasons no quantitative studies have been performed. Intracellular record-ings from pigment epithelial cells in the cat after short flashes (480 msec) demonstrated a linear relationship between stimulus intensity and the ampli-tude of the responses within a range of about 2.5 log units (SCHMIDT & STEINBERG 1971).

Our results show a linear relationship between log stimulus intensity and the c-wave amplitude within a range of 2 log units. This was valid either the c-wave was measured from the base-line or from bottom of the preceding trough. (At stimulus intensities below 3.5 rel. log units it was difficult to measure the c-wave amplitude accurately, while intensities above 5.5 rel. log units often gave rise to disturbing eye movements.)

To avoid too much intereference from the cyclic changes of the c-wave amplitude present on repetitive stimulations, it was necessary to make each series of intensity-amplitude recordings as short as possible. However, it was desirable to use an averaging technique, and thus each series lasted five minutes. Since the series were distributed on different places of the oscilla-tions, the influence of the cyclic alterations was kept under full control.

For the study of the cyclic variations of the c-wave amplitude with time a well tolerable light intensity (4.5 rel. log. units) was chosen. The same kind of 2/hour oscillation of the c-wave amplitude as demonstrated in the present report was also shown in experiments on the sheep (CALISSEN-DORFF et al. 1974). These workers also found a slow, cyclic change with a frequency of 0.3-0.5/hour, upon which the faster oscillation seemed to be superimposed. Such a slow variation could be traced also in our recordings, but the duration of the experiments was not long enough to prove definitely the cyclic character of this process.

The pigment epithelium is considered to be the major source of the standing potential (SP) (NOELL 1954, HECK & PAPST 1957, GOURAS 1969) and to generate the c-wave (NOELL 1954, BROWN & WIESEL 1961, STEINBERG et al. 1970). This may be the reason why oscillations with a frequency of 2/hour occur also in the electroculograms (EOG), which re-flects the SP (KRIS 1958, KOLDER 1960, ARDEN, BARRADA & KEL-SEY 1962, GOURAS 1969, TÄUMER et al. 1974 and others). Very slow changes of the EOG potential were reported by DAVIS & SHACKEL (1960).

It seems likely that the c-wave oscillations are related to changes in pigment epithelial and perhaps retinal metabolism. In their study of the c-wave oscillations in the sheep, CALISSENDORFF et al. (1974) also men-tion as a possibility that the cyclic changes may be due to changes in rod sensitivity. It is known that rod sensitivity may be altered also by relatively small bleachings of rhodopsin. (DONNER & REUTER 1968, DOWLING & RIPPS 1972). However, the oscillations are probably not induced by retinal and retinol molecules released from bleached rhodopsin, since under the stimulus conditions used, only a fraction of a per cent of the available rhodopsin was bleached (CALISSENDORFF et al. 1974).

The magnitude of the c-wave oscillations makes it important to consider them, when repeated registrations of the c-wave are made. A standardized procedure will be needed, if one wishes to measure the c-wave amplitude of a patient. Patients cooperated very well, when a stimulus interval of 30 sec. was used in preliminary tests. For clinical use it seems impracticable to wait for a kind of steady state by stimulating repeatedly for more then one hour. One could choose to measure the c-wave amplitude for instance at the first oscillatory peak. One could also make averages of a large number of responses along the oscillations.

REFERENCES

ARDEN, G.B., BARRADA, A. & KELSEY, J.H. *Brit. J. Opthal.* 46, *449-467* (1962).
ASHER, H. *Acta Facultatis Med. Univ. Brunensis* 4, *101-104* (1960).
BERNHARD, C.G. *Acta physiol. scand. 1, suppl.* 1, *71-77* (1940).
BROSSA, A. & KOHLRAUSCH, A. *Arch. Anat. u. Physiol., Physiol. Abtlg.* (Leipzig) *449-492* (1940).
BROWN, K.T. *Vision Res.* 8, *633-677* (1968).
BROWN, K.T. & WIESEL, T.N. *J. Physiol. (Lond.)* 158, *257-280* (1961).
BRÜCKE, E.Th. v. & GARTEN, S. *Pflügers Arch. ges. Physiol.* 120, *290-348* (1907).
CALISSENDORFF, B., KNAVE, B. & PERSSON, H.E. *Vision Res.* In press (1974).
COOPER, S., CREED, R.S. & GRANIT, R. *J. Physiol. (Lond.)* 79, *185-190* (1933).
DAVIS, J.R. & SHACKEL, B. *Brit. J. Ophthal.* 44, *606-618* (1960).
DEWAR, J. & MCKENDRICK, T.G. *Royal Inst. of Great Britain Proc.* 8, *137-149* (1876).
DODT, E. *Albrecht v. Graefes Arch. Ophthal.* 151, *672-692* (1951).
DONNER, K.O. & REUTER, T. *J. Physiol. (Lond.)* 199, *59-87* (1968).
DOWLING J.E. & RIPPS, H. *J. gen. Physiol.* 60, *698-719* (1972).
EINTHOVEN, W. & JOLLY, W.A. *Quart. J. Exp. Physiol.* 1, *373-416* (1908).
GOTCH, F. *J. Physiol. (Lond.)* 29, *388-410* (1903).
GOURAS, P. In: STRAATSMA, B.R., ed. (1969) *The Retina*, pp. 565-581. University of California Press, Berkeley and Los Angeles (1969).
GOURAS, P. & CARR, R.E. *Invest. Ophthal.* 4, *310-317* (1965).
GRANIT, R. *J. Physiol. (Lond.)* 77, *207-239* (1933).
GRANIT, R. Sensory Mechanisms of the Retina. Oxford Univ. Press, London-New York-Toronto. (1947).
HANITZSCH, R., HOMMER, K. & BORNSCHEIN, H. *Vision Res.* 6, *245-250* (1966).
HARTLINE, H.K. *Amer. J. Physiol.* 73, *600-612* (1925).
HECK, J. & PAPST W. *Bibl. ophthal. (Basel)* 48, *96-107* (1957).
HÖHNE, W. *Acta biol. med. germ.* 27, *307-316* (1971).
HÖHNE, W. *Acta biol. med. germ.* 29, *661-665* (1972).
HÖHNE, W. *Acta biol. med. germ.* 30, *493-498* (1973).
KAHN, R. LÖWENSTEIN, A. *Albrecht v. Graefes Arch. Ophthal.* 114, *304-331* (1924).
KNAVE, B., MØLLER, A. & PERSSON, H.E. *Vision Res.* 12, *1669-1684* (1972).
KNAVE, B., NILSSON, S.E.G. & LUNT, T. *Acta ophthal. (Kbh.)* 51, *716-726* (1973).
KOHLRAUSCH, A. In: BETHE, A. et al., eds. *Handb. der norm. u. path. Physiol.* Vol. 12/2, part 2, 1394-1496. Verlag von Julius Springer, Berlin (1931).
KOLDER, H. *Pflügers Arch. ges. Physiol.* 268, *258-272* (1959).
KRIS, Ch. *Nature (Lond.)* 182, *1027-28* (1958).
MÜLLER-LIMMROTH, H.W. *Z.Biol.* 105, *393-404* (1953).
MÜLLER-LIMMROTH, W. Elektrophysiologie des Gesichtssinns, pp. 61-64. Springer-Verlag, Berlin-Göttingen-Heidelberg. (1959).
NIEMEYER, G. *Vision Res.* 13, *1613-1618* (1973).
NOELL, W.K. *Amer. J. Ophthal.* 38, *78-90* (1954).
RODIECK, R.W. *Vision Res.* 12, *773-780* (1972).
SACHS, E. *Klin. Wschr.* 8, *136-137* (1929).
SACHS, E., cited by Kohlrausch, A. In: BETHE, A. et al., eds. Handb. der norm. u. path. Physiol. Vol. 12/2, part 2, 1463-64. Verlag von Julius Springer, Berlin (1931).

SCHMIDT, R. & STEINBERG, R.H. *J. Physiol. (Lond.)* 217, *71-91* (1971).
SICKEL, W. In: FUORTES, M.G.F., ed. Handbook of Sensory Physiology, VII/2, *667-727*. Springer Verlag. Berlin-Heidelberg-New York. (1972).
SKOOG, K.O. & NILSSON, S,E.G. *Acta ophthal. (Kbh.)* 52, *759-773* (1974a).
SKOOG, K.O. & NILSSON, S.E.G. *Acta ophthal. (Kbh.)* 52, *904-912* (1974b).
STEINBERG, R.H., SCHMIDT, R. & BROWN, K.T. *Nature (Lond.)* 227, *728-730*. (1970).
TÄUMER, R., MACKENSEN, G., HARTMANN, H., MOSER, U., STEHLE, R., WER-NER, W. & WOLF, D. *Albrecht v. Graefes Arch. Klin. Ophthal.* 189, *81-97* (1974).
WIRTH, A. *Albrecht. v. Graefes Arch. Ophthal.* 151, *662-671* (1951).
WIRTH, A. & ZETTERSTRÖM, B. *Brit. J. Ophthal.* 38, *257-265* (1954).
WÜNDSCH, L. & BORNSCHEIN, H. *Experientia (Basel)* 28, *409-410* (1972).
YAMASHITA, E., *Tohoku J. exp. Med.* 70, *221-233* (1959).

THE EFFECT OF BARBITURATE ON THE C—WAVE OF THE ELECTRORETINOGRAM AND THE STANDING POTENTIAL OF THE SHEEP EYE

BENGT KNAVE, HANS E. PERSSON & SVEN ERIK G. NILSSON

(Stockholm, Sweden)

INTRODUCTION

It is a well-known fact that barbiturates influence the functions of the neuroretina (see *e.g.* DANIS 1956, WOHLZOGEN 1956, NOELL 1958, KNAVE & PERSSON 1974 a, b). Thus, the administration of small doses is reported to result in an increase of the *a*- and *b*-wave amplitudes of the conventional electroretinogram (ERG), whereas larger doses depress the *b*-wave.

The pigment epithelial cells of the retina have a specific sensitivity to certain drugs such as rifampicin (BOMAN 1973, KNAVE, PERSSON, CALISSENDORFF & NILSSON 1973), chloroquine (BERNSTEIN & GINSBERG 1964, MONAHAN & HORNS 1964) and chlorpromazine (reviewed by LINDQUIST & ULLBERG 1972).

Two questions were posed in the present study, on the basis of the foregoing facts. 1. Do barbiturates also have an affinity for the pigment epithelial cells and influence their functions? 2. If so, do barbiturates have a dual site of action on the retina, namely on the neuroretina and on the pigment epithelium? These questions were analysed by means of recording of the *c*-wave known to be generated in the pigment epithelium (NOELL 1954, BROWN & WIESEL 1961, STEINBERG, SCHMIDT & BROWN 1970) and the standing potential (SP) which partly originates in the same cells (NOELL 1954, 1963, GOURAS 1969) before and after administration of barbiturate. Furthermore, experiments were made in which the functions of the pigment epithelial cells were selectively blocked by *i.v.* administration of sodium iodate (NaIO$_3$, NOELL 1954). For further details on the effect of barbiturate on retinal functions, see KNAVE & PERSSON 1974 a, b, KNAVE, PERSSON & NILSSON 1974.

METHODS

The experiments were made on the intact sheep eye kept in the dark-adapted state. The method used has recently been described in detail (KNAVE, MØLLER & PERSSON 1972, see also KNAVE & PERSSON 1974 a, b, KNAVE, PERSSON & NILSSON 1974). It should be emphasized that with this method it is possible to record d.c. responses from the intact eye in long-term studies during constant experimental conditions. The SP of the intact eye was recorded between a corneal electrode and an electrode placed subcutaneously at the upper bony margin of the orbit. These electrodes (calomel half-cells) were connected to the differential inputs of a low-drift d.c. amplifier. An ultra-short acting barbiturate, thiopental (Pentothal-Sodium®), which is the thioanalog of pentobarbital (Nembutal®) was used in the present study and administered *i.v.* The effect of barbiturate on the components of the conventional ERG and on the SP was measured in

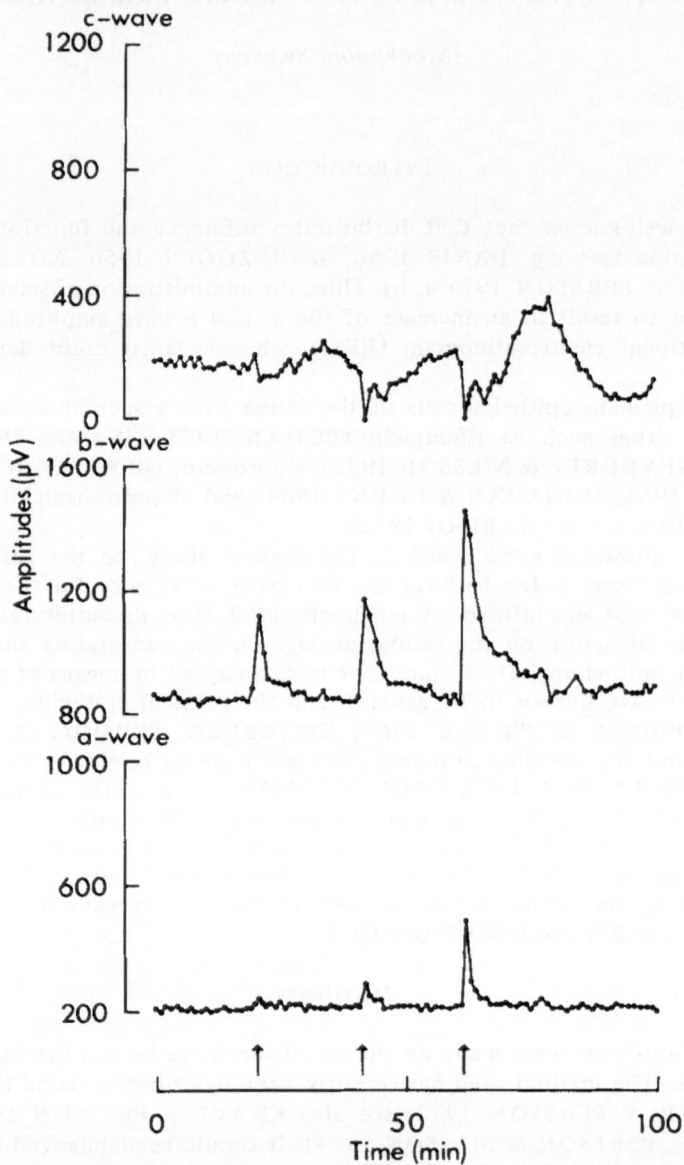

Fig. 1. Effect of thiopental on *a*-, *b*- and *c*-wave amplitudes of the dark-adapted sheep eye. Three *i.v.* injections of 2.5, 5 and 10 mg thiopental per kg body weight, respectively, were given in turns (arrows). Stimulus intensity: 5.0 log units above *b*-wave threshold. Stimulus duration: 0.1 sec.

some experiments after selective blocking of the functions of the pigment epithelial cells by means of *i.v.* administration of sodium iodate (NaIO$_3$; NOELL 1954).

RESULTS

The graphs of Fig. 1 show the amplitudes of the *a*-, *b*- and *c*-waves from an

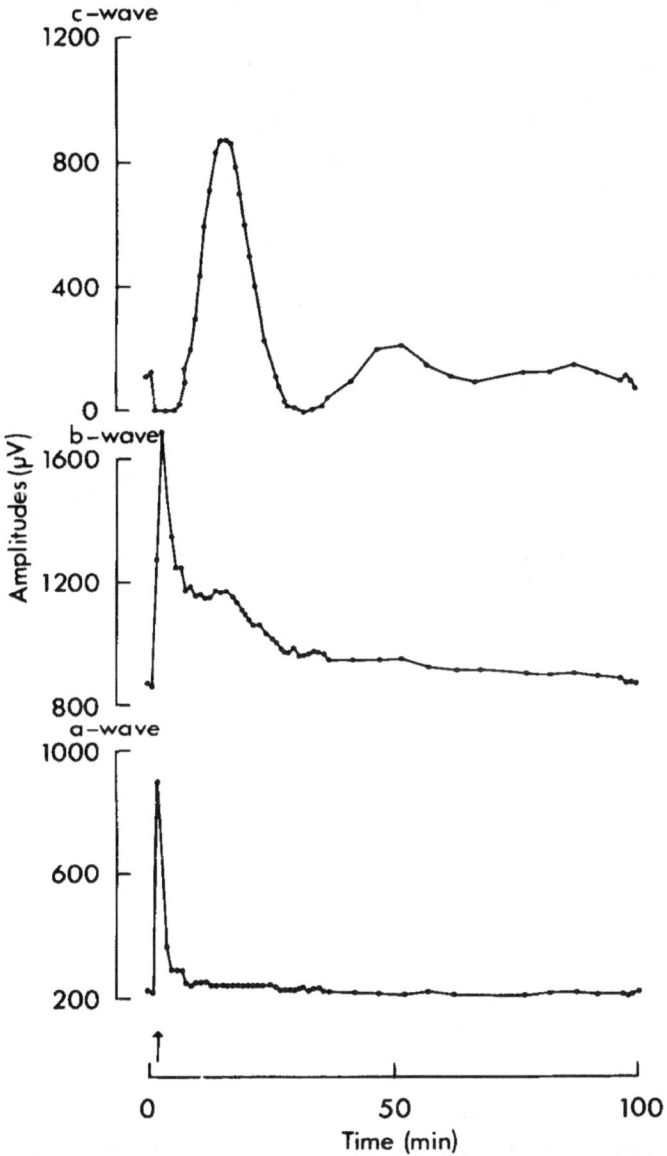

Fig. 2. Effect of thiopental on *a*-, *b*- and *c*-wave amplitudes of the dark-adapted sheep eye. An *i.v.* injection of 20 mg per kg body weight was given (arrow). Stimulus intensity: 5.0 log units above *b*-wave threshold. Stimulus duration: 0.1 sec.

experiment in which *low and moderate* doses of thiopental were administered (2.5, 5 and 10 mg thiopental per kg body weight; arrows). A rapid
dose — related increase of short duration was observed in the *a*- and *b*-waves
after each injection. The *c*-wave, however, immediately decreased or was
abolished after thiopental. The last of these injections resulted in late
changes of the *c*-wave amplitude with a supernormal peak (*vide infra*).

The principal alterations of the *a*-, *b*- and *c*-wave amplitudes after the *i.v.*
administration of a *large* dose of thiopental (20 mg per kg body weight) are
depicted in Fig. 2 (see also Fig. 3). The *c*-wave decreased immediately and
was temporarily abolished. The depression of the *c*-wave was followed by a
slow, transient increase with peak amplitudes about 15 min after the injection (Fig. 2 and Fig. 3, upper trace). The *c*-wave then showed amplitude
variations resembling damped oscillations down to its original value. Note,
the dose related, initial enhancement of the *a*- and *b*-wave amplitudes.
Furthermore, the late oscillatory changes in the *c*-wave were not correlated
in time with any substantial changes in the *a*- and *b*-waves.

In addition to the effects on the *c*-wave, thiopental was found to induce
changes in the standing (resting) potential (SP) of the eye. Following the
administration of *small* doses (≤ 5 mg per kg body weight) a negative d.c.

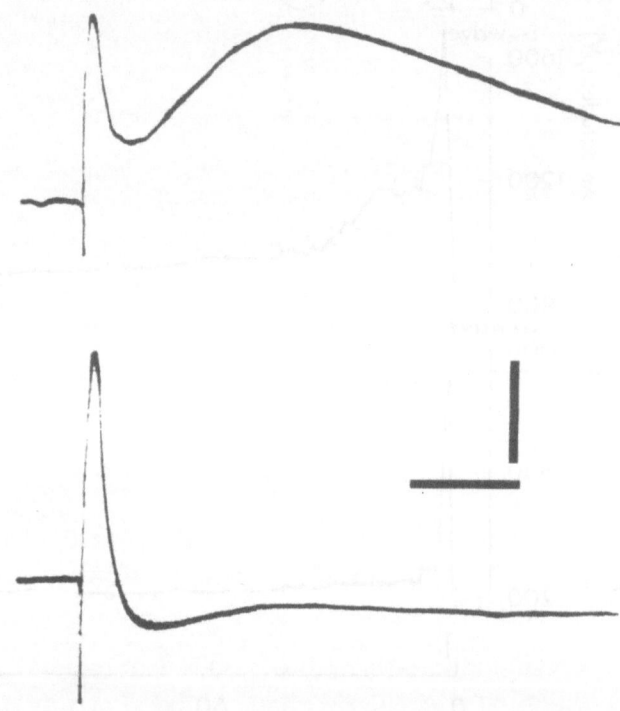

Fig. 3.   ERG of the dark-adapted sheep eye 18 min and 2 min after *i.v.* injection of
20 mg thiopental per kg body weight (upper and lower recording, respectively).
Stimulus intensity: 5.0 log units above the *b*-wave threshold. Stimulus duration:
0.1 sec. Time calibration: 1 sec. Amplitude calibration: 500μV.

shift was recorded consisting of an initial, rapid phase and followed by a slow, sustained one. A dose-related increased in amplitude and duration of the slow negative shift was observed. The alterations of the SP after an *i.v.* administration of a larger dose *i.e.* 10 mg thiopental per kg body weight is illustrated in Fig. 4. The negative d.c. shift was found to be followed by a

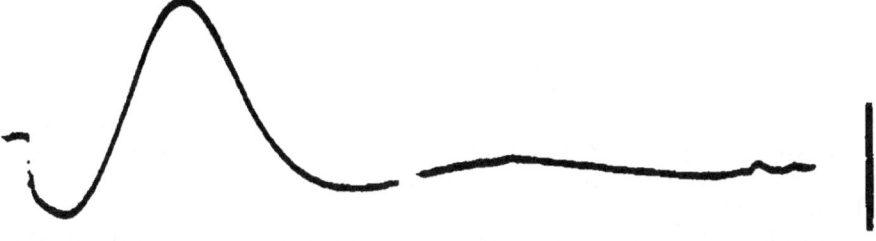

Fig. 4. Effect of thiopental on the standing potential (SP) of the dark-adapted sheep eye. The SP was followed 64 min after *i.v.* injection of 10 mg thiopental per kg body weight. Time calibration: 10 min. Amplitude calibration: 4 mV.

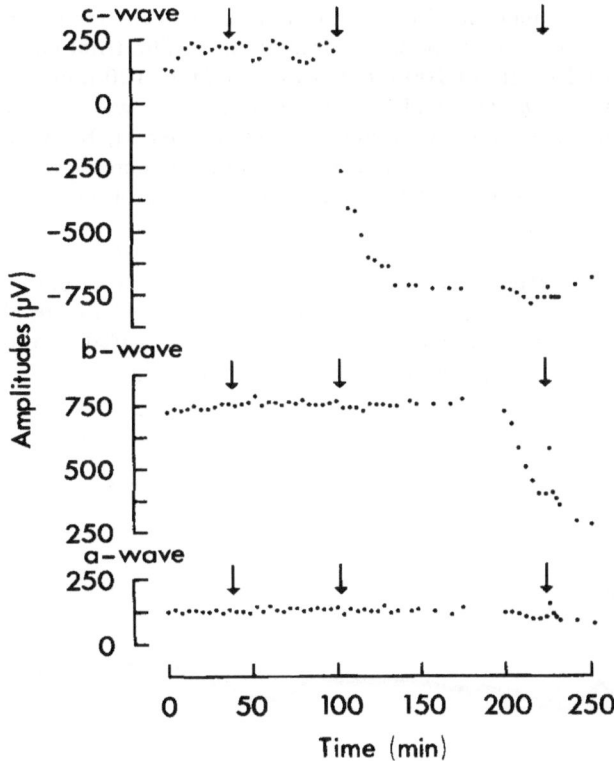

Fig. 5. Effects of sodium iodate on the *a*-, *b*- and *c*-wave amplitudes of the dark-adapted sheep eye. At 40, 100 and 225 min (arrows) *i.v.* injections of 50 ml Ringer's solution, 30 mg $NaIO_3$ per kg body weight and 5 mg thiopental per kg body weight, respectively, were given. Stimulus intensity: 5.0 log units above *b*-wave threshold. Stimulus duration: 0.1 sec.

slow, *positive* d.c. shift with a peak amplitude about 13 min after the injection. The SP then showed smooth variations similar to the oscillations observed in the c-wave amplitude (see Fig. 1). At the end of the recording *i.e.* 64 min after barbiturate administration, the SP was still negative compared to the original isoelectric line.

It should be pointed out, that there is a striking resemblance in time course of the polarity and amplitude changes of the c-wave and the SP in response to a single dose of thiopental. No similarities could be demonstrated, however, between the SP and a- and the b-wave of the ERG.

In order to evaluate whether or not the alterations of the c-wave and the SP after thiopental administration actually originated from the pigment epithelial cells experiments were made in which the functions of these cells were selectively blocked by means of *i.v.* injection of sodium iodate ($NaIO_3$; NOELL 1954).

In Fig. 5 the a-, b- and c-waves were recorded after *i.v.* injection of 50 ml of Ringer's solution (arrow at 40 min), after *i.v.* injection of 30 mg per kg body weight of $NaIO_3$ (arrow at 100 min) and after *i.v.* injection of 5 mg per kg body weight of barbiturate (thiopental; arrow at 225 min).

The a-, b- and c-waves remained unchanged after injection of Ringer's solution. After injection of $NaIO_3$ the a- and b-waves were still not changed, whereas the c-wave was abolished dramatically. The total change in amplitude amounted to about 1000 μV! Approximately 100 min after the $NaIO_3$ injection also the b-wave and, to a less extent, the a-wave began to decrease in amplitude. The thiopental injection (5 mg per kg body weight) given 125 min after the $NaIO_3$ resulted in an amplitude increase of the residual a- and b-waves, but no significant alterations could be observed in the c-waves compared to those recorded from the normal eye (see Fig. 1).

During the time period from 80-95 min after $NaIO_3$ administration the SP was followed after injections of 5 mg thiopental per kg body weight (Fig. 6, arrows). Insignificant negative shifts were obtained in the SP. However, these changes were of a very small magnitude compared to those recorded from eyes with intact pigment epithelium (see Fig. 4).

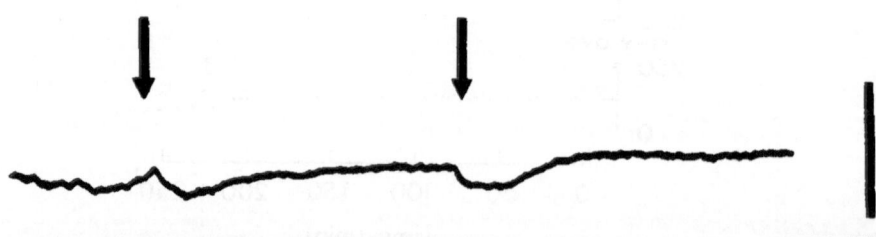

Fig. 6. Effect of thiopental on the standing potential (SP) of the dark-adapted $NaIO_3$ treated sheep eye. Two *i.v.* injections of 5 mg thiopental per kg body weight were given (arrows) 80 min after *i.v.* injection of 30 mg $NaIO_3$ per kg body weight. Time calibration: 2 min. Amplitude calibration: 0.5 mV.

DISCUSSION

The present study shows that barbiturates have an effect on the c-wave of the ERG and on the SP recorded from the intact eye. Furthermore, there was similarity in the time-course of the changes of these potentials. The c-wave is known to be generated in the pigment epithelial cells of the retina (NOELL 1954, BROWN & WIESEL 1961, STEINBERG, SCHMIDT & BROWN 1970) and these cells are considered at least partly to be responsible for the SP (NOELL 1954, 1963, GOURAS 1969). These facts give evidence for the notion that barbiturates in the same way influence the pigment epithelium. A view which is further supported by the observation that the barbiturate effects on the c-wave and the SP were abolished after blocking the functions of the pigment epithelium with sodium iodate.

The functional mechanism of the barbiturate effect on the pigment epithelial cells cannot be explained on the basis of the present results. However, it is interesting to note that the barbiturate induced changes of the a- and b-waves on one hand were not correlated with those of the c-wave and the SP on the other. Furthermore, the a- and b-wave alterations remained after administration of sodium iodate, whereas the changes of the c-wave and the SP were dramatically abolished.

On the basis of these observations, it is tentatively suggested that barbiturates may have a duel site of action on the retina, namely on the neuroretina and on the pigment epithelium cells.

SUMMARY

The c-wave of the sheep electroretinogram was studied in long-term experiments. It was found that the c-wave amplitude changed as a function of time and these alterations were dependent on frequency of the stimulus flash used. A slow oscillation (frequency about 0.3-0.5 per hr) of the c-wave amplitude was observed, using 1 sec light stimuli and long flash intervals (2 min). Shorter flash intervals gave rise to oscillations with a frequency of about 2 per hour. These fast oscillations initially were of relatively large amplitudes but decreased with time and reached a constant level after about 100 min. Shortening of stimulus duration (0.1 sec) resulted in c-waves of less amplitudes, but the cyclic variation pattern described above did not change.

This work was supported by grants from the Swedish Medical Research Council, the Magnus Bergvall Foundation for Scientific Research and Karolinska Institutet.

REFERENCES

BERNSTEIN, H.N. & J. GINSBERG, The pathology of chloroquine retinopathy. *Arch Ophthal.* 71, *238-245*, 1964.

BOMAN, G., Melanin affinity of a new antituberculous drug, rifampicin, investigated by whole body autoradiography. *Acta Ophthal. (Kbh.).* 51, *367-370*, 1973.

BROWN, K.T. & T.N. WIESEL, Localization of origins of electroretinogram components by intra-retinal recording in the intact cat eye. *J. Physiol. (Lond.).* 158, *257-280*, 1961.

DANIS, P., Modifications de l' électrorétinogramme du rat produites par l' injection intra-artérielle proche de potassium, de vératrine et de narcotiques. *J. Physiol. Path. Gén.* 48, *479-483*, 1956.

GOURAS, P., Clinical electro-oculography. In Straatsma, B.R. (Ed.). *The Retina.* University of California Press, Berkeley and Los Angeles. *565-581*, 1969.

KNAVE, B., A.R. MØLLER & H.E. PERSSON, A component analysis of the electroretinogram. *Vision Res.* 12. *1669-1684*, 1972.

KNAVE, B. & H.E. PERSSON, The effect of barbiturate on retinal functions. I. Effects on the conventional electroretinogram of the sheep eye. *Acta physiol. scand.* 91, *53-60*, 1974.

KNAVE, B. & H.E. PERSSON, The effect of barbiturate on retinal functions. III. Effects on the isolated receptor responses and the inner nuclear layer components of the low-intensity electroretinogram in the sheep eye. *Acta physiol. scand.* 91, *187-195*, 1974.

KNAVE, B., H.E. PERSSON & S.E.G. NILSSON, The effect of barbiturate on retinal functions. II. Effects on the *c*-wave of the electroretinogram and the standing potential of the sheep eye. *Acta physiol. scand.* 91, *180-186*, 1974.

KNAVE, B., H.E. PERSSON & S.E.G. NILSSON, A comparative study on the effects of barbiturate and ethyl alcohol on retinal functions with special reference to the *c*-wave of the electroretinogram and the standing potential of the sheep eye. *Acta Ophthal. (Kbh.).* 52, *254-259*, 1974.

KNAVE, B., H.E. PERSSON, B. CALISSENDORFF & S.E.G. NILSSON, Selective effects of a new antituberculous drug, rifampicin, on the *c*-wave of the sheep electroretinogram. *Acta Ophthal. (Kbh.).* 51. *371-374*. 1973.

LINDQUIST, N.G. & S. ULLBERG, The melanin affinity of chloroquine and chlorpromazine studied by whole body autoradiography. *Acta Pharmacol. (Kbh.).* 31. Suppl. II. 1972.

NOELL, W.K., The origin of the electroretinogram. *Amer. J. Ophthal.* 38. *78-90*. 1954.

NOELL, W.K., Cellular physiology of the retina. *J. Ophthalmol. Soc. Amer.* 53. *36-48*. 1963.

NOELL, W.K., Differentiation, metabolic organization and viability of the visual cell. *Arch. Ophthal.* 60. *702-733*. 1958.

MONAHAN, R.H. & R.C. HORNS, The pathology of chloroquine in the eye. *Trans. Amer. Acad. Ophthal. Otolaryng.* 68. *40-44*. 1964.

STEINBERG, R.H., R. SCHMIDT & K.T. BROWN, Intracellular response to light from cat pigment epithelium: origin of the electroretinogram *c*-wave. *Nature (Lond.).* 227. *728-730*. 1970.

WOHLZOGEN, F.X., Beeinflussung des Säuger-ERG durch zentralnervös wirksame Substanzen. *Z. Biol.* 108, *217-233*, 1956.

274

THE EFFECT OF ELEVATED INTRAOCULAR PRESSURE
ON THE HUMAN ERG AND VER

G. BARTL, O. BENEDIKT & H. HITI

(Graz, Austria)

INTRODUCTION

It is well known that the alterations of the ERG and responses of the optic tract at raised intraocular pressure (IOP) are caused by a decrease of the blood supply and damage to the optic disc rather than the retina (HAYREH 1970).

To study the effects of elevated IOP on optic nerve fibers and their function, we monitored the conduction of optic nerve impulses through the optic disc at different levels of IOP by studying the visual evoked responses (VER) of the cortex elicited by light stimulation of the retina. In this manner we were able to observe the diminished electrical responses of optic nerve fibers by the VERs, since diminished optic nerve responses represent diminished VERs.

At the same time ERGs were recorded and compared with the VERs. All electro-physiological responses were correlated to the ophthalmic artery blood pressure.

Such experiments have been done previously in cats, rabbits and monkeys, with different results, as the blood supply of the retina of cats is different from that of monkeys or men (NOELL 1954, BORNSCHEIN 1958, UENOYAMA et al. 1969).

In monkeys and men, some retinal circulation is maintained at IOPs that stop blood flow completely in the choroid and optic disc, while this is not true of cats.

The purpose of our study was to observe the alterations of the ERG and VER in the human eye at elevated IOP, and to correlate the results to the blood supply of the retina and the optic disc.

METHOD

The experiments were performed on ten healthy persons with normal IOP and normal visual function. The systemic and ophthalmic artery blood pressures were also normal. The IOP was elevated in steps by means of a Müller dynamometer. The IOP was maintained at each level for about 80 seconds, and during the first 20 seconds, the responses were not recorded so that we obtained a steady state in the blood circulation.

To record the ERG, a silver-silver chloride electroretinograph lens was placed on the cornea and a reference electrode on the forehead. The scalp electrodes for recording visual evoked responses were located homo- and

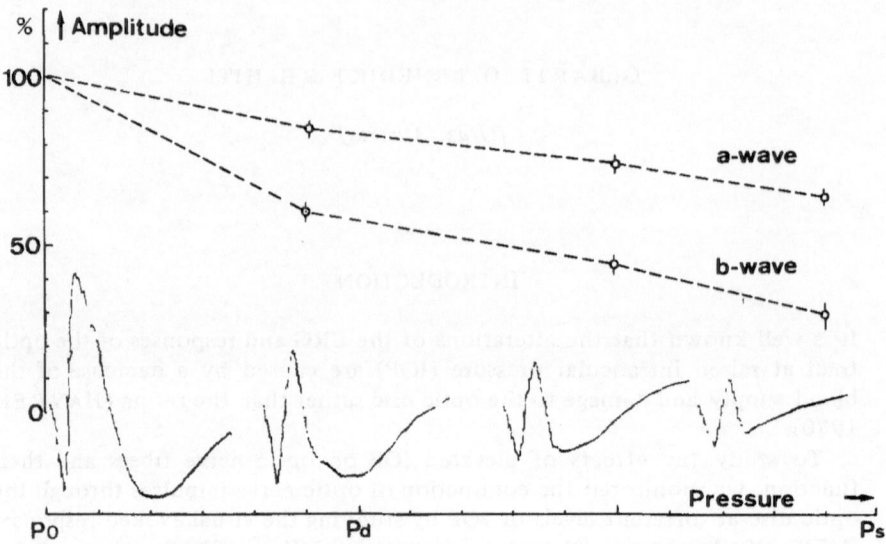

Fig. 1. The relative amplitude of the ERG plotted against the IOP. The broken lines show averaged results of the a-wave and b-wave of ten patients. The vertical lines show the standard deviation of the ten patients. The results obtained with the IOPs at P_o, near Pd, in the middle between Pd and Ps and near Ps. Below the broken lines the orginal responses are shown at normal and steplike elevated level of IOP.

contralateral on protuberantia occipitalis externa.

The eyes were dark adapted for 20 minutes before the recording was started.

In each experiment the second eye was closed to eliminate its potentials. For the same purpose we closed the ears.

In our experiments we examined the ERG and VER at four different levels of IOP. The first recording was without an elevated IOP. In the following four experiments the IOP was chosen so that various levels of IOP were reached from near diastolic to near systolic blood pressure in the ophthalmic artery. Between the different IOPs we waited 5 minutes in the same patient, so that the retina had ample time to recover to its normal physiological function. A short photic stimulus of 10 μsec. duration was delivered through a xenon lamp photostimulator triggered by an electronic stimulator (Knott-Elektronic Strobotest II) with 0,375/J intensity and with a frequence of 1 cps. Responses which were picked up simultaneously from the eyeball and visual cortex were fed into a computer (CAT 400 C) for averaging after amplification (time constant = 0,3 sec.). 60 impulses were averaged and the results were displayed by an x-y-Plotter (Hewlett and Packard).

The amplitude of the b-wave and a-wave of the ERG were measured in the conventional way. The amplitudes of the VERs were measured from the first negative peak to the following first positive peak.

RESULTS

The experimental records obtained from one patient are shown in Fig. 1-2. The results were similar in all patients.

Effect of elevated IOP on ERG

The a-wave and b-wave of the ERG showed first alterations when the IOP reached a level near diastolic blood pressure. Both the a- and b-waves showed a slight decrease in amplitude. When the IOP was elevated steplike, the amplitude of the b-wave was much more altered than the a-wave at each level of change in the IOP. At near systolic blood pressure the amplitude of the a-wave was diminished 35% whereas the amplitude of the b-wave was diminished 70%.

VER at elevated IOP

The amplitudes of the VERs from the homo- and contralateral visual cortex were decreased when IOP was 20% above the diastolic blood pressure. Above this level the VERs decreased much more than the b-wave and the a-wave. In all cases the difference between homo- and contralateral VERs was not significant. When the IOP approached the systolic blood pressure of the ophthalmic artery the VERs were eliminated.

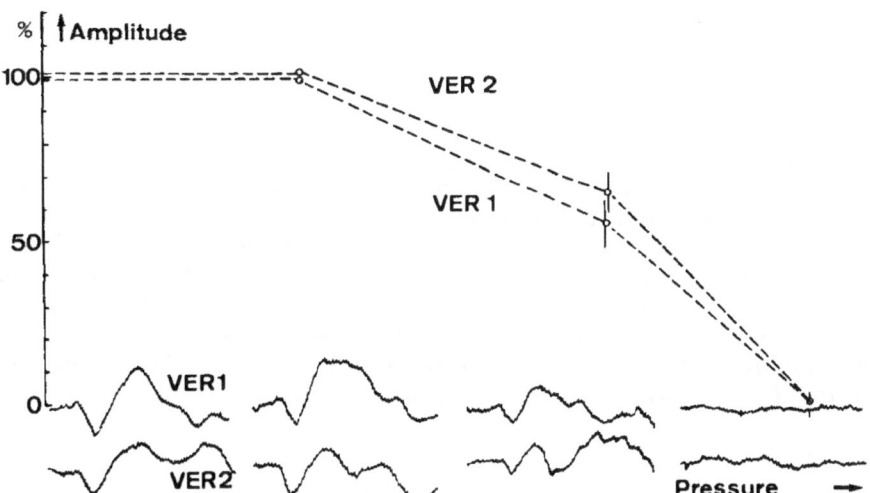

Fig. 2. The relative amplitude of the VER plotted against the IOP. The broken lines show averaged results of the homo- (VER_1) and contralateral (VER_2) visual cortex of ten patients. The vertical lines show the standard deviation of the ten patients. The results obtained with the IOPs at P_o, near Pd, in the middle between Pd and Ps, and near Ps. Below the broken lines the orginal responses are shown at normal and steplike elevated level of IOP.

DISCUSSION

In comparison with previous research we observed the first alteration of the ERG at a pressure near Pd (BORNSCHEIN 1958, NOELL 1952). At continuing elevations of the IOP the a-wave was more resistent than the b-wave. Previous experiments showed that there is a close relationship between the IOP and the blood supply in the eye. It might be that the changes of the ERG induced by elevated IOP resulted from secondary anoxia due to a disturbance of the blood circulation of the retina (GRANIT 1933, BORN-SCHEIN & ZWIAUER 1951-1952, HENKES 1957, BÖCK et al. 1959, BORNSCHEIN 1958, UENOYAMA 1969).

The level of the IOP that caused a change of the amplitudes of the VER was above Pd. From this point the amplitudes of the VERs decreased rapidly and were eliminated long before the IOP reached the Ps, while it was observed that the ERG showed an earlier but more gradual decrease in amplitude. The VER amplitude reacted later to the increased IOP but was the first to disappear.

The reason why the VER disappeared at elevated IOP at a lower level than the b-wave and a-wave could be a different sensitivity of blood circulation in the retina and in the optic disc to raised IOP.

Histological findings after total anoxia of the retinae showed that the ganglion cells were the first to be damaged with a simultaneus decrease in electrical activity (KROLL 1968, HAMASAKI & KROLL 1968). This decrease in electrical activity might be the reason that the impulses of the third neuron diminished correspondingly to the steplike elevation of the IOP, with a gradual decrease of amplitude of the VER at the same time.

SUMMARY

After induced elevations of the intraocular pressure, ERG and VER from the visual cortex of physically healthy persons were examined. The b-wave was more susceptible to elevations of the intraocular pressure than the a-wave. On a certain level of the intraocular pressure the VER also started to decrease. When intraocular pressure reached near systolic blood pressure of the ophthalmic artery the ERG could be recorded but the VER was unrecordable. We believe that these electrophysiological findings are caused by the different blood circulation of the retina and that of the optic disc with different sensitivity to raised intraocular pressure.

BIBLIOGRAPHY

BÖCK, J. BORNSCHEIN, J. & HOMMER, K. Die Überlebenszeit der a-Welle im ERG des Menschen. *Albrecht v. Graefes Arch. Ophthal.* 161, *6-15* (1959).

BORNSCHEIN, H. & ZWIAUER, A. Das Elektroretinogramm des Kaninschens bei experimenteller Erhöhung des intraocularen Druckes. *Albrecht von Graefes Arch. Ophthal.* 152, *527-531*, (1951-1952).

BORNSCHEIN, H. Spontan- und Belichtungsaktivität in Einzelfasern des Nervus opticus der Katze. *Z. Biol.* 110, *210-222*, (1958).

HAMASAKI, D.J. & KROLL, A.J. Experimental Central Retinal Artery Occlusion. (an electrophysiological study). *Arch. of Opthalm.* 80, *243-248* (1968).

HAYREH, S.S. Blood supply of the Optic Nerve Head and its role in Optic Atrophy, Glaucoma and Oedema of the Optic Disc. *British Journ. of Ophthalm.* 53, *721-748* (1969).

HAYREH, S.S. Pathogenesis of visual field defects. *British Journ. Ophthalm.* 54, *289-311* (1970).

HENKES, H. An Evaluation of the Influence of the Retinal and General Metabolic Condition on the Electrical Response of the Retina. *American Journ. Ophth.* 43, *67-86* (1957).

KROLL, A.J. Experimental Central Retinal Artery Occlusion. *Arch. of Ophthalm.* 79, *453-469* (1968).

NOELL, W.K. Electrophysiological study of the retina during metabolic impairment. *American Journ. Ophthalm.* 35, *126-133* (1952).

UENOYAMA, K., MC.DONALD, J.S. & DRANCE, S.M. The effect of intraocular pressure on visual electrical responses. *Arch. Ophthalm. (Chicago)* 81, *722-729* (1969).

PARAVENOUS PIGMENTARY RETINOPATHY

J. FRANÇOIS & A. DE ROUCK

(Ghent, Belgium)

The paravenous pigmentary retinopathy (or pigmented paravenous retino-choroidal degeneration) is a very rare disease. Cases have been published by BROWN (1937), CHI HSIN-HSIANG (1948), MORGAN (1948), LAW (1948), BROGNOLI (1949), WEVE (1957), ZIV & DUNPHY (1964), COLLIER (1965), TASSY et al. (1967), TOTA (1967), ARDOUIN et al. (1967), AMALRIC & SCHUM (1968), BONAMOUR & RAVAULT (1968).

The disease is characterized by perivascular and particularly perivenous pigmentary deposits, localized either around the optic disc or in the periphery. In some cases all the veins are involved, in others only some branches. Peripapillary chorioretinal atrophy with radiated extensions, following the vessels and situated behind the pigmentation, are frequently seen. The retina is greyish and is dystrophic at the level or in the neighbourhood of the lesions, but between the affected zones, the retina as well as the choroid are normal. The disc is mostly normal. The retinal vessels may be narrowed. Both eyes are involved and the lesions are usually symmetrical.

The *retinal functions* are very variable. The visual acuity is normal or only slightly reduced. The visual field may be normal (BROGNOLI, 1948; BONAMOUR & RAVAULT, 1968). The blind spot is sometimes enlarged (AMALRIC & SCHUM, 1968). Cuneiform defects, corresponding to the paravenous dystrophic zones, or more severe alterations of the visual fields may be seen, such as a ring scotoma (TASSY et al., 1967) or a peripheral narrowing of the isopters with enlargement of the blind spot (BROWN, 1937; CHI HSIN-HSIANG, 1948; LAW, 1948; WEVE, 1957; ZIV & DUNPHY, 1964; ARDOUIN et al., 1967).

The dark adaptation curve may be normal (TOTA, 1967; AMALRIC & SCHUM, 1968) or subnormal with elevation of the final scotopic threshold (BROGNOLI, 1948; ZIV & DUNPHY, 1964; TASSY et al., 1967; BONAMOUR & RAVAULT, 1968).

We have little information concerning the ERG and EOG.

BROGNOLI (1948), AMALRIC & SCHUM (1968) were able to follow their cases during respectively 6 and 10 years. There was no change in the ophthalmoscopical aspect or in the functional state.

We have examined 5 cases of paravenous pigmentary retinopathy particularly on the bioelectric point of view.

The visual field was tested at the Goldmann perimeter. For the subjective dark adaptation curve we have used the Goldmann-Weekers adaptometer: after 5 min light adaptation at 2000 asb, the final threshold was determined after 15 min; the normal threshold is $\overline{5},0$ with an upper limit of $\overline{5},7$. Colour vision was tested with the Ishihara and AO-HRR pseudoisochromatic plates, the panel D15, the tritan plate and the Naegel anomaloscope.

For the ERG recording the xenon stroboscope Van Gogh was placed 10 cm in front of the patient. Neutral filters were used in order to obtain intensities varying up to 3 logarithmic units. After preamplification a direct inscription on an Elema Mingograph and a recording of the resulting summation of 5 to 10 ERG responses on a cathodic oscilloscope were made (analysing time 250 msec, time constant 0,3 msec).

The ERG was recorded on the following way:
I.   After dark adaptation,
1.   Response in red light.
2.   Responses with single flashes of increasing intensities (from $\overline{3},0$ to $0,0$ relative log units).
3.   Low flicker (frequency of 1,5 c/s) obtained at the same intensity levels of stimulation as the single responses.
II.   After light adaptation (300 Lux), single flashes with increasing intensities (from $\overline{3},0$ to $0,0$ relative log units).

For the interpretation of the ERG the following data were taken into account: amplitude of the a and b-waves in darkness and in light, ratio a_1/a_2, oscillatory potentials and late photopic oscillatory complex, latency and culmination times of the components.

The normal photopic b wave has $100\,\mu V$ (m-2S: $70\,\mu V$) and the normal scotopic b wave $320\,\mu V$ (m-2S : $240\,\mu V$).

For the EOG we used the technique of FRANÇOIS et al. (1966). We have mainly taken into account the L/D ratio of Arden. This ratio is normally between 210 and 180, although lower values between 180 and 165 may be found in normal subjects.

RESULTS

The results obtained in our 5 cases are summarized in table I.

All our cases show common features. The pigment deposits are localized around some peripheral venous branches in the equatorial area. They are associated with small zones of chorioretinal atrophy. Outside these zones the retina is normal, as is proven by the fluorescein angiography.

Other ophthalmoscopical signs are inconstant. The disc is either normal or discoloured. The retinal vessels are either normal or rather narrow. Case I is a bilateral vitreoretinal degeneration with microfibrillar vitreous alterations, peripheral retinoschisis and unilateral inferior detachment of the retina. Case II shows an aspect of peripapillary choroidal sclerosis. In case III there are macular lesions and only the veins of the inferior half of the retina are involved in both eyes. In case V the right eye shows a paravenous pigmentary retinopathy of the inferior half, while the left eye shows

TABLE I

Sex	Age	V	Vis. Field	Dark adaptation	Colour Vision	ERG Phot. b wave μV	ERG Scot. b wave μV	EOG L/D ratio %	Clinical features
1 M	33	RE 1/50	superotemporal defect	4,2	Blue-yellow defect	15	20	115	Vitreoretinal degeneration with retinoschisis. R.E.: inferior retinal detachment
		LE 12/10	enlarged blind spot	5,6	no	60	210	150	
2 F	44	RE 2/10	concentric narrowing	3,3	no	30	50	120	Peripapillary choroidal atrophy. Most of the peripheral veins surrounded by pigment clumps
		LE 2/10	no	3,0	no	85	230	150	
	46	RE 1/10	tubular 5°	2,2	?	20	40	115	
		LE 1/10	tubular 15°	2,2	?	90	240	140	
3 M	57	RE 1/10	superior defect	4,0	blue-yellow defect	40	245	160	Paravenous pigmentations in the inferior half of the retina. Macular degeneration. Involvement of the cone function
		LE 10/10	superior defect	4,0	idem	30	170	154	
4 M	61	RE 1/50	central scotoma. Peripheral narrowing	3,2	?	10	20	115	Peripheral paravenous pigmentary retinopathy
		LE 10/10	no	4,3	no	60	130	126	
5 M	26	RE 10/10	ring scotoma	5,6	no	110	180	124	RE: peripheral inferior veins surrounded by pigment clumps LE: disseminated pigmentations in the fundus, but particularly around the veins. Narrow arteries.
		LE 1/10	tubular	4,3	blue-yellow defect	30	60	100	

a diffuse retinal involvement with yellow spots in the peripapillary area and disseminated pigment clumps, although more concentrated around the veins.

Visual functions. — They are very variable.

The visual field is sometimes normal (case IV), but mostly parthologic. Enlargement of the blind spot (case I), ring scotoma (case V) narrowing of the peripheral isopters (case II, fig. 1, case IV), localized peripheral defect (cases I and III) and tubular fields (cases II and V) have been seen.

The dark adaptation curve (fig. 2) was either normal (cases I and V) or slightly subnormal with elevation of the final threshold. Case II showed a monophasic curve with absence of the Kohlrausch kink.

The colour vision was either normal or abnormal (blue-yellow deficiency).

The bioelectric tests were mostly severely disturbed (Fig. 3 and 4). In opposition to the findings in the classical pigmentary retinopathy, the ERG was, however, never abolished, even not in the left eye of case V, where the retina was diffusely involved (fig. 5). The reduction of the ERG varied widely. Sometimes only residual potentials were found. In one case the ERG was normal (case II, left eye, fig. 6). Usually the response was subnormal, the temporal characteristics being normal or abnormal. The reduction of the ERG was not the same in both eyes, while in classical pigmentary retinopathy an asymmetric behaviour is rare.

In case III (fig. 7) the reduction of the ERG involved particularly the photopic components. This case was also characterized by macular alterations, a paravenous pigmentary retinopathy of the inferior half of the retina

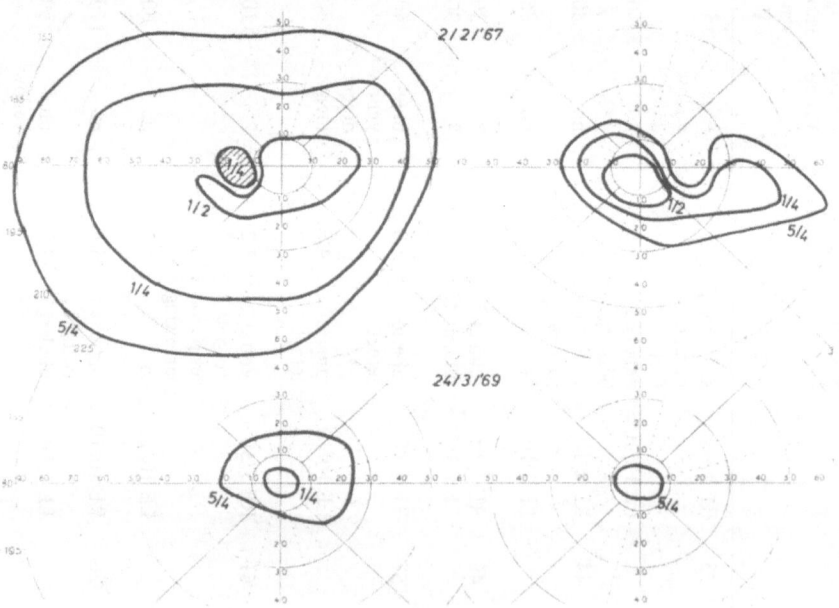

Fig. 1.   Case II. Progressive deterioration of the visual field.

284

and a monophasic dark adaptation curve. It is closely related to the cases of progressive cone dysfunction associated with a sector shaped retinopathy, as described by SLOAN & BROWN (1962), THALER et al. (1972), FRANÇOIS et al. (1973).

The EOG was obviously subnormal or abnormal. It seemed less involved in case III (cone dystrophy) and was completely extinguished in the left eye of case V (diffuse retinopathy).

There was no correlation between the bioelectrical results and the functional state of the retina. So, for instance, in case IV the retinal functions were nearly normal, but the ERG and the EOG were very much reduced. In case II the EOG was subnormal, but the ERG was normal and remained so, although the visual functions were progressively and severely impaired.

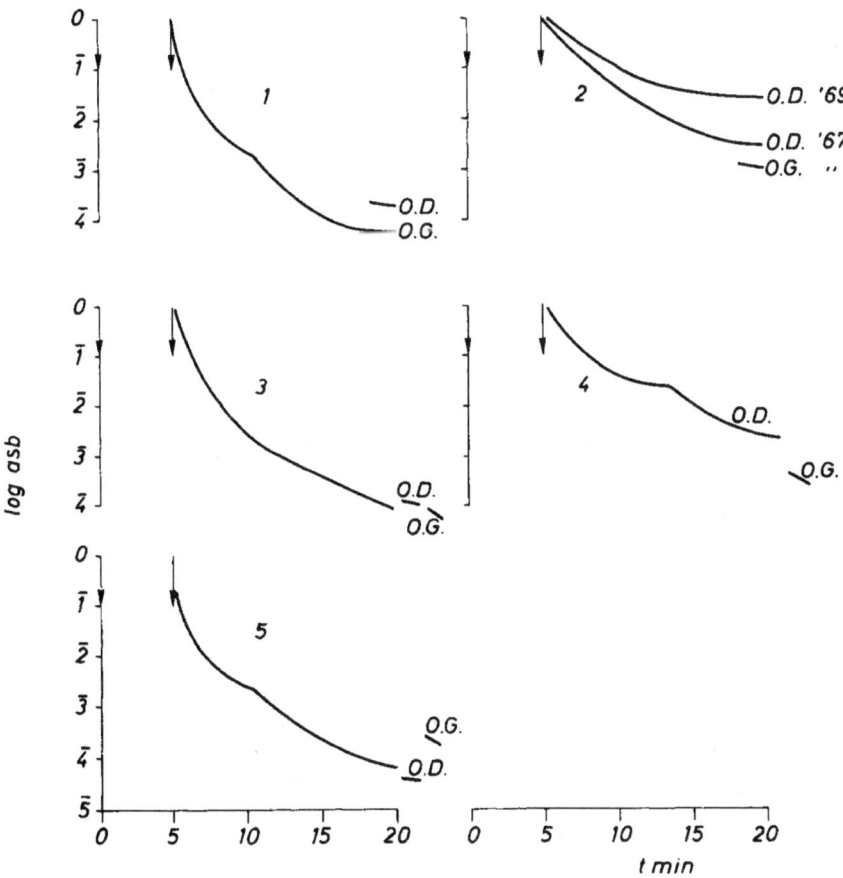

Fig. 2. Dark adaptation curves of the 5 cases. Goldmann-Weekers adaptometer. Preadaptation of 2000 asb during 5 min.

285

CONCLUSIONS

Our 5 cases represent a heterogenous group of atypical tapeto-retinal dystrophies of the paravenous type. The chorioretinal and pigmentary lesions were localized around some peripheral venous branches ophthalmoscopically as well as fluoroangiographically.

The visual functions were severely impaired, just as in classical pigmentary retinopathy. The EOG was obviously abnormal and even extinguished in all the cases. The ERG was involved in a very irregular way. It may be normal, but sometimes only residual potentials remain. The results are not

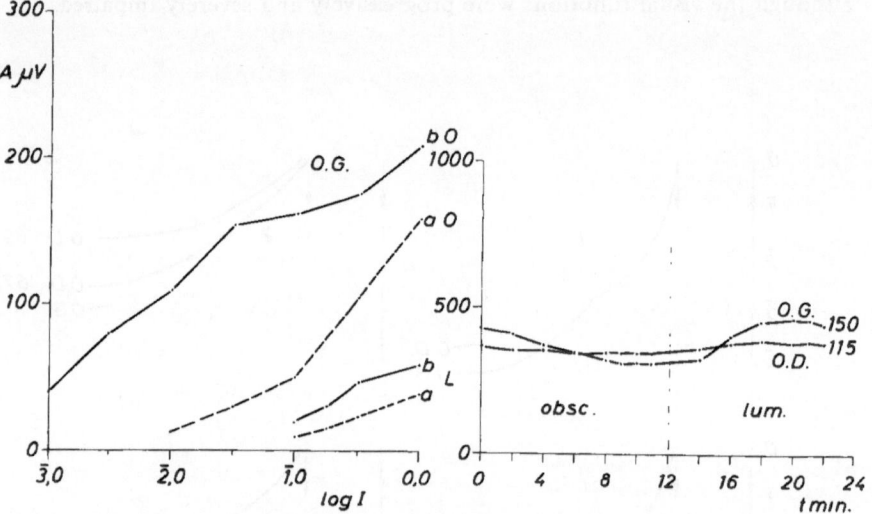

Fig. 3. Case I. At the left, ERG (L.E.): amplitude curves of the *a* and *b* waves. O: dark-adapted, L: light adapted. At the right: amplitude of the EOG of both eyes during dark and light adaptation (the numbers refer to the L/D ratio x 100).

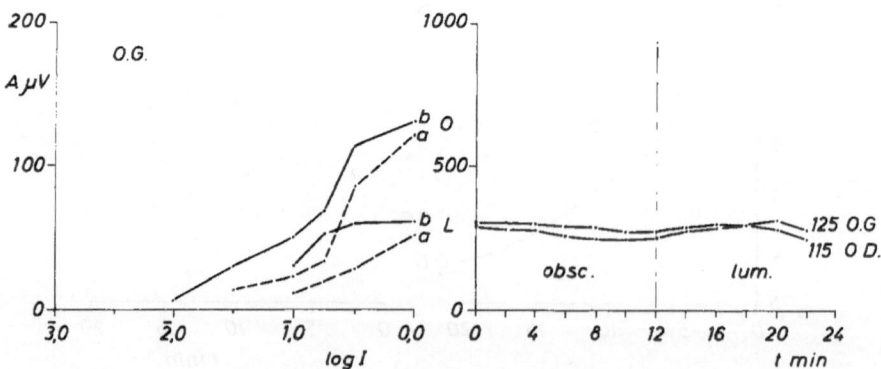

Fig. 4. Case IV. At the left, amplitude curves of the *a* and *b* waves of the L.E. in darkness (O) and light (L). At the right amplitude of the EOG of both eyes during dark and light adaptation.

286

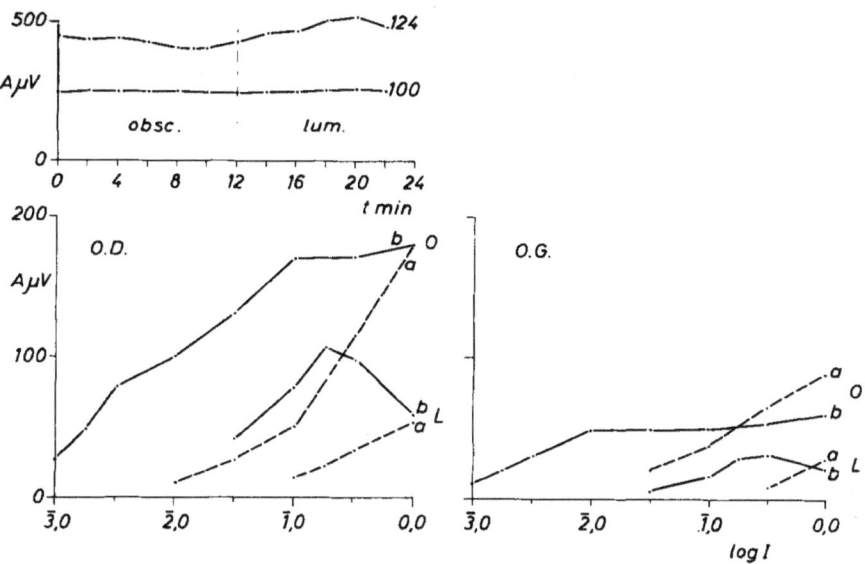

Fig. 5. Case V. Upper record: amplitude of the EOG of both eyes during dark and light adaptation. Below, amplitude curves of the *a* and *b* waves in darkness (O) and light (L); at the left right eye, at the right left eye.

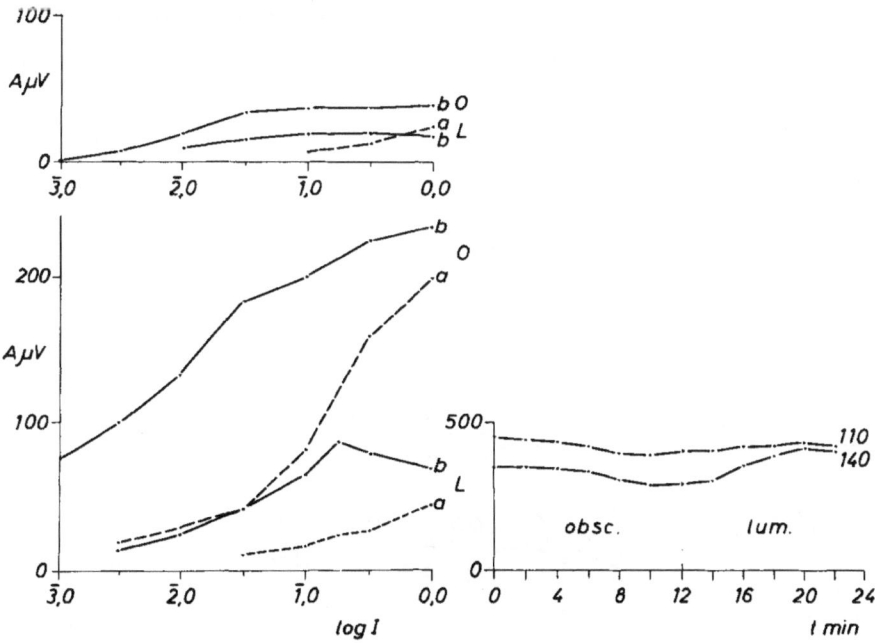

Fig. 6. Case II. At the left, amplitude curves of the *a* and *b* waves in darkness (O) and light (L): above right eye, below left eye. At the right, amplitude of the EOG of both eyes during dark and light adaptation.

symmetrical in both eyes and are very different from these seen in classical pigmentary retinopathy.

One has to distinguish between, on the one hand, the true stationary paravenous pigmentary retinopathy, where the alteration of the visual functions is minimal and related to the areas of paravenous dystrophy, and, on the other hand, the progressive paravenous pigmentary retinopathy, characterized by a localized dystrophy, as proven ophthalmoscopically and fluoroangiographically, a peculiar behaviour of the ERG and a severe and progressive deterioration of the visual functions. These cases are, nevertheless, to be differentiated from some atypical chorioretinal degenerations, which show the ophthalmoscopical aspect of a paravenous retinopathy, but where the fluorescein angiography reveals a diffuse involvement of the pigment epithelium (BABEL et al., 1972).

SUMMARY

Five cases of atypical paravenous pigmentary retinopathy are discussed particularly on the bioelectrical point of view.

REFERENCES

AMALRIC P. & SCHUM U. Pigmentierte, paravenöse Netz- und Aderhautatrophie. *Klin. Mbl. Augenheilk.*, 153, 770-775, 1968.

ARDOUIN M., BEAUCHAMP, CHANTEAU Y. & URVOY M. Dégénérescence retino-choroïdienne paraveineuse pigmentée. *Bull. Soc. Ophtal. France*, 67, 742-744, 1967.

BABEL J., STANGOS N., SPIRITUS M. & KOROL S. Dégénérescences chorio-rétiniennes du pôle posterieur. *Bull. Soc. Franç. Ophtal.*, 85, 479-494, 1972.

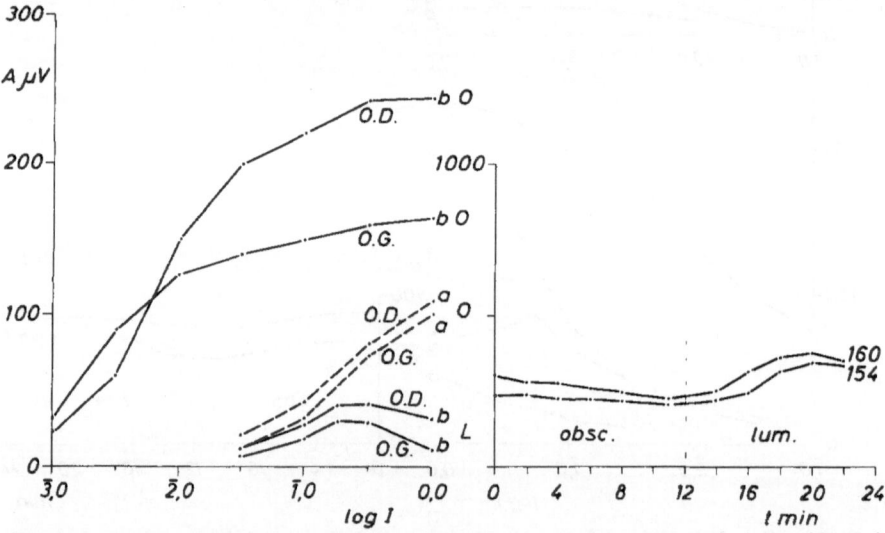

Fig. 7. Case III. At the left, amplitude curves of the *a* and *b* waves in darkness (O) and light (L). OD: right eye, OG: left eye. At the right, amplitude of the EOG of both eyes (reduction of the photopic components).

288

BONAMOUR G. & RAVAULT M. Dégénérescence chorio-rétinienne paraveineuse pigmentée. *Bull. Soc. Ophtal. France* , 68, *681-684*, 1968.

BROGNOLI C. Sopra un caso di pigmentazione anomala del fondo oculare (melanosi della retina). *Arch. Ottal.*, 53, *99-119*, 1949.

BROWN T.H. Retino-choroiditis radiata. *Brit. J. Ophthal.*, 21, *645-648*, 1937.

CHI-HSIN-HSIANG. Retinochoroiditis radiata. Amer. *J. Ophthal.*, 31, *1485-1487*, 1948.

COLLIER M. Dégénérescence choriorétinienne paraveineuse pigmentée. *Bull. Soc. Ophtal. France*, 65, 775-782, 1965.

FRANCESCHETTI A., FRANÇOIS J. & BABEL J. Les hérédo-dégénerescences chorio-rétiniennes. Ed. Masson, Paris, 1963.

FRANÇOIS J., DE ROUCK A., CAMBIE E. & ZANEN A. L'électro-diagnostic des affections rétiniennes (Etude des potentiels de repos et d'action rétiniens). Ed. Masson, Paris, 1974.

FRANÇOIS J., DE ROUCK A., VERRIEST G., DE LAEY J.J. & CAMBIE E. Cone dysfunctions. Proc. XI ISCERG Symp., Bad-Nauheim, 1973 Doc. Ophthal. Proc. Series 4, *99-105*, 1973.

FRANÇOIS J., DE ROUCK A., VERRIEST G. & SZMIGIELSKI M. An extended clinical test of the ocular standing potential and its results in some cases of retinal degeneration. Proc. IV ISCERG Symp., Hakone, *Jap. J. Ophthal., suppl.*, 10, *257-268*, 1966.

LAW F. Discussion of the paper of Morgan O.G. *Proc. Roy. Soc. Med.*, 41, *727*, 1948.

MORGAN O.G. Congenital pigmentation of the retina. *Proc. Roy Soc. Med.*, 41, *726-727*, 1948.

SLOAN L. & BROWN D.J. Progressive retinal degeneration with selective involvement of the cone mechanism. *Amer. J. Ophthal.*, 54, *629-641*, 1962.

TASSY A.F., JAYLE G.E. & SAROCCO J.B. A propos d'un cas d'engaînement noir des veines rétiniennes. *Bull. Soc. Ophtal. France*, 67, *690-692*, 1967.

THALER A., HEILIG P. & SLEZAK H. Kombination einer angeborenen Achromatopsie mit sektorenformiger Degeneration pigmentosa retinae. *Graefes Arch. Ophthal.*, 183, *310-316*, 1972.

THALER A., HEILIG P. & SLEZAK H. Sectorial retinopathia pigmentosa. Involvement of the retina and pigment epithelium as reflected in bioelectric response. Proc. X ISCERG Symp., Los Angeles, 1972, Doc. Ophthal. Proc. Series, 4, *237-244*, 1973.

TOTA G. Retinite pigmentosa juxtapapillare. *Ann. Ottal.*, 93, *575-582*, 1967.

WEVE J. Degeneratio retinae paravenosa. *Mod. Probl. Ophthal., Karger, Basel*, 1, *664-667*, 1957.

ZIV B. & DUNPHY E. Pigmented retinal arteries in retinitis pigmentosa. *Amer. J. Ophthal.*, 57, *132-133*, 1964.

A COMPARISON OF ELECTRORETINOGRAPHIC AND DARK ADAPTATION STUDIES IN RETINITIS PIGMENTOSA

GEORGE W. WEINSTEIN, GEORGE G. LOWELL &
ROBERT R. HOBSON

(San Antonio, Texas)

INTRODUCTION

Electroretinography and studies of dark adaptation are both frequently used laboratory tests for retinitis pigmentosa (R.P.). Until the past decade, a complete absence of the electroretinogram (ERG) was thought to be pathognomonic for R.P. (FRANÇOIS, 1961) but RUBINO & PONTE (1962) documented the presence of a subnormal ERG in 30 patients reported by 8 different authors. All of these patients showed decreased dark adaptation, whatever the evolution or seriousness of their disease. This high correlation between abnormal dark adaptation and electroretinography in the diagnosis of R.P. has been found by other authors. (CAMPBELL, 1965; GOURAS & CARR 1964, GOURAS, ARMINGTON, KROPFL & GUNKEL 1964) This raises the question of whether studies of dark adaptation (DA) are of equal or greater diagnostic value than electroretinography.

METHODS

The present report is a retrospective analysis of 2 groups of R.P. patients studied. with a variety of retinal function tests: a San Antonio (S.A.) group of 100 patients and a Baltimore group of 60 patients. Patients were selected for study if they had a history of night blindness, fundus findings typical of R.P., or a strong family history of R.P. The diagnosis of R.P. was made on the basis of personal or family history, fundus findings, and visual fields. ERG and dark adaptation studies were used as confirmatory tests.

The ERG studies of all patients used the previously reported constant amplitude method (WEINSTEIN, WEINBERG & HOBSON 1970) where a light stimulus is varied in intensity by use of neutral density filters, in both light and dark adaptation, using a translucent contact lens electrode. For the S.A. group, conventional Goldmann-Weekers dark adaptometry (GWDA) was used to test an 11 degree area, 11 degrees superior to fixation. Dark adaptation in the Baltimore group was studied using the Tubingen perimeter to examine the absolute profile visual field (TAPF). (LINDQUIST, WEINSTEIN & FEIOCK 1970, FORSTOT, WEINSTEIN & FEIOCK 1970). This method tests the visual field of the dark adapted eye in a given meridian with multiple stationary stimuli of variable intensity.

Of a total of 100 patients in the S.A. group, 52 had both ERG and GWDA.
Of 60 patients in the Baltimore group, 40 had both ERG and TAPF.
    The results were assorted according to the following scheme:
I.   Agreement between ERG and DA
    A.   Normal ERG/normal DA (Fig. 1)
    B.   Subnormal ERG/subnormal DA (Fig. 2)
    C.   Non-recordable ERG/abnormal DA (Fig. 3)
II.   Disagreement between ERG and DA
    A.   Normal ERG
        1.   Normal ERG/mildly abnormal DA (Fig. 4)
        2.   Normal ERG/markedly abnormal DA (Fig. 5)

NORMAL ERG

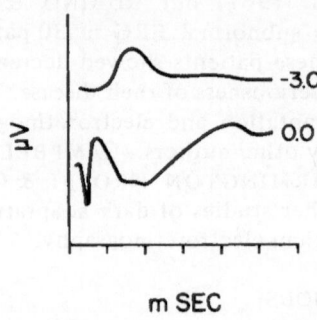

NORMAL DA

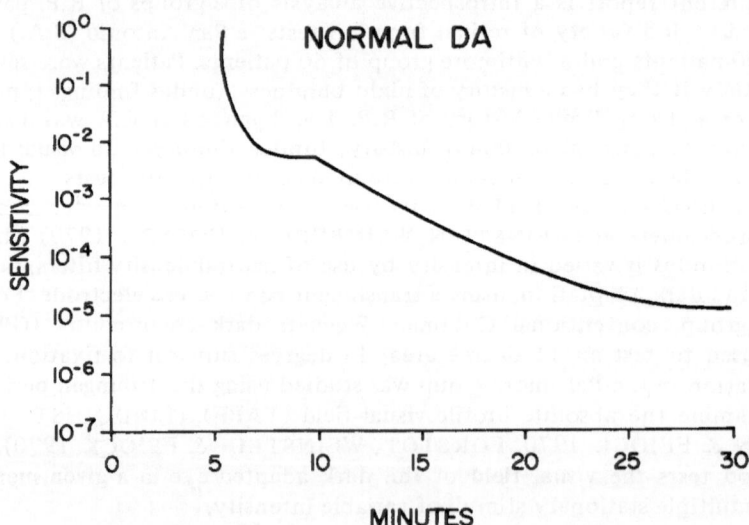

Fig. 1.   A normal ERG above and a normal D.A. below, both from the same patient
with retinitis pigmentosa

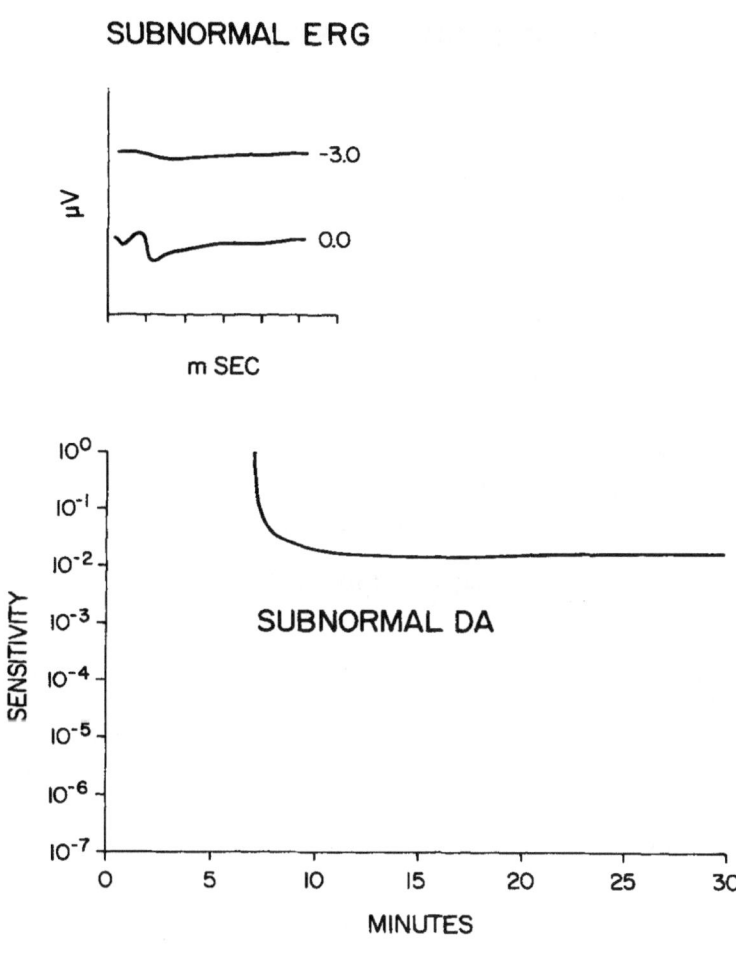

Fig. 2. A subnormal ERG above and a subnormal D.A. below, both from the same patient with retinitis pigmentosa

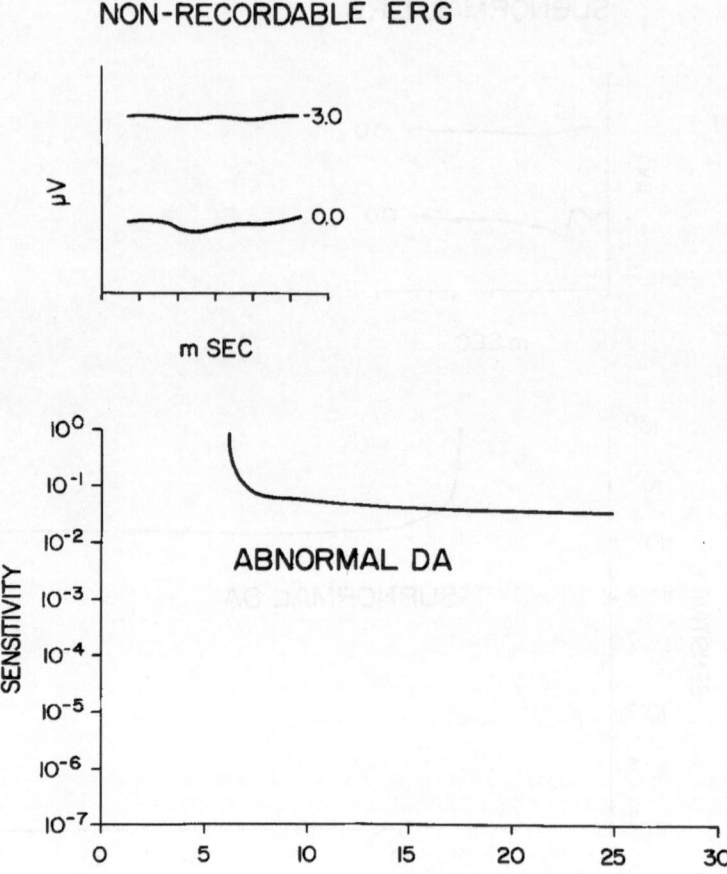

Fig. 3. A non-recordable ERG above and an abnormal D.A. below, both from the same patient with retinitis pigmentosa

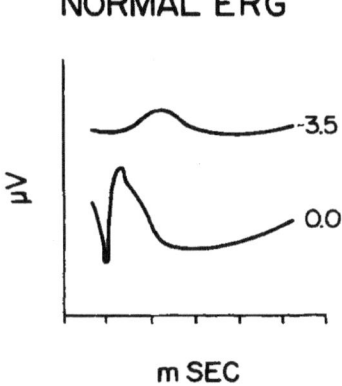

NORMAL ERG

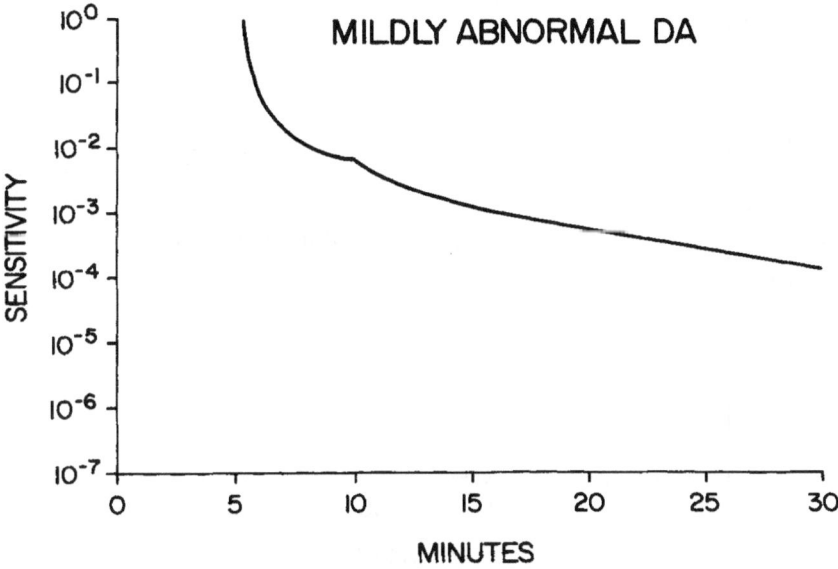

Fig. 4. A normal ERG above and a mildly abnormal D.A. below, both from the same patient with retinitis pigmentosa

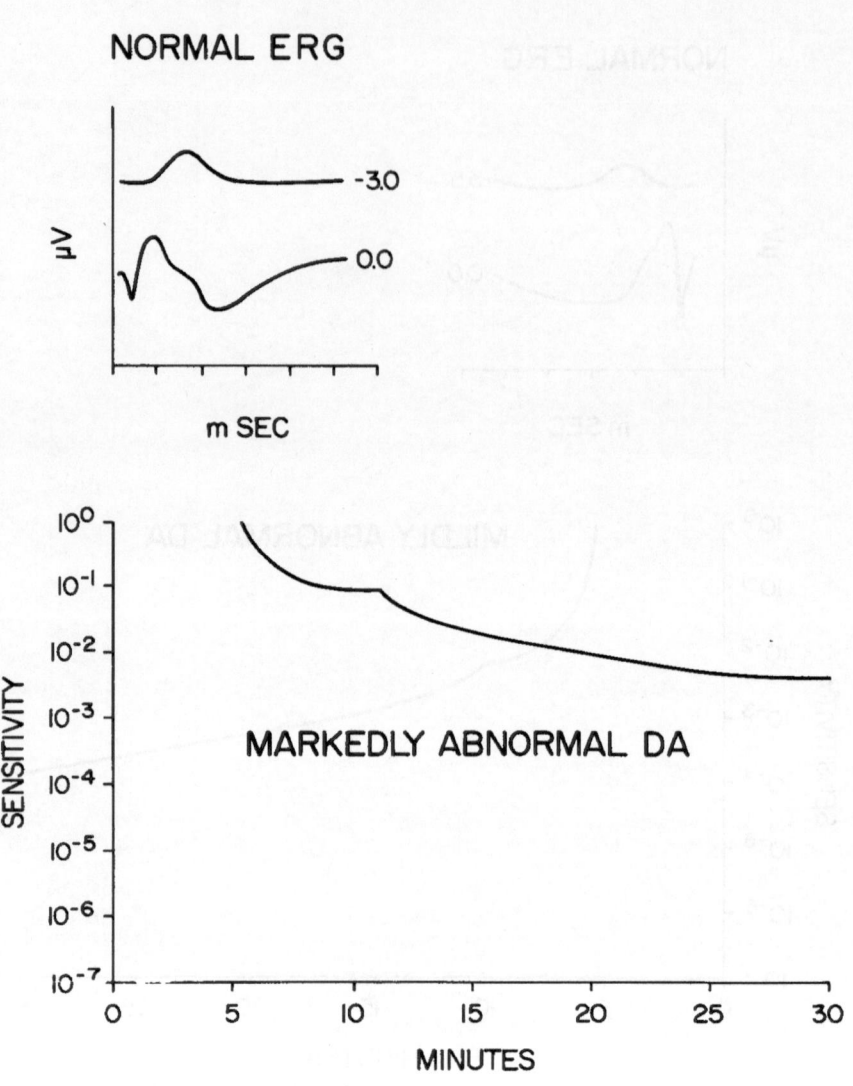

Fig. 5. A normal ERG above and a markedly abnormal D.A. below, both from the same patient with retinitis pigmentosa

SUBNORMAL ERG

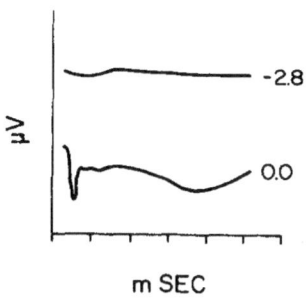

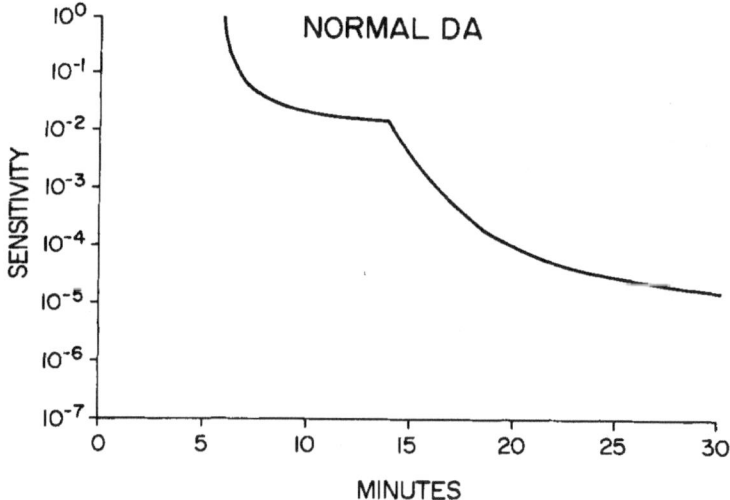

Fig. 6. A subnormal ERG above and a normal D.A. below, both from the same patient with retinitis pigmentosa

B.   Normal DA
  1.   Subnormal ERG/normal DA (Fig. 6)
  2.   Non-recordable ERG/normal DA (Fig. 7)

Figures 8, 9, and 10 show the results of this data for the S.A. group, Baltimore group, and the 2 groups combined, respectively. The S.A. group, comparing ERG with GWDA showed 71% agreement, 23% mild disagreement and 6% marked disagreement. The Baltimore group comparing ERG and TAPF showed 90% agreement, 3% mild disagreement, and 7% marked disagreement. In the combined patients, 79% showed agreement of ERG and DA, 16% mild disagreement, and 7% marked disagreement.

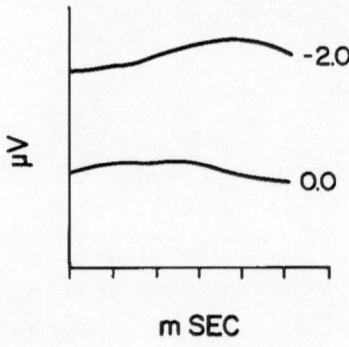

NON-RECORDABLE ERG

-2.0

0.0

μV

m SEC

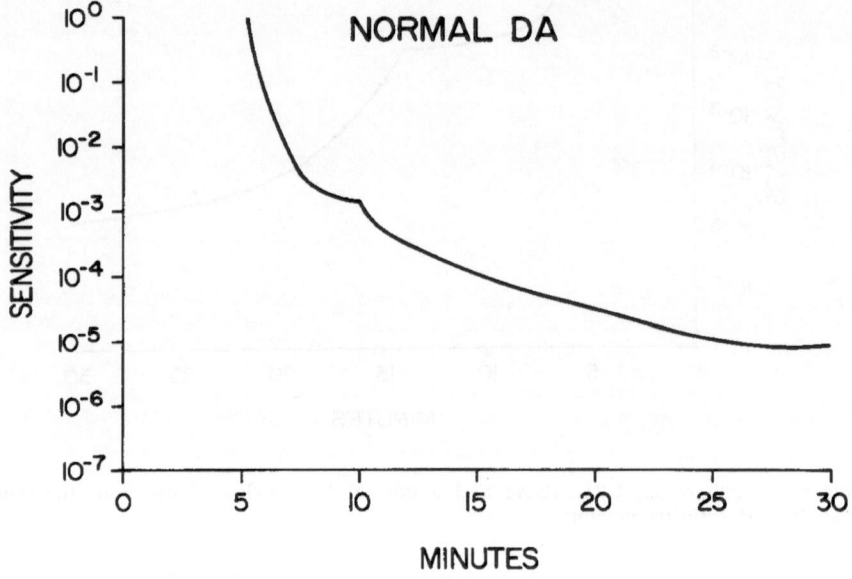

NORMAL DA

SENSITIVITY

10^0
10^{-1}
10^{-2}
10^{-3}
10^{-4}
10^{-5}
10^{-6}
10^{-7}

0   5   10   15   20   25   30

MINUTES

Fig. 7. A non-recordable ERG above and a normal D.A. below, both from the same patient with retinitis pigmentosa

In both series, most patients showed close agreement between ERG and DA studies, implying that either test would suffice to confirm the diagnosis. The fact that there were no normal dark adaptation examinations in the Baltimore R.P. patients in sub-group II-B (normal DA, with subnormal or non-recordable ERG) suggests that the TAPF is the most sensitive test, compared to the ERG and GWDA. However, this method has the disadvantages of being expensive and time consuming, and it requires a specially trained technician. Of the disagreement in the S.A. group, the 12 patients with mild disagreement were divided evenly, 6 in II-A-1 (normal ERG/mildly abnormal DA) and 6 in II-B-1 (subnormal ERG/normal DA). The 3 patients with marked disagreement were divided, with 2 in II-A-2 (normal ERG/ markedly abnormal DA) and 1 in II-B-2 (non-recordable ERG/normal DA). This suggests that the ERG and GWDA are of equal value in the diagnosis of R.P.

The higher sensitivity of the TAPF as compared to GWDA can be explained by referring to a case described previously (LINDQUIST, WEINSTEIN & FEIOCK 1970). In that report, Case 2 is a 30 year old female, the

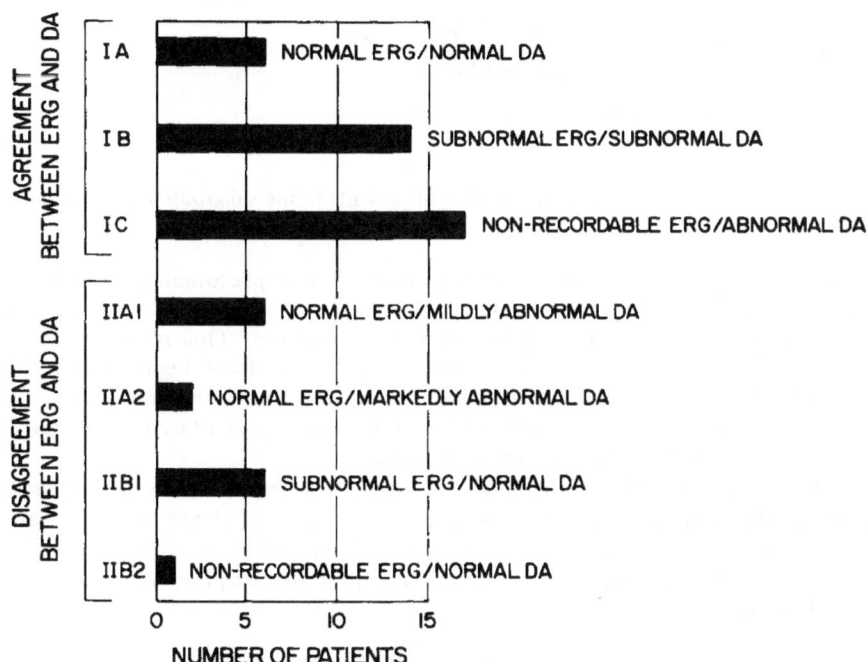

Fig. 8. A histogram depicting the number of patients in the subgroup of the San Antonio study

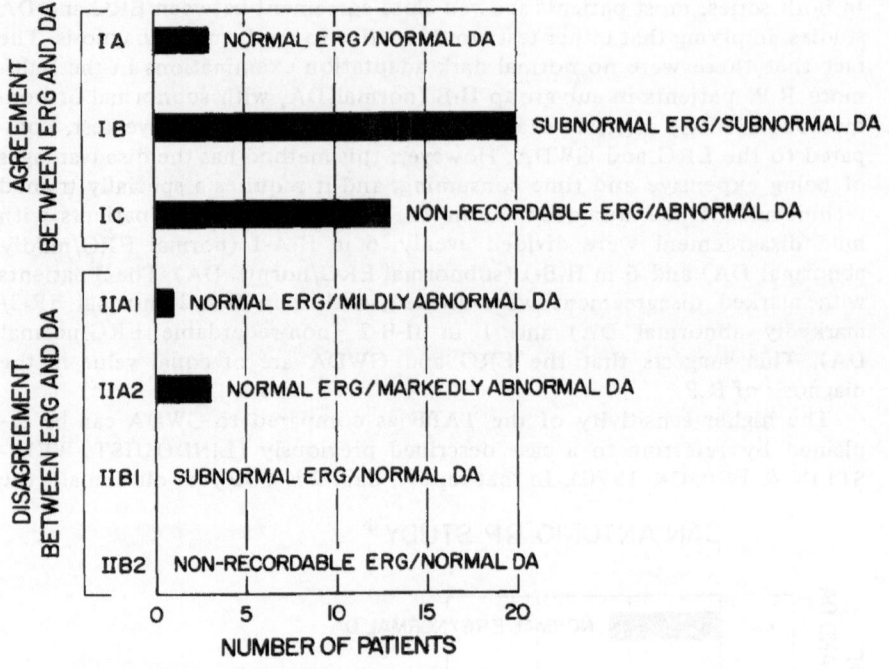

Fig. 9. A histogram depicting the number of patients in the subgroup of the Baltimore study

mother of a severely affected R.P. patient. She is presumably a carrier of X-linked disease. Her TAPF is slightly abnormal everywhere in the horizontal meridian except 9-15 degrees nasal to the fovea. This relatively small island of normal scotopic sensitivity might well have been chosen for GWDA. If so, the patient would have been considered normal. Thus, the GWDA assumes that the 1 retinal locus tested is representative of all areas, when, in fact, this might not always be true.

It appears that the single most sensitive test for the early diagnosis of R.P. is the Tubingen absolute profile field. Next best are the ERG and Goldmann-Weekers dark adaptometry which are of equal value when performed separately, but when combined, equal the diagnostic value of the TAPF alone.

SUMMARY

Both ERG and DA are usually abnormal in patients with retinitis pigmentosa (R.P.) With improvements in electroretinography (ERG), it had been established that not every patient with R.P. has an extinguished ERG.

300

To determine the relative diagnostic value of the ERG and studies of dark adaptation (DA), the data from 92 patients with R.P. was analyzed retrospectively. ERG was done with the constant amplitude method. DA was tested in 52 patients with the Goldmann-Weekers dark adaptometry (GWDA) and in 40 patients with the Tubingen absolute profile field (TAPF).

Although TAPF appears to be somewhat superior diagnostically, it is technically difficult, time consuming, and expensive. ERG and GWDA are separately of equal diagnostic value, and when used together are equal to the TAPF.

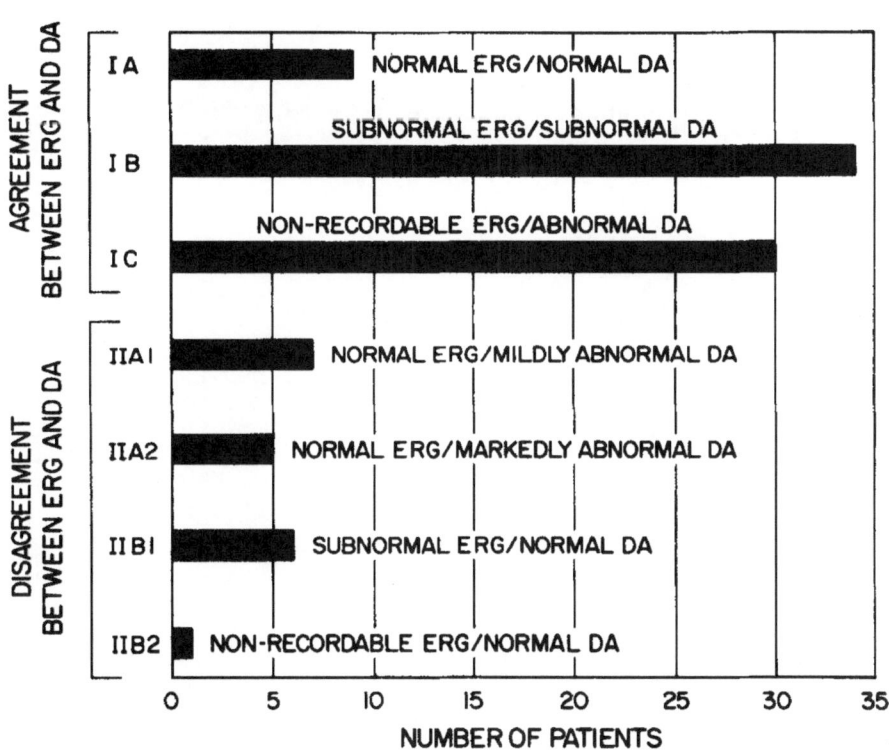

Fig. 10. A histogram depicting the number of patients in the subgroups of the San Antonio and Baltimore studies combined

REFERENCES

CAMPBELL, D. Some Physiological Aspects of Retinitis Pigmentosa in Man and in Animals. *Trans. Ophthalmol. Soc. Uk* 82: *667-702*, 1965.

FORSTOT, S., WEINSTEIN, G. & FEIOCK, K.: Studies with the Tübingen Perimeter of Harms and Aulhorn. *Annals of Ophthal.* 2: *843-54*, 1970.

FRANÇOIS, J. Chorioretinal Heredo-degeneration. *Proc. R. Soc. Med.* 54: *1109-15*, 1961.

GOURAS, P. & CARR, R. Electrophysiological Studies in Early Retinitis Pigmentosa. *Arch. Ophthalmol.* 72: *104-10*, 1964.

GOURAS, P., ARMINGTON, J., KROPFL, W. & GUNKEL, R.: Electronic Computation of Human Retinal and Brain Responses to Light Stimulation. *Ann N.Y. Acad. Sci.* 115: *763-75*, 1964.

LINDQUIST, C., WEINSTEIN, G. & FEIOCK, K.: Absolute Profile Visual Field Studies with the Tubingen Perimeter in Normal Subjects and in Patients with Early Retinitis Pigmentosa. *Eye Ear Nose Throat Mon.* 49: *497-502*, 1970.

RUBINO, A. & PONTI, F. The Role of Electroretinography in the Diagnosis and Prognosis of Retinitis Pigmentosa. *Acta Ophthalmol. (suppl)* 70: *232-7*, 1962.

WEINSTEIN, G., WEINBERG, R. & HOBSON, R.: Constant Amplitude Electroretinography for the Determination of Retinal Sensitivity in Normal and Abnormal Subjects. *Am. J. Ophthal.* 69: *836-49*, 1970.

TAPETO-CHOROIDAL ATROPHY

J.G.H. SCHMIDT

(Cologne, West Germany)

It is the exception among those diseases labelled 'primary choroidal sclerosis' to detect arteriosclerotic changes. According to histological investigations by ASHTON, BABEL, KLIEN, HOWARD & WOLF it is more often the case to find atrophy of muscular vessel-wall portions and of remaining intravascular tissue, together with fibrosis. Thus, the designation 'primary choroidal atrophy' is much more to the point. However, ophthalmoscopically it is sometimes extremely difficult to distinguish this from genuine arteriosclerotic processes, or, in rare cases, from conditions following widespread chorio-retinitis.

As many observations show, these slow, advancing processes carry with them a high degree of hereditary taint. This would seem to justify the term choroidal dystrophy, currently being used more and more. Several examinations in the early stage of choroidal atrophy indicate that initial damage occurs in the pigment epithelium and spreads to the choriocapillaris (PAMEYER; WAARDENBURG; KURSTJENS; DEUTMAN) while the retina is effected only in the later stages. For this reason, a relatively slight change in the electro-retinogram (ERG) and a severe damage in the electro-oculogram (EOG) can be expected. Only in the final stage the ERG may be highly reduced or extinguished beside a flat EOG.

In cases of retinal dystrophy — especially central and pericentral retinopathia pigmentosa — zones of choroidal dystrophy may also be detected ophthalmoscopically, making diagnosis difficult. The differential diagnosis between choroidal dystrophy and choroidal atrophy can be especially difficult if — as in the following cases — there is no possibility of examining members of the patient's family.

CASE HISTORIES

Case 1: Peripapillary and pericentral choroidal atrophy.

Fig. 5 shows the ophthalmoscopic picture of peripapillary retinal and choroidal atrophy. On the right side, an extension of this atrophy has reached

This research was supported by Deutsche Forschungsgemeinschaft, Bonn/Bad Godesberg, Germany.

the macula and caused considerable reduction of visual acuity (27-3-73). This functional deterioration can also be seen in the decrease of the ERG potentials. During treatment with Cosaldon (Fig. 1c), the patient regained completely normal functional capacity. There remained on the right side a paracentral scotoma and on the left a peripapillary scotoma. Dark adaptation was bilaterally normal in all examinations. During the period of observation, no changes were found in the repeatedly photographed ophthalmoscopic findings.

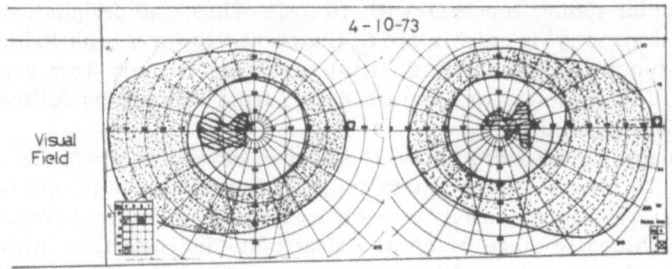

Fig. 1a-c. (Case 1): Peripapillary and pericentral choroidal atrophy.

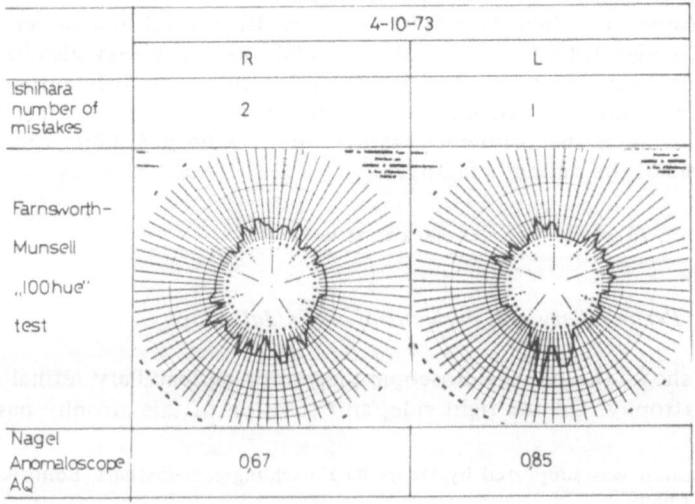

	4-10-73	
	R	L
Ishihara number of mistakes	2	I
Farnsworth– Munsell „100hue" test		
Nagel Anomaloscope AQ	0,67	0,85

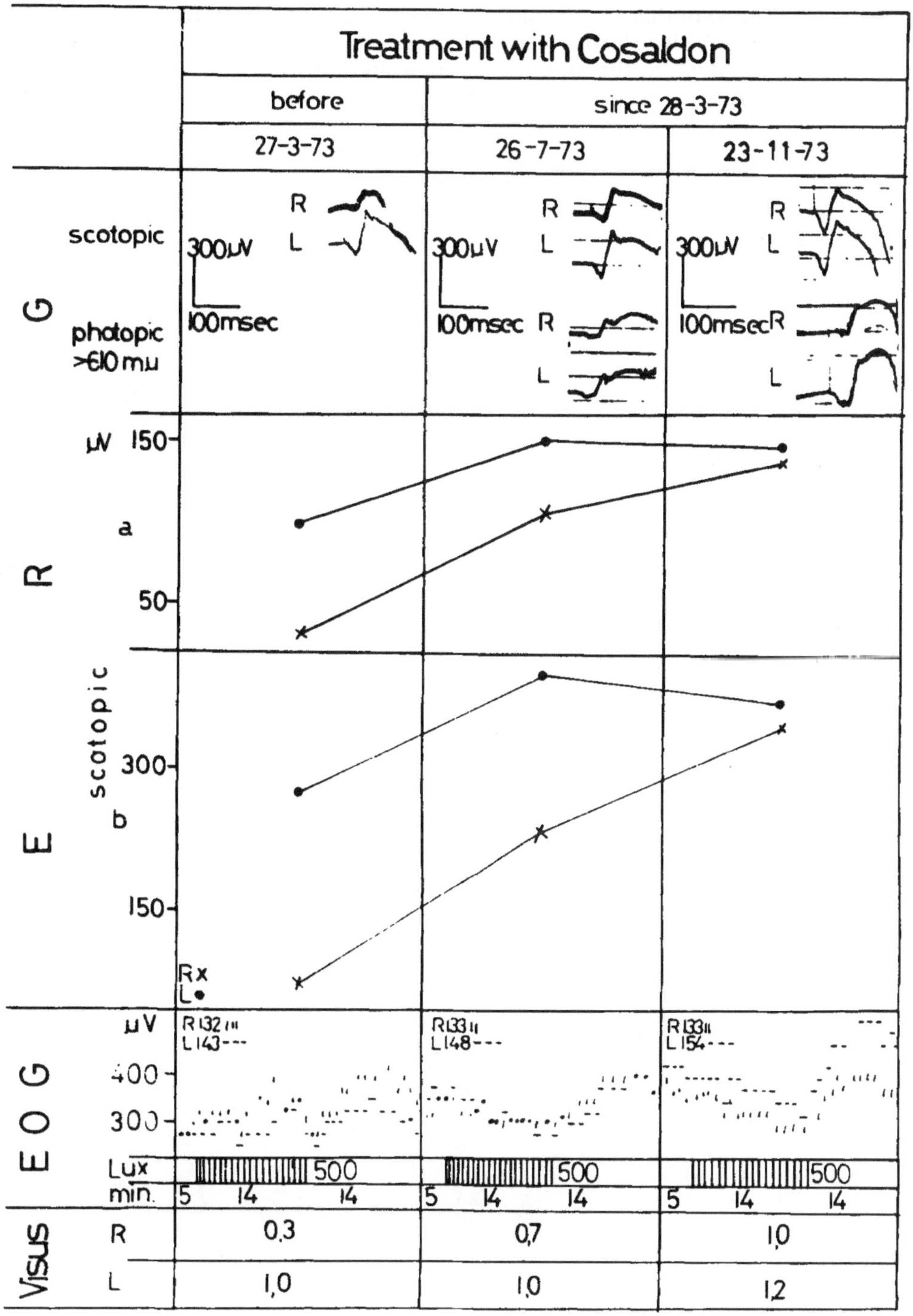

	Treatment with Cosaldon		
	before	since 28-3-73	
	27-3-73	26-7-73	23-11-73

G

scotopic — R, L — 300μV — 100msec
photopic >610 mμ

R — scotopic **a**
μV 150— 50—

E — scotopic **b**
300— 150—
Rx L•

E O G
μV — R 132 ᶦᵐ / L 143---
400— 300—
R 133 ᵢᵢ / L 148---
R 133 ᵢᵢ / L 154---

	Lux min.								
	5	14	500 14	5	14	500 14	5	14	500 14

Visus

R	0,3	0,7	1,0
L	1,0	1,0	1,2

In the case of this 38-year-old man we considered the differential diagnosis of chorioretinitis. However, the fluorescence angiography on 27-3-73 revealed no dye in the ophthalmoscopically affected region (Dr. PAUL-MANN). A repetition on 4-10-73 demonstrated no changes. A very thorough otologic and internal examination, including a toxoplasma and Lues reaction, revealed no pathological findings. Only the serum cholesterine was above normal, at 345 mg %. Thus, there was no evidence of inflammation. The family history likewise gave us no clues.

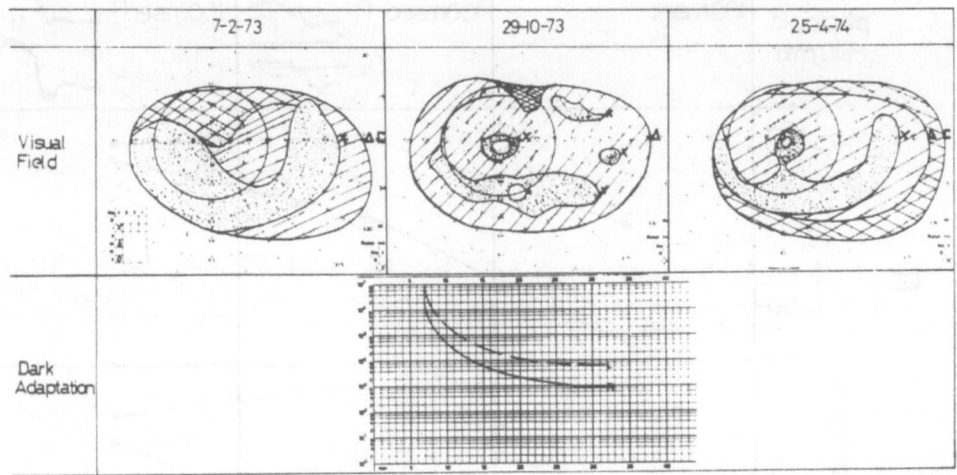

	7-2-73	29-10-73	25-4-74
Visual Field			
Dark Adaptation			

Fig. 2a-c. (Case 2): Peripapillary and pericentral choroidal atrophy.

	29-10-73	25-4-74
	R	R
Ishihara number of mistakes	11	9
Farnsworth-Munsell „100 hue" test		
Nagel Anomaloscope AQ	0,55	0,75

306

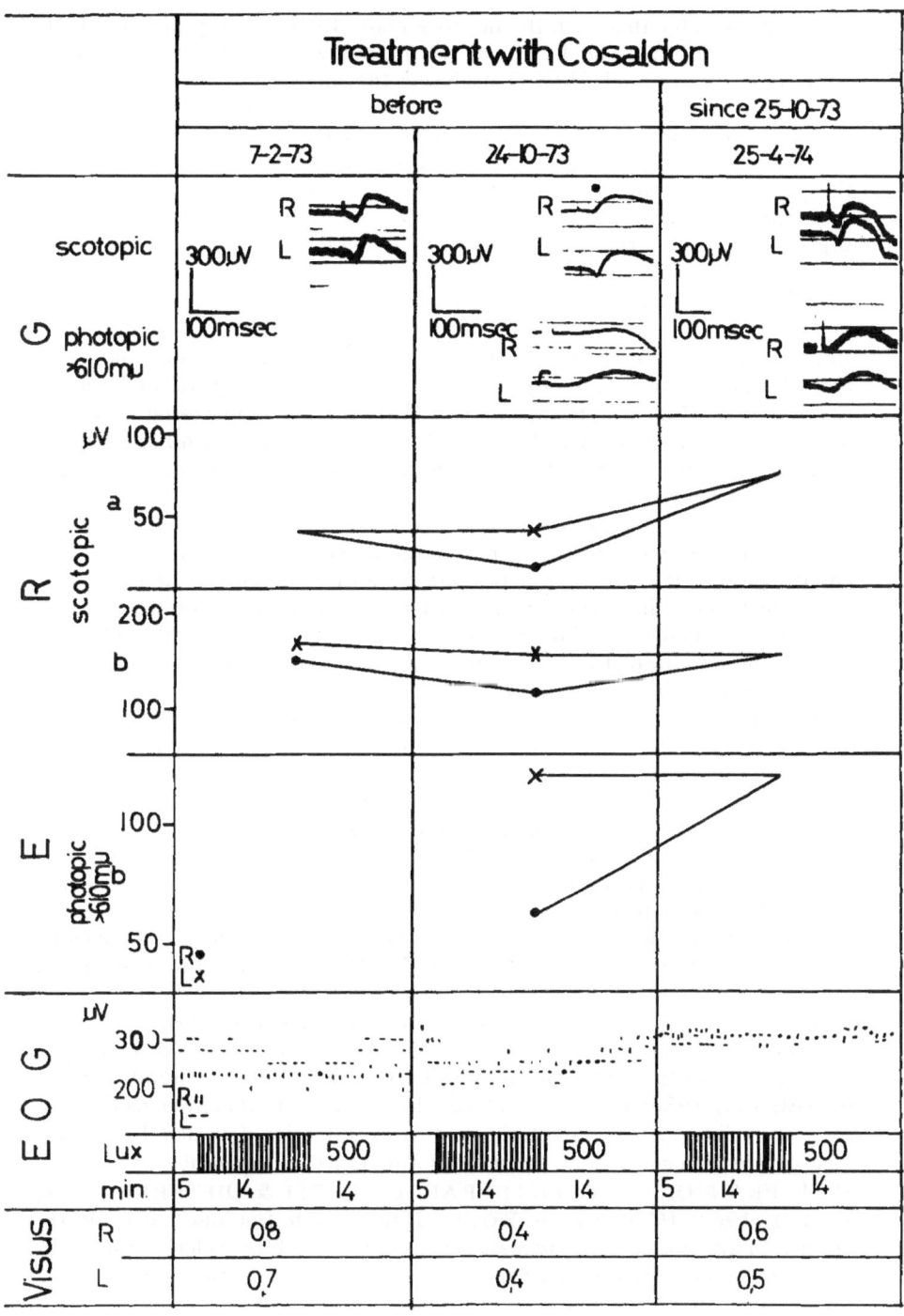

	Treatment with Cosaldon		
	before		since 25-10-73
	7-2-73	24-10-73	25-4-74

scotopic

G photopic >610mμ

R scotopic a / b

E photopic >610mμ b

EOG

Lux	500	500	500
min.	5 14 14	5 14 14	5 14 14

Visus				
R	0,8	0,4	0,6
L	0,7	0,4	0,5

307

It is remarkable that with the improvement of visual acuity only the ERG returned to normal. The EOG was still pathological on 23-11-73, in sharp contrast to the normal ERG. Considering the sharp reduction of the light/dark ratio, we must assume extensive damage of the pigment epithelium, which possibly goes beyond the changes recognized ophthalmoscopically. According to the electrophysiological findings, we can see that damage of the pigment epithelium and perhaps also of the choriocapillaris remains very constant, while that of the retina is still to a great extent reversible. This supports the theory that retinal damage is secondary.

Case 2: Peripapillary and pericentral choroidal atrophy.

Here we find a very distinct retinal choroidal atrophy, peripapillary and arch- formed in the mid-periphery, with extensive pericentral invasion on the left side. (Fig. 6) The atrophic zone is sharply demarcated from the periphery and the undamaged central parts and is spotted with bone-corpuscular pigmentations. The retinal vessels show attenuation of the calibre, the optic disc is normal.

The degree of the present damage is shown by the ERG, which lies on the border between normal and pathological. The EOG is especially effected. In spring, 1972, the outer borders of both visual fields (GOLDMANN perimeter) were still normal. One year later, a very sharp lesion was discernible with a tendency to ring-scotoma formation (Fig. 2a). On 29-10-73 this formation was complete. Fig. 2c shows the values of the visual acuity, after correction for a slight hypermetropy.

During the treatment with Cosaldon (twice daily 1 tablet Cosaldon retard) no functional deterioration was to determine. We even had the impression that visual acuity and ERG showed a certain improvement. The Farnsworth dichotomous (D-28 panel) test revealed no clear axis in the right eye, while, in the left eye (distinct ophthalmoscopic change in the macula), massive disturbance similar to the Tritan-axis was revealed. By the way, the more time-consuming Farnsworth-Munsell '100 hue' test showed no advantage over the D-28 test.

These findings lead us to suspect a tapeto-choroidal atrophy. The lack of familial appearance of this case makes classification under the dystrophies impossible without further evidence.

Considering the age of this female patient (70 years old), we should question whether we are not perhaps dealing with a purely sclerotic process. Comparable ophthalmoscopic findings have been described as senile processes (BIETTI, 1937; PILLAT, 1950). These older reports either lacked the electrophysiological examination, or this examination revealed frequently high degree changes in such a fundus picture (ERG extinguished: BOUNDS, 1954; FRANCOIS et al, 1956; FRANCESCHETTI & DIETERLE, 1957; BIETTI, 1962; HOWARD & WOLF, 1964). Such findings speak clearly against an arteriosclerotic process. On the other hand, considering the existing ERG potentials, we cannot exclude a dystrophy in these cases, since intact zones can still be detected ophthalmoscopically.

The histological examination of comparable ophthalmoscopic cases revealed no arteriosclerotic choroidal changes (ASHTON, 1953: 56-year-old woman; KLIEN, 1964: 71-year-old man; HOWARD & WOLF, 1964: 56-year-old woman). Furthermore, we must take into account that retinal and choroidal atrophies generally progress slowly and the beginning of the changes is seldom detected. In Case 2, the fundus changes were noted accidentally 5 years ago during an examination for eye glasses. It is also noticeable in this case that the retinal periphery is intact. There are no polygonal pigmentations or other changes generally recognized as typical senile symptoms.

Case 3: Pericentral retinopathia pigmentosa.

The parenchyma changes of the retina in the posterior pole correspond to the typical picture of peripapillary and central areolar choroidal atrophy. Next to this, there is a bilateral circular atrophy of pigment epithelium in the mid-periphery, with some bone-corpuscular pigmentations. On the left eye, we find in addition a sharply demarcated zone with many typical bone-corpuscular pigmentations. Considerable attenuation of the retinal vessels can be detected throughout the fundus (Fig. 5), which is typical for retinopathia pigmentosa. The optic discs, however, are not pale.

The ophthalmoscopic results give us already the characteristic symptoms of tapeto-choroidal and tapeto-retinal dystrophy. Also severe damage of the retina is indicated here by the results of the ERG, which, contrary to cases 1 and 2, are at least as abnormal as the EOG values. In connection with the ring scotoma the classification retinopathia pigmentosa would seem correct here (SCHMIDT 1973). Central vision — bilaterally 0.7 — is remarkably good, despite morphologic macular changes. The test results of the Ishihara tables, the Farnsworth-Munsell '100 hue' test and the Nagel anomaloscope were, however, for each eye highly pathological. This is due to the high degree of limitation of the central island of the visual field. We could not detect an achromatopsia. Also in this case the electrophysiological changes preceed the subjective dark adaptation disturbances.

Casuistical contributions show that pigmentations in the case of central and pericentral retinopathia pigmentosa are often combined with atrophy of the choriocapillaris and the choroid (FRANCESCHETTI, FRANCOIS & BABEL 1963, 351). This fact alone indicates that we will be confronted with great difficulties in typifying the dystrophies, especially of this group; all the more so, since pericentral retinopathia pigmentosa has been observed together with retinopathia albipunctata (FRANCESCHETTI, FRANCOIS & BABEL, 1963; PILLAT, 1930). In addition, this case shows ophthalmoscopically a combination of pericentral with sectorial retinopathia pigmentosa (left eye background).

We have not yet observed improvement in this patient with the Cosaldon treatment.

Case 4: Progressive choroidal atrophy.

When we first examined this male patient (born 1932) in 1971, we found on both sides a distinct retinal choroidal atrophy surrounding the optic disc, with finger-like extensions into the mid-periphery (Fig. 5). The intact

309

pigmentary epithelium covered the choriocapillaris only at the outer periphery. The calibre of the retinal arteries was already at that time attenuated. Pigmentations were visible, sometimes surrounding the arteries and the intact veins.

During the following years, the photo control showed a slow increase of changes, in particular, several zones became larger through complete atrophy of retinal tissue. Some pigmentations disappeared only to be replaced by new. Judging from the slow progress during this observation period, we assume that the patient has suffered for a long time.

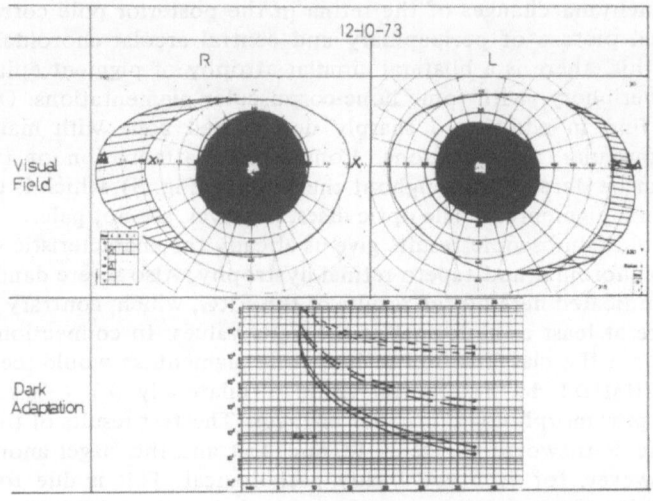

Fig. 3a-c. (Case 3): Pericentral retinopathia pigmentosa.

	12 – 1 0–73	
	R	L
Ishihara number of mistakes	12	10
Farnsworth– Munsell „100hue" test		
Nagel Anomaloscope AQ	0,51	0,27

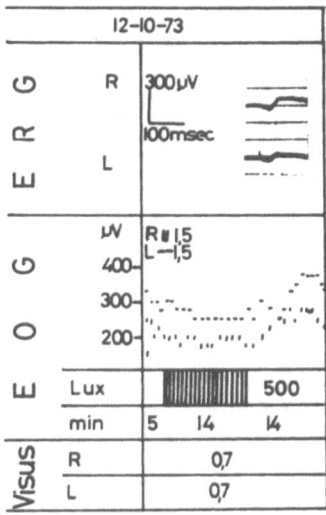

The visual fields, dark adaptation and the electrophysiological findings indicate a diffuse process. We have here a progressive diffuse choroidal atrophy. Since we could not obtain reliable data from the members of the family, we could not determine whether a X-chromosomal (choroideremia: GOEDBLOED; WAARDENBURG) or an autosomal transmission is involved.

The neurological findings were normal. There were no dermatological changes and no deafness. Ophthalmoscopically comparable findings have been reported by SORSBY et al., NEUBAUER, J.C. and R.J.P. MCCULLOCH, PÖLLOT respectively JAEGER & GRÜTZNER, KURSTJENS, KRILL & ARCHER. The discrepancy between the electrophysiological results is important in this case: in the ERG we still find clear potentials, while the EOG in all examinations is completely flat. Thus we have to look for the primary, or at least, the major damage in the pigment epithelium. Another point to notice: in 1971 dark adaptation was still considered normal, while in the EOG, the light rise was completely missing. The absolute threshold of dark adaptation increased only after further decrease of the ERG potentials, which points to a connection between these two functions (WEINSTEIN, LOWELL & HOBSON). A dyschromatopsia in the blue-yellow axis was revealed even more clearly in the Farnsworth dichotomous (D-28 panel) test than in the Farnsworth-Munsell '100 hue' test shown here (Fig. 4b). FRANCESCHETTI, FRANCOIS & BABEL (1963) and VERRIEST (1964) have reported the same findings in advanced cases.

In such severe cases, therapeutic effects can hardly be expected. We can only report that during the treatment with Cosaldon no further change for the worse in either the electrophysiological findings or visual acuity (R c−4,5 sph, L c−6,0 sph) was observed.

311

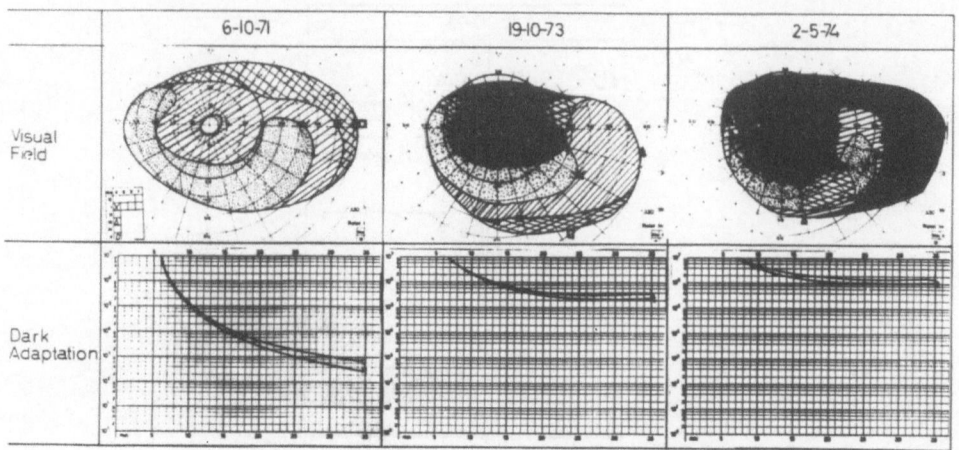

Fig. 4a-c.   (Case 4): Progressive choroidal atrophy.

| | 2-5-74 | |
	R	L
Ishihara number of mistakes	5	8
Farnsworth– Munsell „100 hue" test	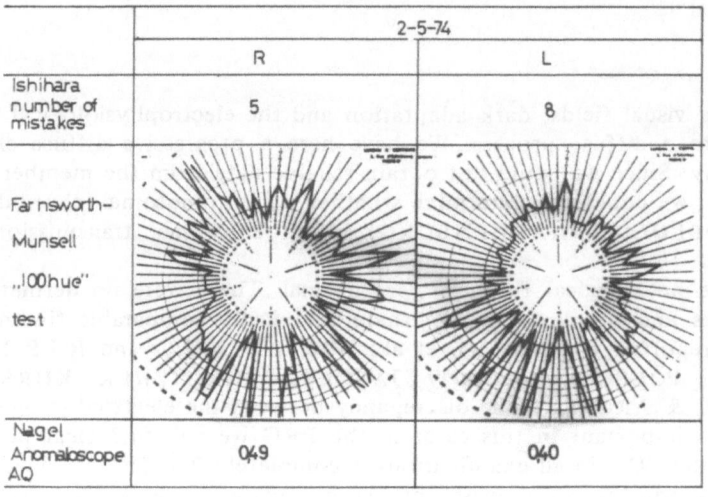	
Nagel Anomaloscope AQ	0,49	0,40

METHODS

The recording procedures for the ERG and the EOG were identical to those described at an other place (SCHMIDT 1972, 1976). ERG: 4000 Lux Osram-L 20 W 15 'day-light'; 1 msec.—200 Luxi, Schottfilter RG 630; 20 msec.

SUMMARY

In conclusion, I would like to single out the following observation:
1. Reporting about 4 cases with different forms of tapeto-choroidal atro-

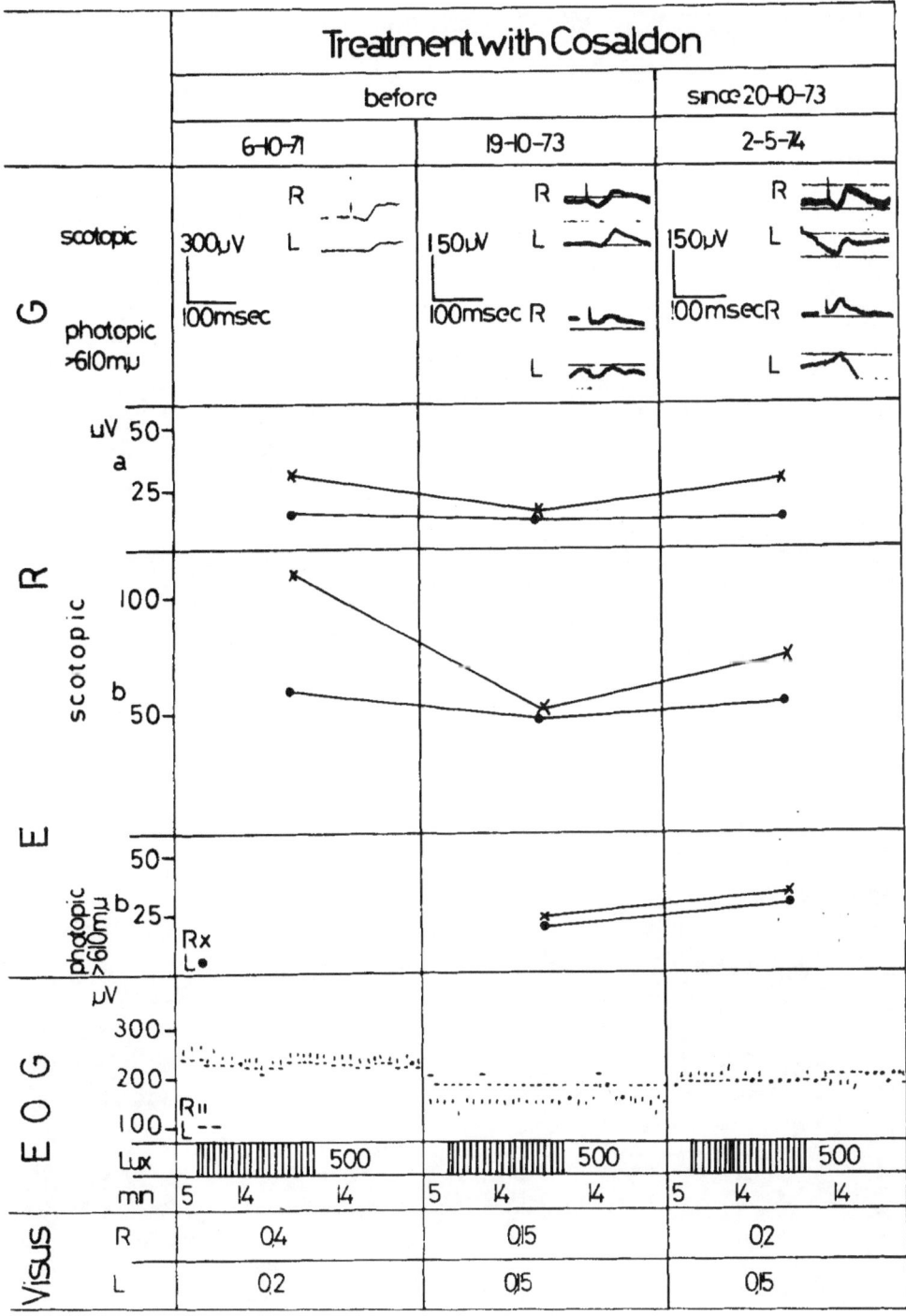

		Treatment with Cosaldon		
		before		since 20-10-73
		6-10-71	19-10-73	2-5-74

(figure rows as shown in image)

Visus	R	0,4	0,15	0,2
	L	0,2	0,15	0,5

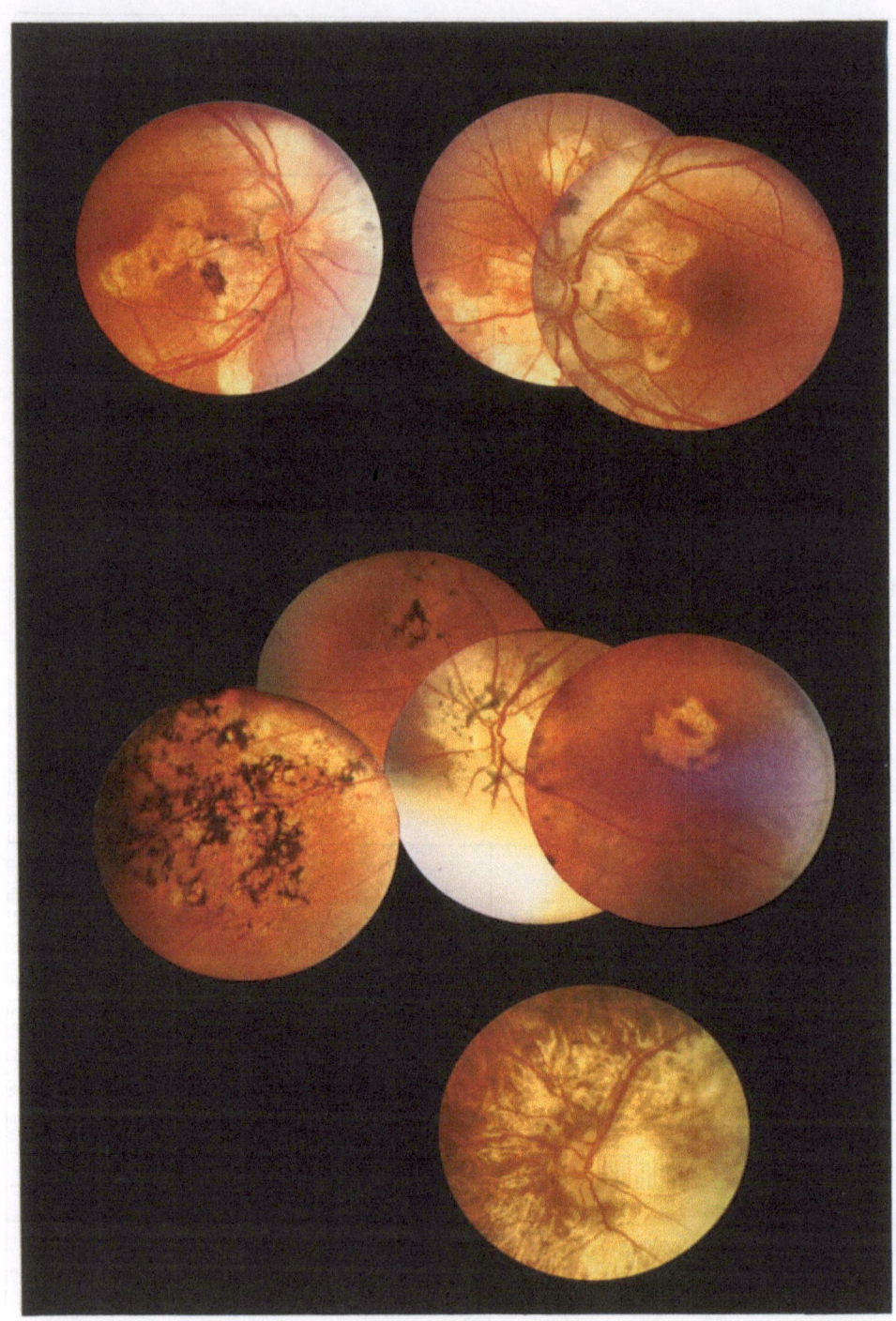

Fig. 5: Case 1, 3 and 4.

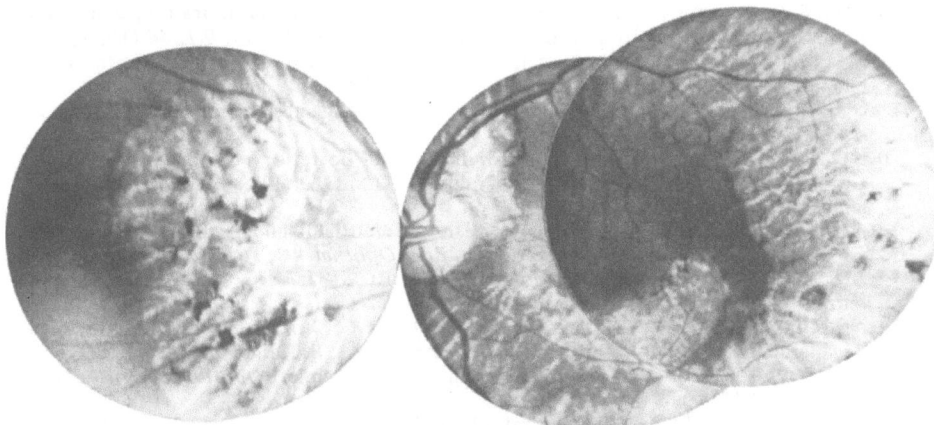

Fig. 6: Case 2.

phies, we have discussed the symptomatology of this group and the differential diagnosis of ophthalmoscopically similar retinal choroidal diseases.

2. In cases 1, 2 and 4 the ERG is far less damaged than the EOG. This finding concurs with the histological results of various authors, indicating that the greatest changes are to be found in the choriocapillaris and in the pigment epithelium. Damage of the retina appears only in advanced stages.

3. In case 3 we also find a peripapillary and central atrophy. However, in this patient we state a sharp reduction of the ERG whereas the EOG still shows a moderate light rise. This indicates a distinct atrophy of the retina and makes, in connection with other symptoms, the diagnosis of a pericentral and sectorial retinopathia pigmentosa.

4. We could determine no connection between the functions of dark adaptation and of the EOG. Thus, in cases 2 and 4, the absolute threshold of dark adaptation was in the normal range, while the EOG was flat. However, there is a parallel between dark adaptation and the ERG. Disturbance was detected earlier, however, in the ERG than in the test on the Goldmann-Weekers apparatus.

5. During treatment with Cosaldon, we observed a favourable course in cases of restricted tapeto-choroidal atrophies.

ACKNOWLEDGEMENT

I am indebted to Mrs. MARLIES MÄURER for her excellent technical assistence. Miss ANGELA PETERS and Mrs. ILSE FISCHER provided the photographs.

REFERENCES

ASHTON, N. Central areolar choroidal sclerosis. A histopathological study. *Brit. J. Ophthal.* 37, *140-147* (1953)
BABEL, J. La rôle de la choriocapillaire dans les affections dégénératives du pôle posterieur. *Bull. Mém. Soc. franç. Opht.* 70, *389-398* (1958)

315

BIETTI, G.B. Su alcune forme atipiche o rare di degenerazione retinica (degenerazioni tappetoretiniche e quadri morbosi similari). *Boll. Oculist.* 16, *1159-1244* (1937)

BIETTI, G.B. Atrofia girata senile della coroide e della retina. Contributo morfologico ed elettroretinografico. *Doc. Ophthal.* 16, *11-20* (1962)

BOUNDS, G. Disc. in RIGGS, L.A.: Electroretinography in cases of night blindness. *Amer. J. Ophthal.* 38, *70-78* (1954)

DEUTMAN, A.F. The hereditary dystrophies of the posterior pole of the eye. Van Gorcum & Comp. N.V. – Dr. H.J. Prakke & H.M.G. Prakke. Assen, The Netherlands, 1971

FRANCESCHETTI, A. & DIETERLE, P. Die differentialdiagnostische Bedeutung des ERG bei tapetoretinalen Degenerationen. *Bibl. Ophthal.* 48, *161-181* (1957)

FRANCESCHETTI, A., FRANCOIS, J. & BABEL, J. Les hérédo-dégénérescences chorio-rétiniennes Masson et Cie, Paris 1963

FRANCOIS, J., DE ROUCK, A. & VERRIEST, G. Les fonctions visuelles dans les dégénérescences tapeto-retiniennes. *Bibl. Ophthal.* 43, S. Karger 1956

GOEDBLOED, J. Mode of inheritance in choroideremia. *Ophthalmologica* 104, *308-315* (1942).

HOWARD, G.M. & WOLF, E. Central choroidal sclerosis: Clinical and pathologic study. *Trans. Amer. Acad. Ophthal. Otolaryng.* 68, *647-660* (1964).

KAPUSCINSKI, W. sen. Über familiäre Aderhautentartung mit ataktischen Störungen. *Ber. Dtsch. Ophthal. Ges.* 30, *13-19* (1934).

KLIEN, B.A. Heredodegeneration of the macula lutea: diagnostic and differentialdiagnostic considerations and a histopathologic report. *Amer. J. Ophthal.* 33, *371-379* (1950).

KLIEN, B.A. Some aspects of classification and differential diagnosis of senile macular degeneration. *Amer. J. Ophthal.* 58, *927-939* (1964).

KRILL, A.E. & ARCHER, D. Classification of the choroidal atrophies. *Amer. J. Ophthal.* 72, *562-585* (1971).

KURSTJENS, J.H. Choroideremia and gyrata atrophy of the choroid and retina. *Doc. Ophthal.* 19, *1-125* (1965).

MCCULLOCH, J.C. & MCCULLOCH, R.J.P. A hereditary and clinical study of choroideremia. *Trans. Amer. Acad. Ophthal. Otolaryngol.* 52, *160-190* (1948).

NEUBAUER, H. Progressive Aderhautatrophie. *Graefes Arch. Ophthal.* 156, *577-589* (1955).

PAMEYER, J.K., WAARDENBURG, P.J. & HENKES, H.E. Choroideremia. *Brit. J. Ophthal.* 44, *724-738* (1960)

PILLAT, A. Tapetoretinal degeneration of the central fundus region. A combination of retinitis pigmentosa centralis and retinitis punctata albescens. *Amer. J. Ophthal.* 13, *1-12* (1930)

PILLAT, A. Die senile Pigmentierung der Netzhaut. *Graefes Arch. Ophthal.* 150, *1-27* (1950)

POLLOT, W. Atypische Chorioretinitis pigmentosa hereditaria. *Graefes Arch. Ophthal.* 80, *379-394* (1912)

SCHMIDT, J.G.H. Stargardt'sche Makuladegeneration oder Makula-Typ der diffusen tapeto-retinalen Degeneration? *Ber. Dtsch. Ophthal. Ges.* 72, *235-242* (1972)

SCHMIDT, J.G.H. and MÄURER, M. On the differentiation of heredo-macular degenerations. 2nd South African Intern. Ophthal. Symposium, Johannesburg 1973

SCHMIDT, J.G.H. and MÄURER, M.: The value of electro-oculography for the diagnosis of tapeto-retinal degenerations. Bibl. Ophthal. *85*, 1976.

SORSBY, A., FRANCESCHETTI, A., JOSEPH, R. & J.B. DAVEY Choroideremia. Clinical and genetic aspects. *Brit. J. Ophthal.* 36, *547-581* (1952)

VERRIEST, G. Les déficiences acquises de la discrimination chromatique. Memoires IV. Impr. Med. et Scientifique, Bruxelles 1964.

WAARDENBURG, P.J. Chorioideremie als Erbmerkmal. *Acta ophthal. (Kbh)* 20, *235-274* (1942)

WEINSTEIN, G.W., LOWELL, G.G. & HOBSON, R.R. A comparison of electroretinographic and dark adaptation studies in retinitis pigmentosa. XIIth ISCERG Symposium, Clermont-Ferrand 1974

316

THE OSCILLATORY POTENTIALS OF
THE ERG IN OGUCHI'S DISEASE

YASUO KUBOTA

(Chiba, Japan)

As is well known, the ERG of Oguchi's disease composed of an a-wave and oscillatory potentials, and the ERG lacks a b-wave. Its is also reported that the a-wave is diminished compared to that of a normal ERG. However, the oscillatory potentials of the ERG in this disease are not yet fully studied.

Recently 3 cases of Oguchi's disease were evaluated in our clinic. These cases were examined, and the ERGs were recorded. The amplitudes and the peak times of the oscillatory potentials were measured and compared to those of a normal subject.

CASE REPORTS

Case 1. 22-year-old-man. His chief complaint was congenital nightblindness. The vision of the both eyes were 1.2. The color sense was normal. Constriction of the visual field was seen when using dim objects. With regard to dark adaptation, the first curve was slightly disturbed, and the second curve was not seen within 30 minutes.

Examination of the fundi revealed the typical characteristic changes, these are, especially in the peripheral region of the fundus, specific phosphorescent change. The vessels were blackish. After 3 hours of dark adaptation Mizuo's phenomenon was seen. (This case has been reported previously by us.) (Kubota 1965)

Case 2. 6-year-old boy. The chief complaint was also nightblindness. The visual acuity of the both eyes was 1.2. The visual field seemed to be normal. However, exact examinations were not possible because of the patient's age.

The fundi were very similar to those of the first case. The specific changes were observed. Mizuo's phenomenon was observed after 2 hours dark adaptation (Fig. 1a, 1b).

Case 3. 2-year-old boy. Recently his mother discovered that he could not see w ll at night. He was too young to be evaluated with exact ophthalmological examinations. Visual acuity, visual field, and light sense were not examined.

Examination of the fundi revealed typical specific fundus changes, similar to those of the above two cases.

METHODS OF ERG EXAMINATION

Details about the methods of ERG examination used in our clinic have been descrived in previous reports. (Kubota 1965, 1966) In brief, a contact lens

317

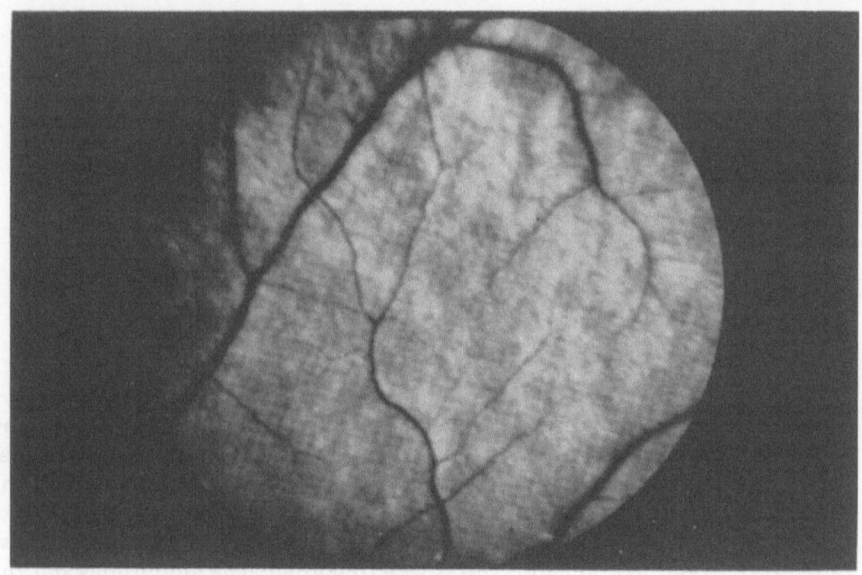

Fig. 1a. The fundus photograph of case 2.

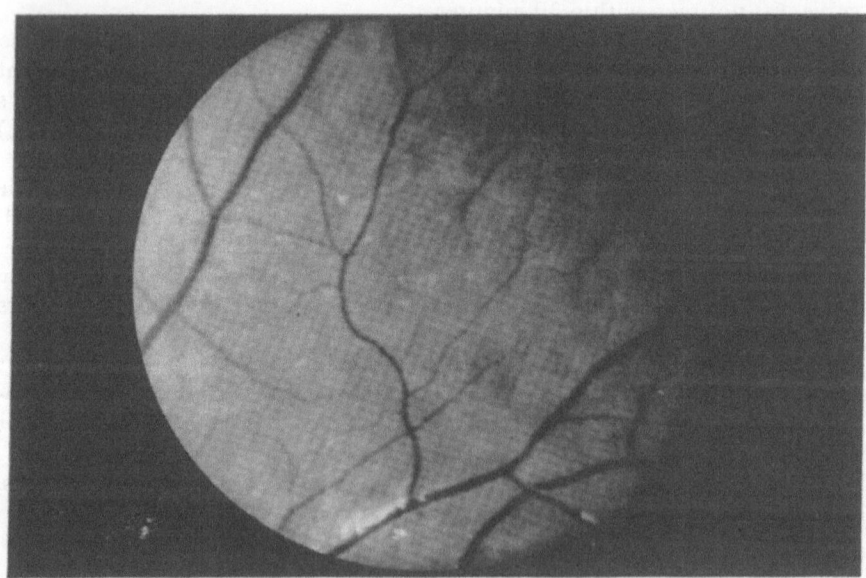

Fig. 1b. After 2 hours dark adaptation mizuo's phenomenon was seen.

318

electrode was used. As the light stimulus, the flash stimulus from a Xenon discharge lamp was employed. To obtain the light stimulus of lower intensity, neutral filters were used. The ERGs recorded on the films were projected on millimeter paper in order to measure the amplitudes and the peak times (Fig. 2, 3).

MEASUREMENTS OF THE AMPLITUDES
AND THE PEAK TIMES
(NORMAL)

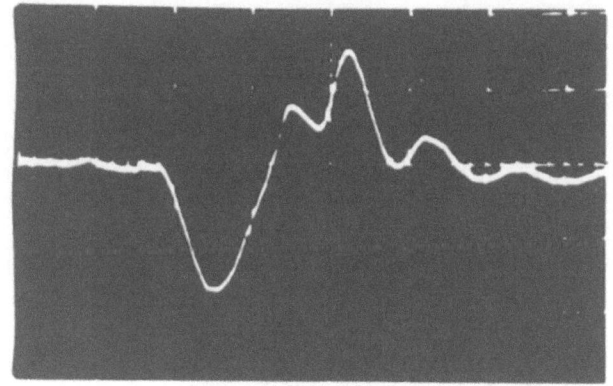

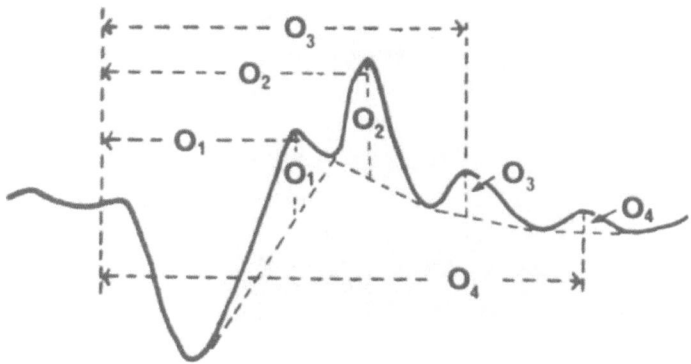

Fig. 2. The methods of the measurement of the amplitudes and the peak times (normal subject).

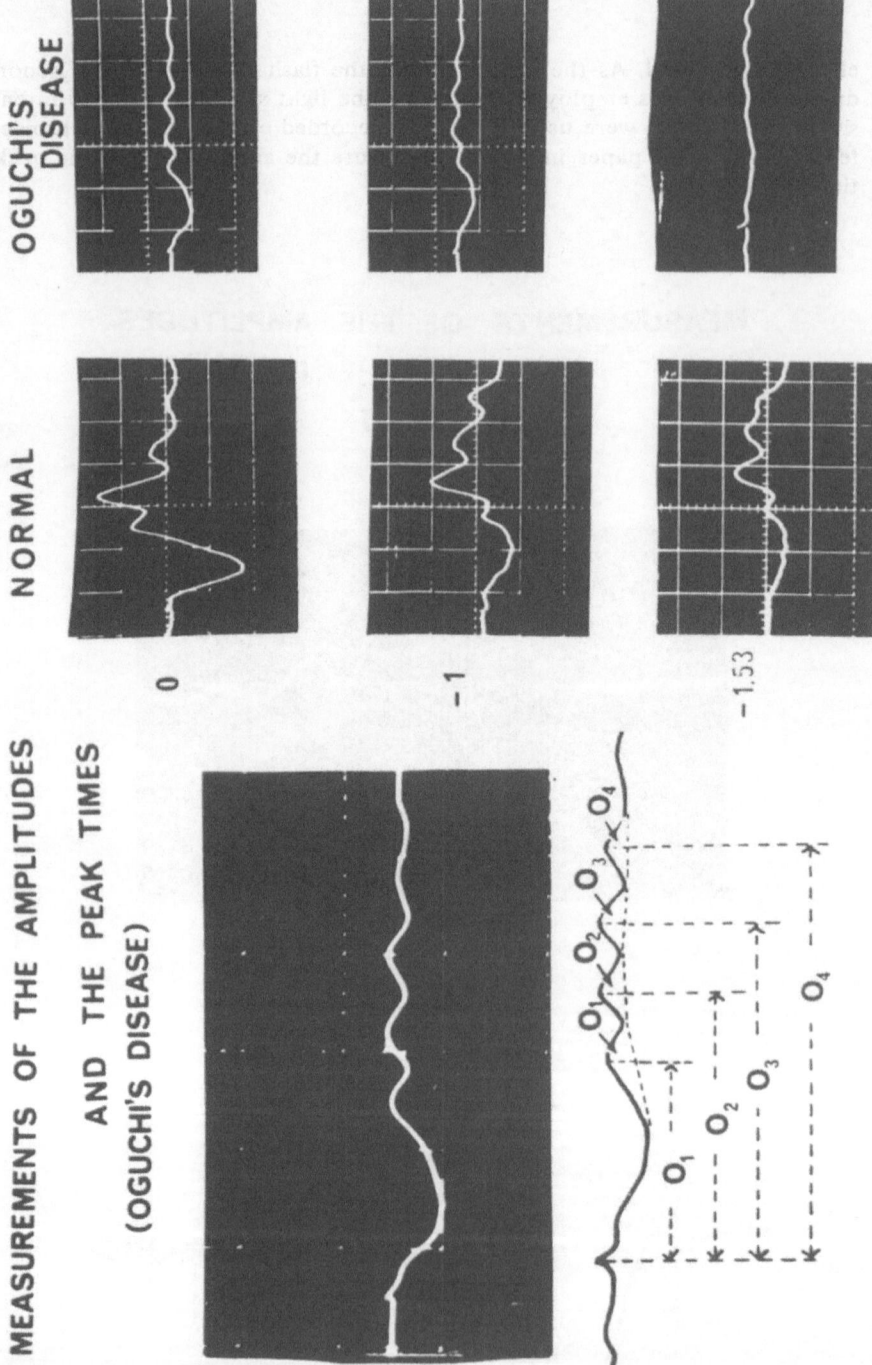

Fig. 3. The methods of the measurement of the amplitudes and the peak times (Oguchi's disease).

Fig. 4. The ERGs of case 1. and a normal subject recorded by the same conditions (time constant: 0.003 sec.).

Figure 4, 5 shows the ERG of case 1 and a normal subject recorded by the same conditions. In the ERG of Oguchi's disease b-wave is not seen. The a-wave of the case is reduced. The oscillatory potentials are clearly seen. However, the amplitudes are diminished compared to those of a normal subject. The peak times of the waves are nearly the same as a normal ERG (Fig. 6, 7).

Figure 8 shows the ERGs of the second and the third cases. In these cases the amplitudes of the oscillatory potentials are also weakened.

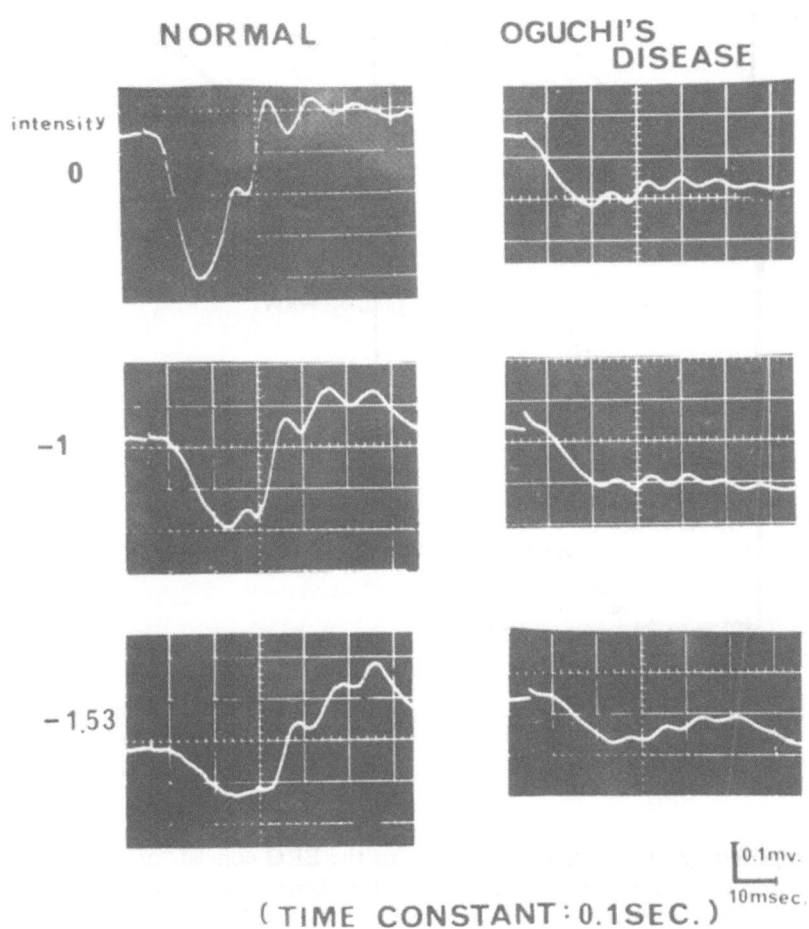

Fig. 5. The ERGs of case 1. and a normal subject recorded by the same conditions (time constant: 0.01 sec.).

AMPLITUDES OF THE OSCILLATORY POTENTIALS

NORMAL   OGUCHI'S DISEASE
- - - ◦   ● ——

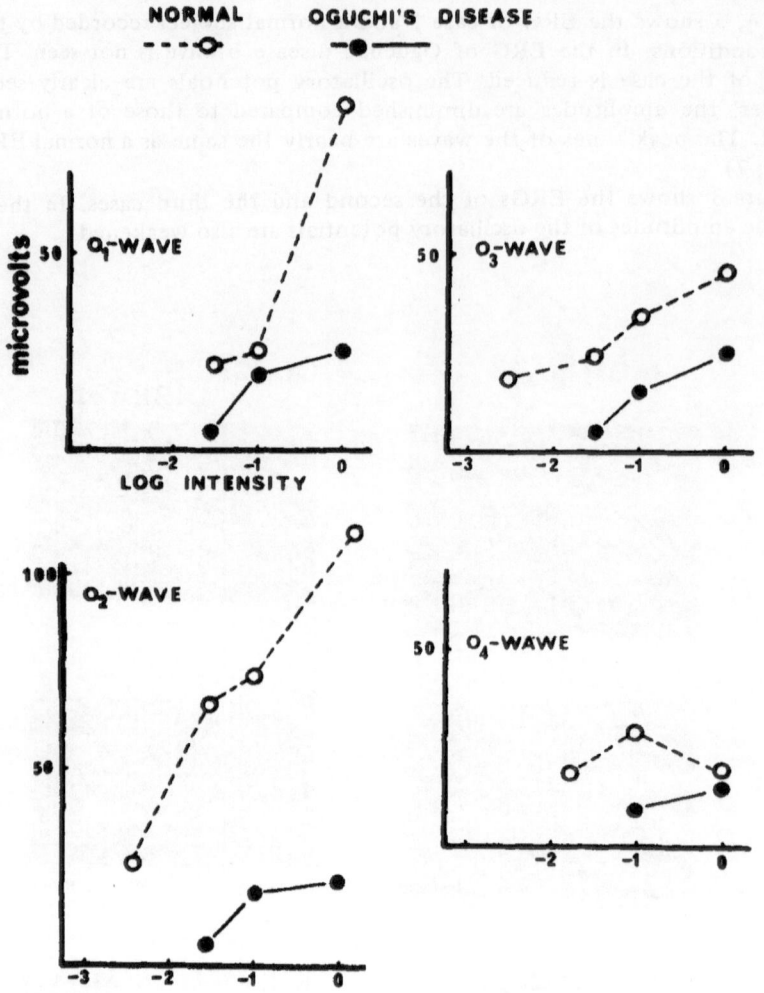

Fig. 6. The amplitudes of the oscillatory potentials of case 1 and a normal subject.

DISCUSSION

It is generally known that the a-wave of the ERG consists of both photopic and scotopic components, and that the b-wave consists of a scotopic component. However, the mechanismus of the oscillatory potentials are not yet fully explained.

They may not be the scotopic component, because they are not seen in the ERG of monochromatismus, which has only a scotopic component. Besides, they may be not purely a photopic component, because they also not seen in congenital stationary nightblindness, which has only a photopic component.

It might be thought that the oscillatory potentials are the responses composed of both photopic and scotopic functions. The photopic function of Oguchi's disease is almost normal, and the scotopic function of this disease is lacking.

From these facts it may be concluded that oscillatory potentials, as well as the a-wave, were composed of both photopic and scotopic components. In Oguchi's disease the scotopic function is lacking, therefore, the b-wave (scotopic component) is not seen, the a-wave as well as the oscillatory potentials (scotopic and photopic components) are reduced.

PEAK TIMES OF THE OSCILLATORY POTENTIALS

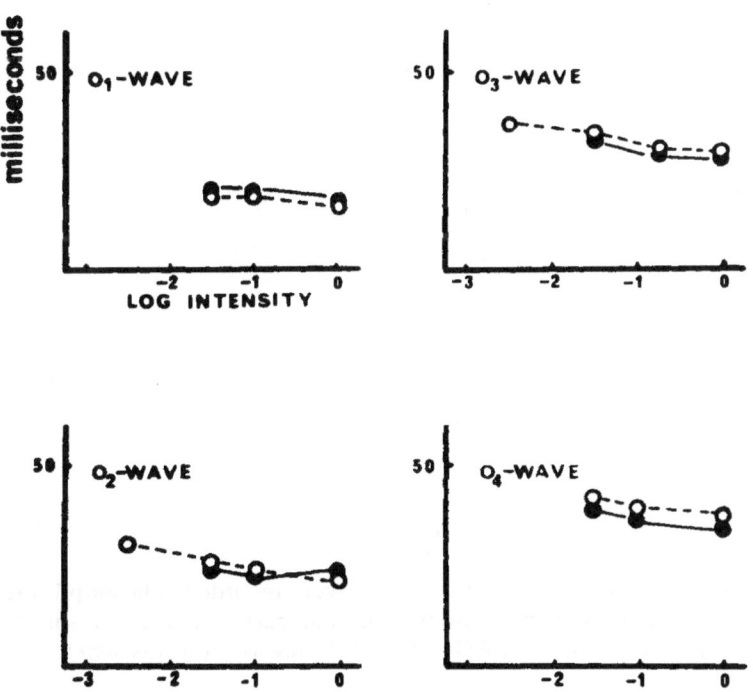

Fig. 7. The peak times of the oscillatory potentials of case 1 and a normal subject.

OGUCHI'S DISEASE
(CASE 2)

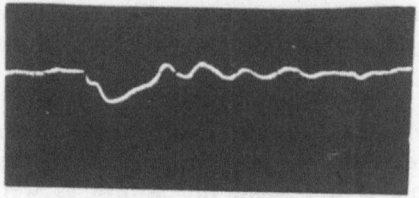

OGUCHI'S DISEASE
(CASE 3)

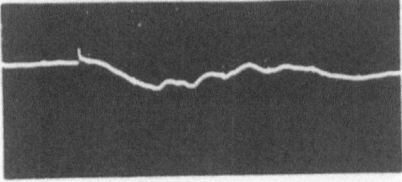

NORMAL

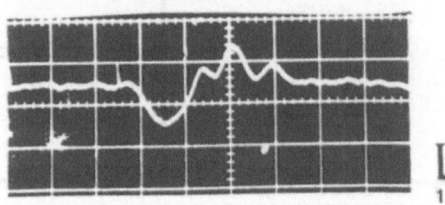

0.1mv.
10msec.

(TIME CONSTANT: 0.003 SEC.)

Fig. 8.   The ERGs of case 2 and case 3.

SUMMARY

The ERGs of 3 cases of Oguchi's diseases were recorded. The amplitudes of the oscillatory potentials were weakened in all cases. The mechanisms of the oscillatory potentials of the ERG in Oguchi's deseases was discussed.

REFERENCES

KUBOTA, Y. *Jap. J. Ophth.* 9: *31*, 1965.
KUBOTA, Y. *Jap. J. Ophth.* Supplement. 10: *317*, 1966.

324

THE INFLUENCE OF MYOPIA ON THE EOG

A. THALER, P. HEILIG, V. SCHEIBER & P. TILL

(Vienna, Austria)

ABSTRACT

The influence of myopia on the EOG was studied in 20 unilateral cases. An inverse relationship could be proven between light peak as well as light trough and the axial length of the globe. No correlation was obtained between dark trough and axial length.

One of the factors responsible for the wide range of variability in electro-oculography is myopia. It was the purpose of this study to find out if there exists any correlation between the axial length of the eye and the reduction of amplitudes in the EOG.

METHODS

To reduce the influence of interindividual variation only cases of unilateral myopia were used for this study. The myopic eye could be compared direct-ly with the normal fellow eye. In 20 subjects (19 to 60 years) the EOG was carried out in front of an Ulbricht sphere. Silver-silver chloride electrodes (Beckman 16 mm, Beckman electrode paste) were fixed near the inner and outer canthi by collodium. The potential was DC amplified and displayed on an oscilloscope (Tektronix 3A9, RM 565) and filmed from the screen (Nihon Kohden PC-2A). After a preadaptation of 35 minutes to 20 asb the recording in darkness lasted for 12 1/2 minutes. Every minute the subject had to perform eye movements of 30 degrees for 15 to 20 seconds. Each fixation light was illuminated for 2 1/2 seconds. The dark adaptation was followed by 30 minutes of light adaptation to 2100 asb. At the light peak recording was continous. No mydriatics were used. The degree of myopia was measured by retinoscopy controlling the axial length by ultra-sonography (1 mm = 3 dptr.). Patients with distinct changes of the posterior pole or with extensive peripapillary atrophy as well as patients with strabis-mus were excluded from this examination. Only patients with axial myopia were used.

The myopic eyes of the patients were corrected by contact lenses or spectacles. In all cases an improvement of visual acuity could be obtained (0.3-1.0).

The statistical analysis tested for a correlation between axial length of the eye and amplitudes of the EOG. A linear or quadratic regression anlysis was computed, based on the difference of dark trough, light peak, and light trough* in relation to the steady state between normal and myopic eyes:

$$\frac{\text{light peak-steady state}}{\text{steady state}} \text{ (myopic eye)} - \frac{\text{light peak-steady state}}{\text{steady state}} \text{ (normal eye)} \quad .100$$

The hypothesis was tested that there is no linear correlation between the axial length of the eye and the EOG.

RESULTS

1. Dark trough

No significant deviation from slope zero could be proven for linear or quadratic regressions by comparing normal and myopic eyes.

2. Light peak (fig. 1)

Linear regression equation:

$y = -0.46 - 1.86 \, x$ $y =$ difference of the normalized reduction of amplitudes

$t = 5.21$ (d.f. 18) $x =$ myopia in dioptries (absolute value)

The above mentioned hypothesis can be rejected with an error probability of 0.001.

    The regression coefficient of the quadratic component was not significantly different from zero.

3. Light trough (fig. 2)

Linear regression equation:

$y = 1.86 + 0.65 \, x$
$t = 2.60$ (d.f. 18)

Quadratic regression equation:

$y = -50.64 + 5.37 \, x - 0.27 \, x^2$
$t = 2.51$ (d.f. 17)

The linear regression coefficient as well as that of the second order are significantly different from zero with an error probability of 0.05.

DISCUSSION

When FRANÇOIS and coworkers introduced electrooculography to clinical ophthalmology they observed normal EOG amplitudes in myopia. ARDEN and coworkers obtained a reduced light-dark ratio. BLACH and coworkers as well as GEIJER-MANNERFELT & PALLIN could not prove any correlation between axial length of the eye and light-dark ratio. GLIEM stated that

* light trough: the lowest amplitude in light following the first light peak.

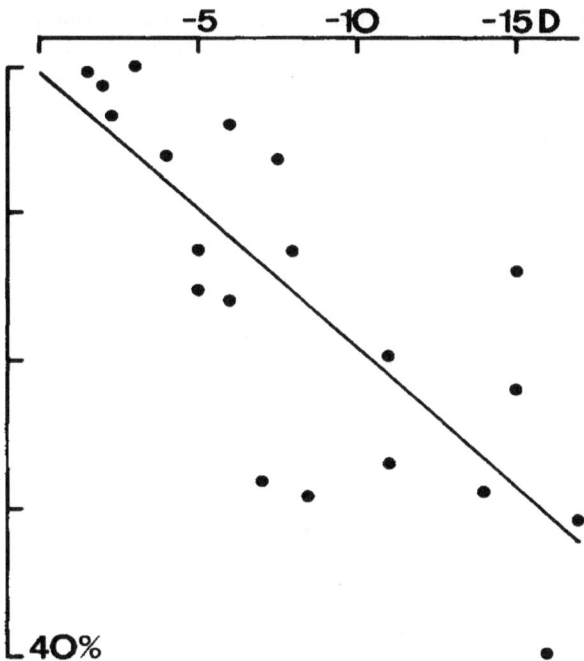

Fig. 1. Linear regression equation of the difference of the normalized reduction of light peak amplitudes in myopia.

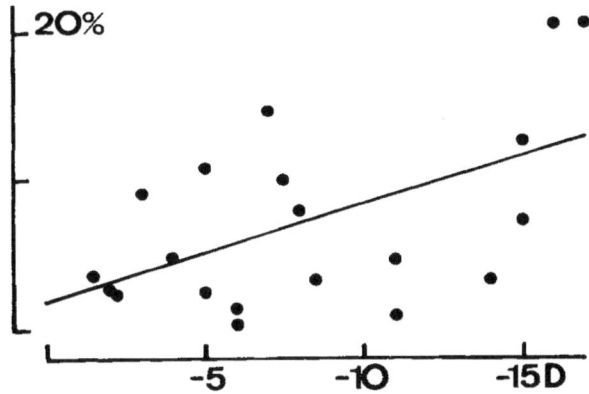

Fig. 2. Linear regression equation of the difference of the normalized reduction of light trough amplitudes in myopia.

in myopia the light rise is reduced whereas the dark trough is normal. In the present study no correlation could be proven between axial length of the globe and dark trough amplitude. This result is in accordance with GLIEM's findings. The linear decrease of light peak with increasing axial length of the eye is highly significant ($P < 0.001$).

The use of a correcting term for myopia makes possible the examination of EOG amplitudes less influenced by the axial length of the eye. Under the above mentioned experimental conditions (steady state, 12 1/2 minutes darkness followed by light (2100 asb)) this additive correcting term for the light peak was found to be:

$0.46 + 1.86 \ x$

$\qquad x = $ dioptries of myopia (absolute value)

ACKNOWLEDGEMENT

The authors are grateful to Prof. Dr. H.J. KOLDER (University of Iowa) for the critical reading of the manuscript.

REFERENCES

ARDEN, G.B., BARRADA, A. & KELSEY, J.H. New clinical test of retinal function based upon the standing potential of the eye. *Brit. J. Ophthal.* 46: *449-467* (1962).

BLACH, R.K., JAY, B. & KOLB, H. Electrical activity of the eye in high myopia. *Brit. J. Ophthal.* 50: *629-641* (1966).

FRANÇOIS, J., VERRIEST, G. & DE ROUCK, A. L'electrooculographie en tant qu'examen fonctionnel de la rétine. *Progr. Ophtal. S. Karger* 7: *1-67* (1957).

GEIJER-MANNERFELT, T. & PALLIN, O. On the correlation between ERG and EOG in normal eyes. In: SCHMOGER, E. Advances in electrophysiology and pathology of the visual system. VEB G. Thieme (Leipzig): 47-52 (1968).

GLIEM, H. Das Elektrookulogramm. VEB G. Thieme, Leipzig (1971).

WILLIAMS, E.J. Regression analysis. J. Wiley & Sons Inc. London (1959).

ERG IN CASES OF THERAPEUTIC LIGHT COAGULATION

E. SCHMÖGER, W. MÜLLER & E. HAASE

(Erfurt, DDR)

Light coagulation of the retina is often carried out in the treatment of diabetic retinopathy although the reason for the therapeutic effect is as yet uncertain. One of the theories is that the reduction in oxygen requirement which follows the extensive scarring is the beneficial factor (MEYER-SCHWICKERATH & SCHOTT, 1968). These changes might be expected to alter the ERG and as such investigations have not previously been carried out, as far as we know, we performed the ERG in patients with diabetic retinopathy before and after therapeutic light coagulation. We were also able to use a stimulus of such high intensity that it has never been used previously as it may coagulate the retina. That is to say, we used the therapeutic coagulation stimulus as the ERG stimulus.

Our investigations are a pilot study. In ten patients with diabetic retino-

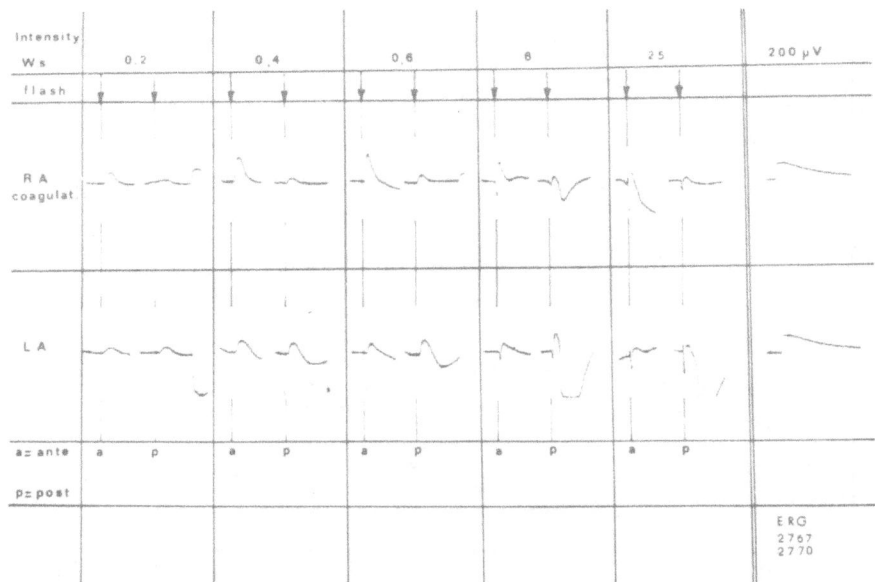

Fig. 1. Comparison between ERG before (a) and one day after (p) light coagulation. Reduction of a- and b-amplitudes in ERG of the right (coagulated) retina. Nearly unchanged ERG from left eye.

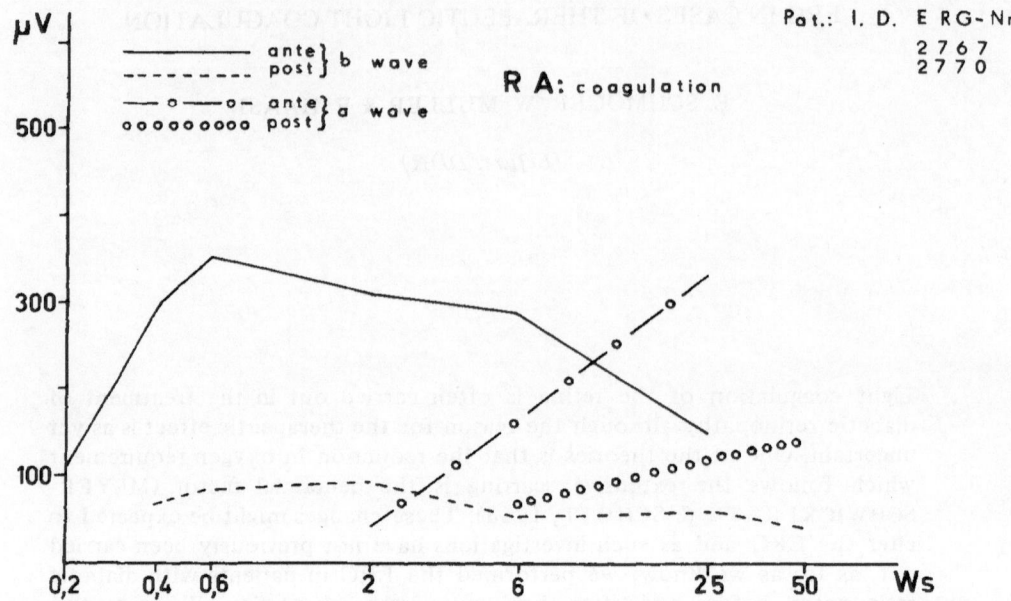

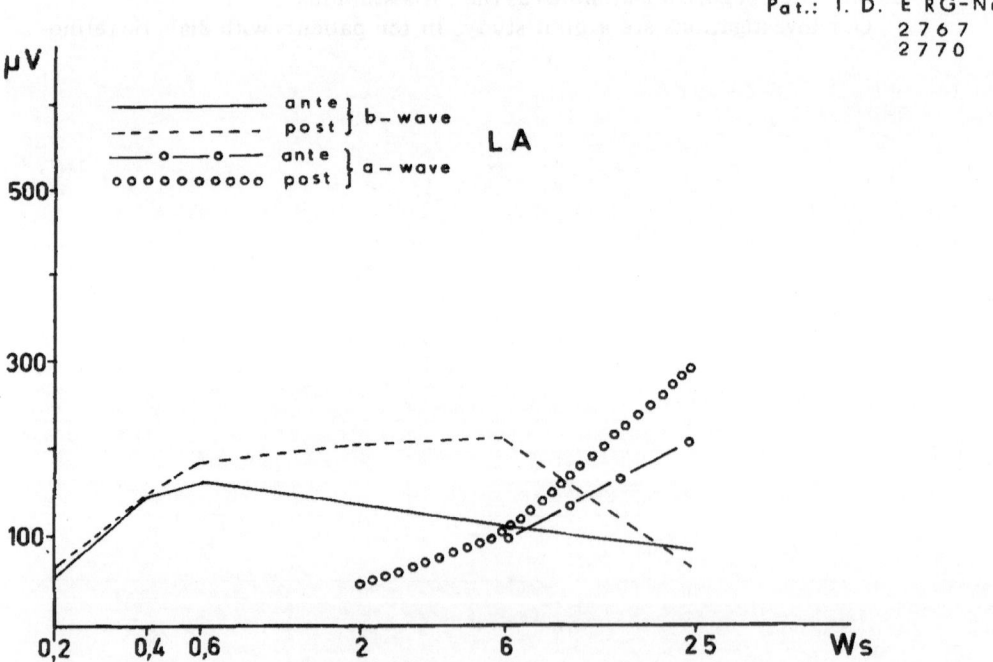

Fig. 2 and 3. The diagrams show the amplitudes of a- and b-waves in the case of fig. 1. Ws = stimulus intensity (Joule) a- and b-amplitudes measured from isoelectric line.

pathy three ERGs were performed, these being before, during, and after the therapeutic coagulation. As a rule the last one was the day after the coagulation. The method for ERG registration before and after the coagulation was the same as used for dark adaptation ERG in the routine techniques of our laboratory. The ERG registration during the light coagulation was technically difficult. We used a contact lens electrode or a skin electrode and another skin electrode as reference. In the first case the light coagulation was accomplished through the contact lens. The coagulator machine was the Lichtkoagulator 5000 from Carl Zeiss, Jena. The field of illumination given by the ophthalmoscope of the apparatus extends about 30 degrees in diameter around the focussed point and is present before and during the coagulation. It has a luminance of about 2,500 or 3,000 lux. The intensities for coagulation used to be between 2,000 and 3,500 Joule and about 60 coagulations of 5 degrees each were the rule. However, we started with the lowest intensity of 700 Joule, which seldom caused a visible coagulation but was always able to elicit an ERG potential. These potentials, always of a photopic character, are passed through an amplifier to an analogue tape recorder for further evaluation.

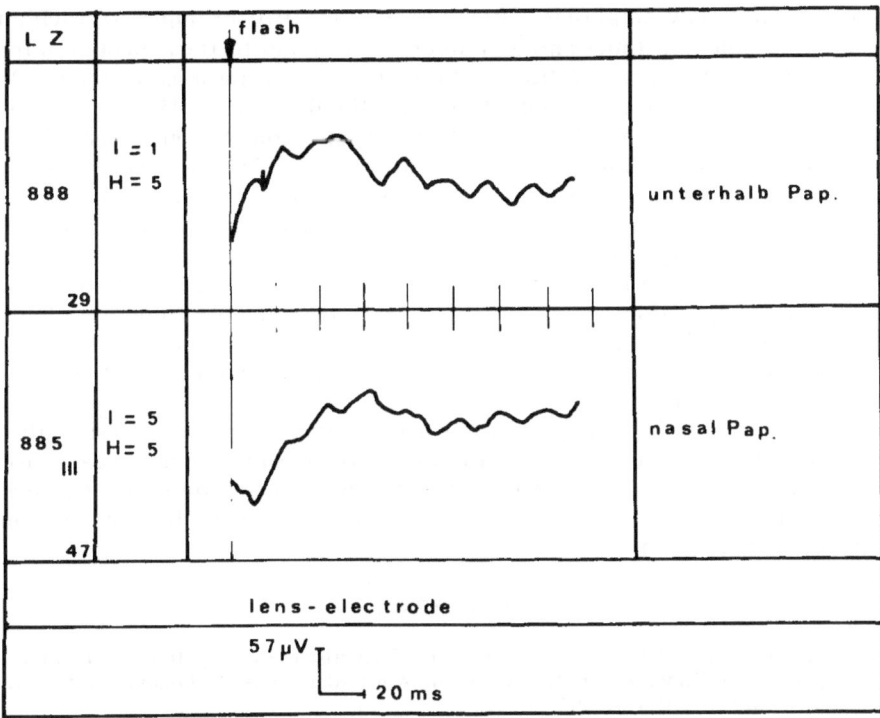

Fig. 4. Two examples of localized photopic ERG elicited by light coagulation flash. LZ means no. of ERG

I = 1 means intensity 700 Joule
I = 5 means intensity 3500 Joule
H = 5 means light spot of 5 degrees focussed to the retina

1.) Comparison of the ERG before and one day after light coagulation:

In 7 of 10 cases there was a distinct reduction of the b-wave amplitude on the day after coagulation, such a reduction of the a-wave amplitude we saw in 5 cases only. Fig. 1 shows as an example the ERG of a 27 year old woman. b- and a-waves are markedly reduced in amplitude from the coagulated eye. The fellow eye shows an unchanged curve (see Figs. 2 and 3). The time relations are unchanged in both eyes. We did not perform an analysis of oscillatory potentials.

In 3 of 10 cases the ERG was of the same pattern before and after the light coagulation. In one of these cases it may have been that the retinopathy was so advanced that the gross reduction in ERG amplitude was not further reduced by the light coagulation. The other two cases had a less severe retinopathy in which only 25 to 30 spot coagulations were carried out.

2.) It was not possible to evaluate all the ERG potentials elicited by the light coagulation flash because of the high level of 'noise' in the curves. Furthermore, because of the stimulus we may expect a photopic ERG and this means a low amplitude ERG. Fig. 4 shows two examples of such an ERG. Culmination times and amplitudes correspond to the expectation for a photopic ERG. The question is; do we have a sum response of the whole retina or is it a focal response from the stimulated area? The background illumination is due to the ambient light adaptation, the intensity of the stimulus is strong enough to cause a stray effect. On the other hand the stimulus is narrowly focussed on the desired spot of the retina by the ophthalmoscope of the apparatus, so that we may presume to have a mainly localised focal response of the retina.

Summarising the first part of our investigations we may state that extensive light coagulation of the retina causes a measureable reduction of the amplitudes of the dark adapted ERG. This affects mainly the b-wave, less so the a-wave. Further investigations are necessary to show possible recovery of the ERG with time.

Concerning the second part of our investigations we are able to state that it is possible to elicit a photopic ERG using the flash of the light coagulator as a stimulus. We believe this ERG to be a localised response of the retinal area which is to be coagulated. The usefulness of this finding depends on further investigations.

REFERENCES

G. MEYER-SCHWICKERATH & K. SCHOTT. Diabetische Retinopathie und Lichtkoagulation. 3. Kongr. europ. Ges. Ophthal., Amsterdam 1968, *Ophthalmologica additamentum ad vol.* 158, 605-614 (1969).

ERG AND EOG-RESULTS IN TOXOCARA CANIS RETINO CHORIOIDITIS

A. DENDEN

(Göttingen, West Germany)

Since WILDER (1950) observed an exceptional case of nematode Endoph-thalmitis and NICHOLS (1956) was able to identify it as ocular toxocariasis, fully authenticated cases have been described by several authors. Besides the symptoms of visceral larva migrans (BEAUTMAN & WOOLF 1951, BEAVERS et al 1952, BRAIN & ALLAN 1964) lesions of the eye can be conceived as isolated (DUGUID 1961, LAQUA 1972, SIAM 1973) or mul-tiple granulomata located in the posterior region of the fundus and in a massive extension of the infestation as a chronic disseminated endophthal-mitis (PERKINS 1968).

The clinical diagnosis is usually difficult and depends on the characteris-tic lesions in the fundus, the occurrence of severe visual disturbances, taken generally with positive intra-dermal-test (SPRENT & ENGLISH 1958), but the more effective serological test (Agar-Gelprecipitation by OCHTER-LONY with complete toxocara antigen and the immediate precipitation with living Toxocara-larven by Lamina) permits a more accurate differential diagnosis of infestations with nematodes in its varying stages.

We have the opportunity to examine 3 cases of toxocararetinochorio-ditis and we would like in this paper to refer to our ERG and EOG — results. At first the clinical picture:

Case no 1: A girl aged 12 complained of gradual loss of vision in her right eye. In the macular region of the right eye was a greyish-reddish blistery exudation measuring two and a half to three optic disc diameters. Temporally there were several fresh greyish spots of retinitis surrounded by older hemorrhages. The left eye was healthy (Fig. 1).

Case no 2: A girl aged 9 complained of gradual visual loss on the right eye within a period of 3 months. Finding right eye: anterior segment normal; optic disc slightly pale temporally. In the macular area there was a horizontal dumb-bell-shaped granulomatous focus surrounded by a greyish area and radial retinal folds. The left eye was normal functionally and morphological-ly (Fig. 2).

Case No 3: A woman aged 21 was referred because of recurrent chorioditis in her right eye since 1966. Finding right eye: the globe was slightly injected at the limbus. Anterior chamber: slight Tyndall-phenomen and some cells. Vitreous body shows cellular infiltration. Fundus: optic disc margin blurred, temporally pale, macula: prominent retinochorioditis lesions measuring 3-3½ optic disc diameters the margins being distinctly separable from the healthy

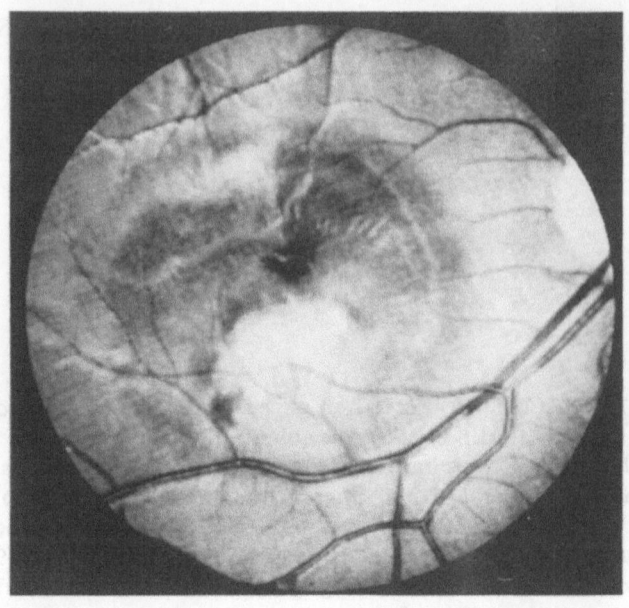

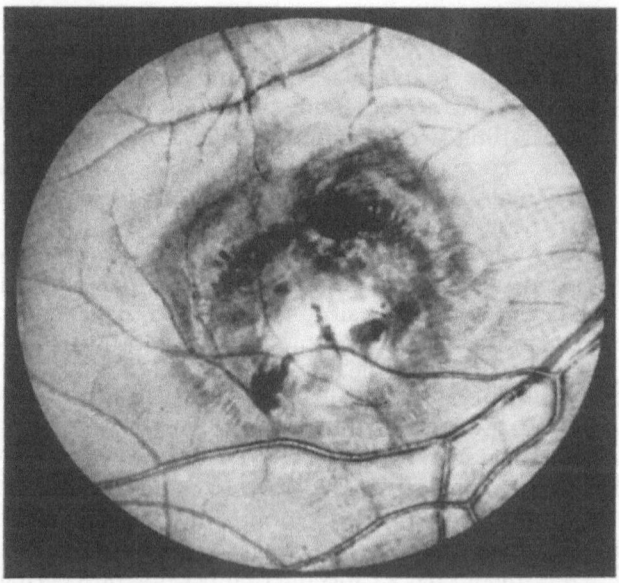

Fig. 1. Fundus photograph showing the granuloma changes in the posterior pole of the right eye. (Case No 1); a) before; b) after the treatment.

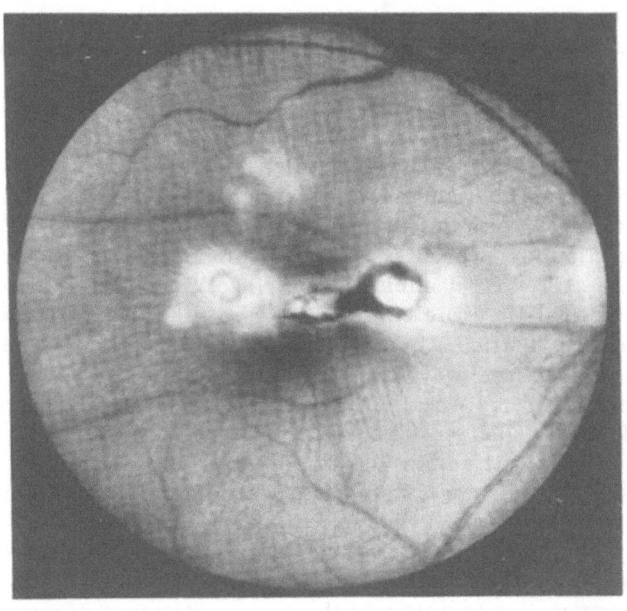

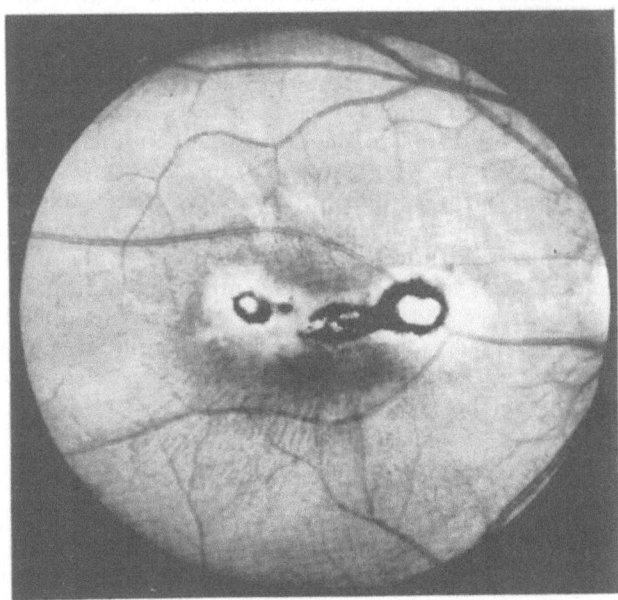

Fig. 2. Fundus photograph showing the toxocaracanis — retinochorioiditis in the affected right eye, (Case No 2); a) before; b) after the treatment.

retina. There were no pathological changes in the left eye (Fig. 3). The serological tests were positive in all 3 cases with special serological proof for toxocara canis.

The figure 4 shows the ERG of case No 1. This ERG was performed in the acute stage of the disease, above the right eye, below the left eye, with marked stimuli at increasing light intensities. This parasitic retinopathy is characterized in the right as well as in the left eye by particularly high amplitudes of all components, which even increase during dark adaption at increasing stimulus intensities. Although the amplitudes of the photopic a_1 and x wave at low flash intensities of 0,125 Wsec are still within the upper range of normal they rise considerably above normal with the next higher flash intensity. Particularly high amplitudes occur in b_1 and b_2 waves, which dominate the b-wave-complex alternately. The b_1-wave at maximum flash intensity of 2,5 Wsec with 475.5 μV forms the highest amplitude of the whole ERG. The scotopic a_2-Wave however shows at all five stimulus intensities the lowest amplitudes of all waves, it does not rise considerably beyond the normal range. Latencies, peak times and duration of photopic (a_1-, x- and b_1-) waves as well as scotopic (a_2 and b_2) waves decrease with increasing stimulus intensities. They show no abnormalities except a few within the positive wave-complexes.

It was interesting to note that there is no difference of size of amplitudes of a- and b-waves in the clinically normal left eye. It is remarkable as well, that amplitudes in case 2 and 3 were just as supernormal as in the first patient, the retino-chorioditis lesions in the macula region apearing approximately the same. This is demonstrated in the Figures 5 and 6.

However, it is interesting that the EOG from the contralateral normal eye were evidently normal whereas the EOG — time curve obtained in the damaged eye — ranged from the pathological in case 1 and subnormal in cases 2 and 3 in proportion to the degree of the retinal degeneration in the fundus as illustrated in the Figures 7, 8 and 9. After the treatment with Menzulon[1], an efficient antihelminthiasis drug the lesions of the posterior pole to the fundus improved a great deal in the three cases and degenerative changes took place as shown in the figures 1b, 2b and 3b. The serological tests became more or less negative. It is interesting to note that the ERG of both the affected eye and the healthy eye became completely normalised, there was a generalised reduction of response amplitude. On the other hand the EOG, according to the degree of the pathological changes in the macular region, remained unchanged.

DISCUSSION

The ERG and EOG-results, which we found in Toxocara canis retino chorioditis do not seen to make much sense. If changes in ERG- and EOG are considered as being due to ganglion or pigmentary cell activity, a larger circumscribed ocular lesions would be expected to reduce the potential and thus give an idea about the retina-chorioidal damage.

1. 2-/4- Thiazolyl-benzimidazol, Dosis: 25 mg/kg, 2 x die. Merck et Co. Inc. Rahway. N.Y. (USA).

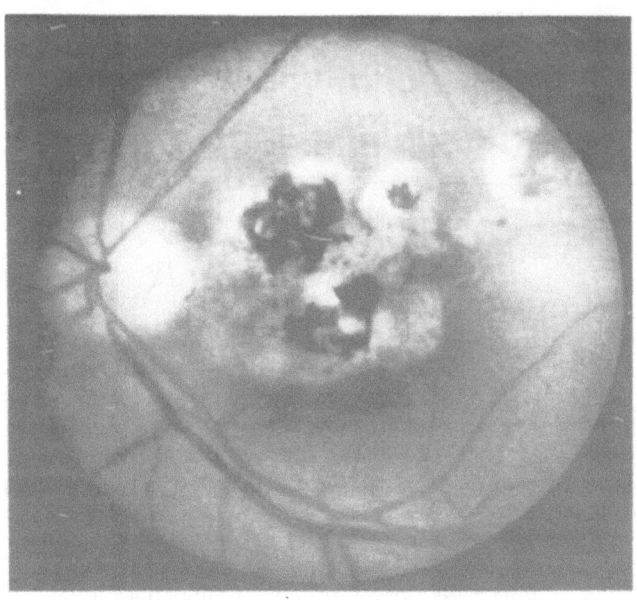

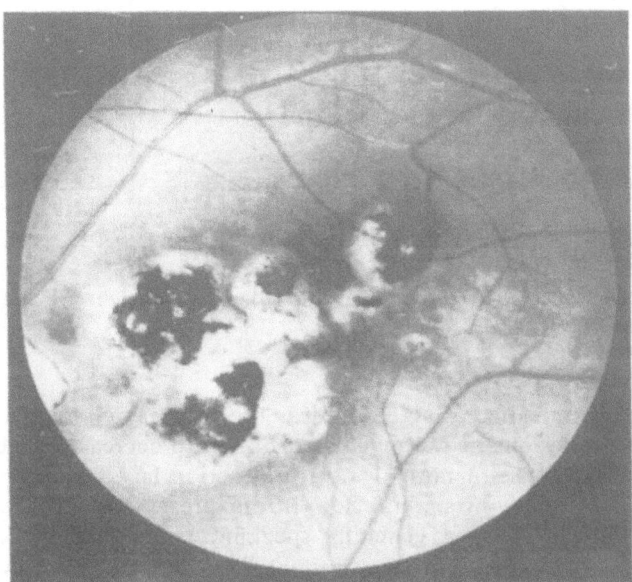

Fig. 3. Fundus photograph showing the granuloma changes in the macular region of the right eye, (Case No 3); a) before; b) after the treatment.

ERG - bei Toxocara-canis Retinochorioïditis

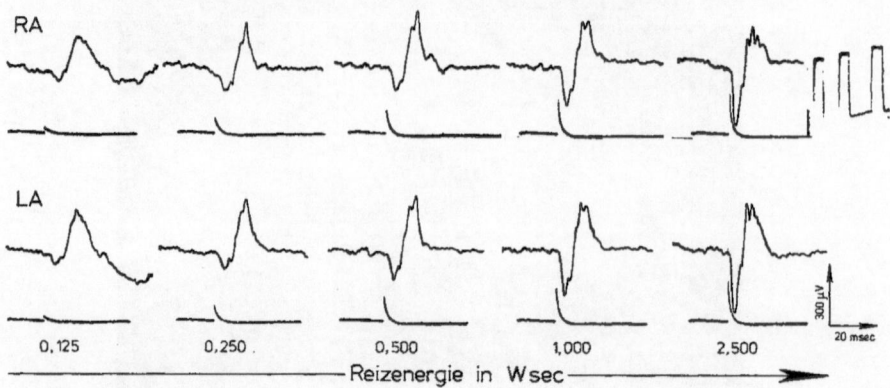

Fig. 4. Single flash ERG – recording from the damaged right eye and the fellow left eye from Case No 1.

ERG - bei Toxocara-canis Retinochorioïditis

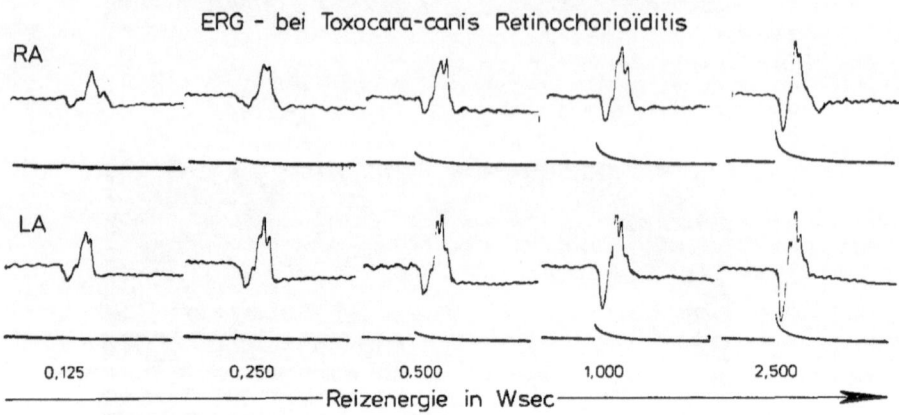

Fig. 5. Single flash ERG – recording from the affected right eye and the fellow left eye from Case No 2.

In toxocara canis retino-choriodits however as opposed to the extensive degenerative lesions of the macular region with decrease of the ERG-waves, there is an increase of normal wave production larger even on the affected side then on the contralateral side. In our present results, the ERG in this disease showed changes, generally speaking earlier than EOG. We can also state, that in this disease supernormal ERG was observed even when the pathologic changes were only small or the EOG was only slightly lowered. These considerations would induce us to think that the increased ERG-potentials particularly in the acute stage of the disease may be an increased irritability of the whole Retina, which possibly means a defense mechanism against larva or its antibodies. The super-normal ERG and the pathological

338

or subnormal EOG-potentials do not contradict our knowledge about the kind of retino-chorioditis affection in toxocara canis infestation.

However, the question remains unanswered why the unaffected, contralateral healthy eye produces similar ERG responses without similar morphological and functional changes. It may be assumed, from ophthalmoscopic

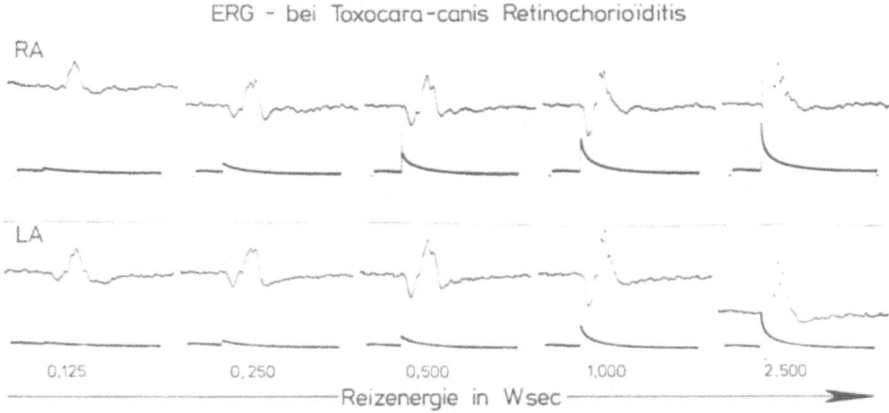

Fig. 6. Single flash ERG – recording from the damaged right eye and the fellow left eye.

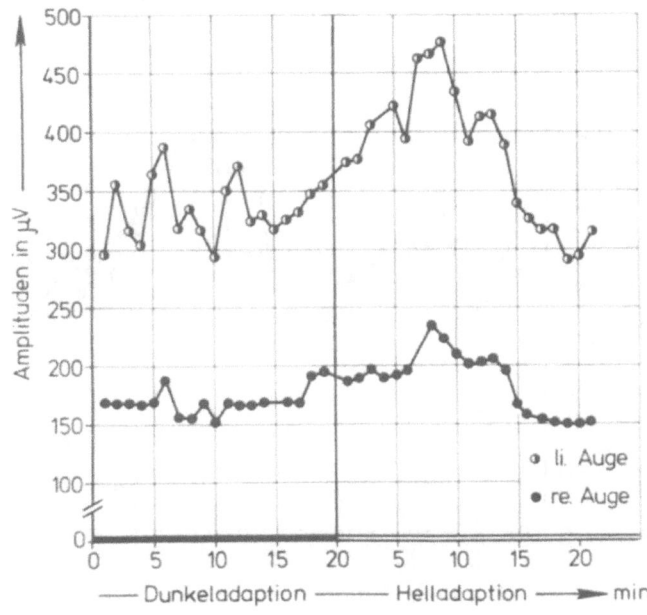

Fig. 7. EOG – graph showing pathological light peak/dark trough ratio in the affected right eye from Case No 1.

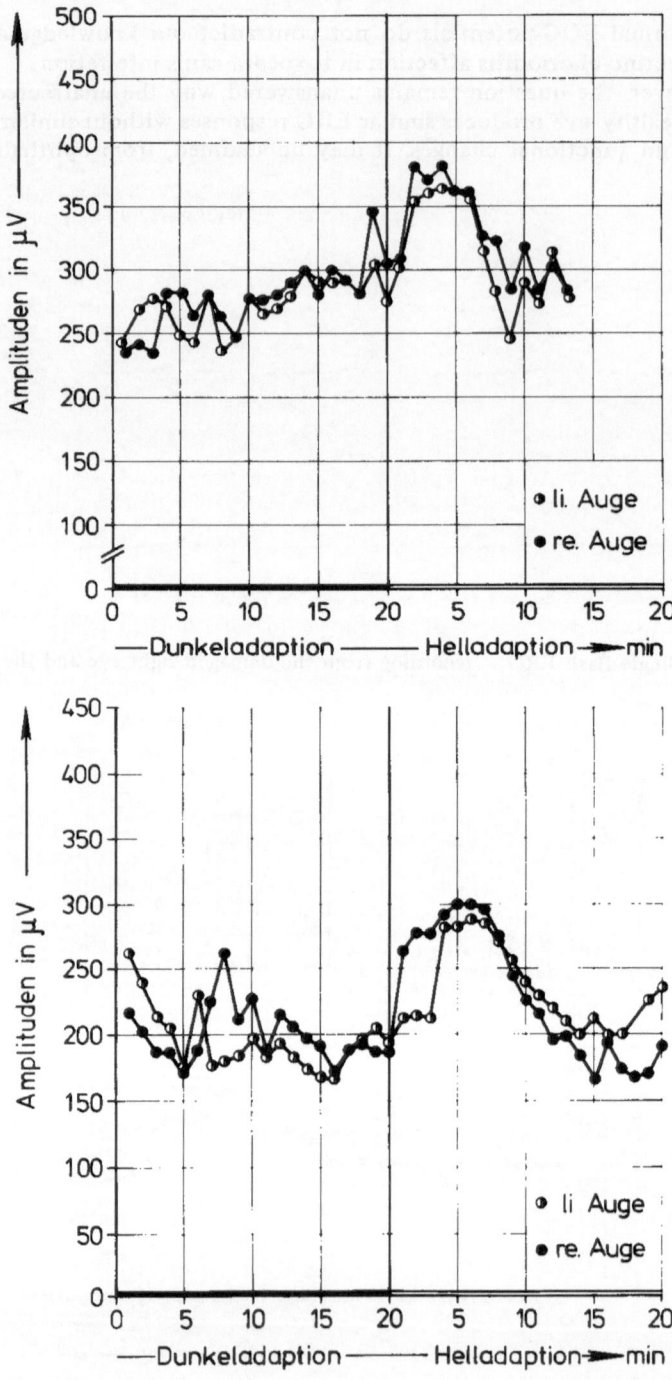

Fig. 8 and 9. EOG – time curve with subnormal Arden – ratio in the affected right eye (Case 2 and Case 3) and a just normal – ratio in the fellow left eye.

340

and histological results (DUGUID 1961), that ocular toxocariasis usually occurs monolaterally and only rarely bilaterally but that the obviously normal eye is affected allergo-toxically. Thus the ERG-wave-form is explained as an unspecific kind of reaction in a prediposed eye. The general reduction of the ERG-amplitude in the latter stages of this disease is also the results of the therapie and the manifestation mainly of a decrease in the excitable area of the retina. Finally, if one considers experimental and clinical findings about the origin of the EOG, the subnormal or pathological EOG indicates a possible migration of toxocara larva via central retinal artery into the inner layers of the pathological process only in an indirect manner resulting in retino-chorioditis degenerations and not chorioretinis lesion.

EFFECT OF STIMULUS DURATION ON THE OSCILLATORY POTENTIALS OF THE HUMAN ELECTRORETINOGRAM

(Preliminary report)

LILLEMOR WACHTMEISTER

(Stockholm, Sweden)

It has been shown psychophysically that in the human darkadapted eye there is a critical duration of the light stimulus below which the relationship I x t = C, the Bunsen-Roscoe law, holds if I is the stimulus intensity and t the duration of light stimulus. In light adaptation this critical duration decreases i.e. the temporal summation is less. The same temporal characteristics of the b- and a-wave of the human electroretinogram have previously been shown by JOHNSON & BARTLETT 1955, ALPERN & FARIS 1956 WIRTH 1956 and VAN LITH 1966.

At the Department of Ophthalmology Karolinska Hospital, Stockholm, we have studied the duration effect of the oscillatory potentials of the human electroretinogram. The apparatus recording system and methods of measurements previously described by ALGVERE, WACHTMEISTER & WESTBECK 1972 and WACHTMEISTER 1974 were used. A pulse generator regulated a electromagnetic shutter, which controlled the duration of light stimulus. The duration varied from about 4 to about 400 msec.

The ERG was recorded after dark adaptation of 30 minutes of 3 young and healthy subjects. Two procedures were used to study the threshold of the potentials.

I. Three consecutive stimulus light of the same intensity were given at an interval of 15 seconds and the ERG in response to the third light was studied. The intensity of all three lights increased logarithmically. The first two stimuli in each series induced a comparatively strong state of light adaptation at the point of time when the third stimulus light was delivered. The procedure was repeated with duration of light stimulus varying over a range of 2 log units.

II. In another series of experiments the procedure was very similar to the described above, light stimuli were given with longer intervals i.e.2 min. The retinal state of light adaptation caused by previous stimuli was then comparatively weak when the next stimulus appeared.

Using the first procedure a b-wave appeared in response to stimulus intensity of log I_s = −4.0 with the shortest duration of stimulus light (4 msec) (Fig. 1). With stimulus of longer duration (400 msec) the b-wave was recorded at stimulation intensity of log I_s = −4.3 of the shortest as well as the longest duration. An a-wave was recordable to stimulus light of log I_s = −2.3 of the shortest as well as the longest duration. The oscillations were elicited when stimulus intensity of log I_s = −2.3 and of the shortest (4 msec)

DURATION

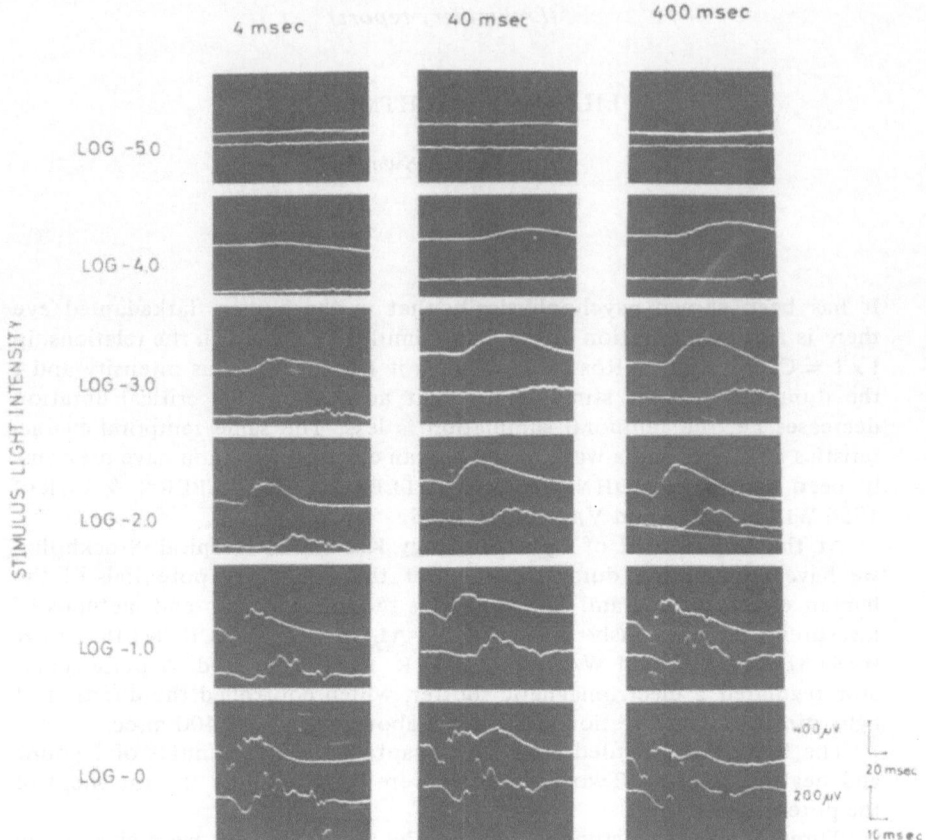

4 msec   40 msec   400 msec

STIMULUS LIGHT INTENSITY

LOG -5.0

LOG -4.0

LOG -3.0

LOG -2.0

LOG -1.0

LOG - 0

400 μV

200 μV

20 msec

10 msec

Fig. 1. Threshold and relation to stimulus light intensity of the amplitude of the slow (a- and b-wave) and the oscillatory potentials for three different durations of stimulus. The duration was varied over a range of 3 log units. A series of three light stimuli of the same intensity was given. The intensity of all three light stimuli increased in a logarithmic scale. There was 15 sec between each stimuli although the intensity of the stimulus varied. Each ERG was displayed in a slow cathode ray sweep speed and low amplification (0.2 mV/cm, 20 msec/cm) (upper trace) and, simultaneously, in a rapid cathode-ray sweep speed and high amplification (0.1 mV/cm, 10 msec/cm) (lower trace). The ERG in response to the third stimulus light in each series of three is illustrated in each picture.

or the longest (400 msec) duration were used. Consequently, the threshold of the a-wave and the oscillatory potentials did not show any significant change when duration light stimulus was changed over a range of 2 log units (Fig. 2). There was a tendency of temporal summation of the b-wave up to 10 msec duration. Using longer stimulus duration the threshold only seemed to be determined by stimulus intensity.

344

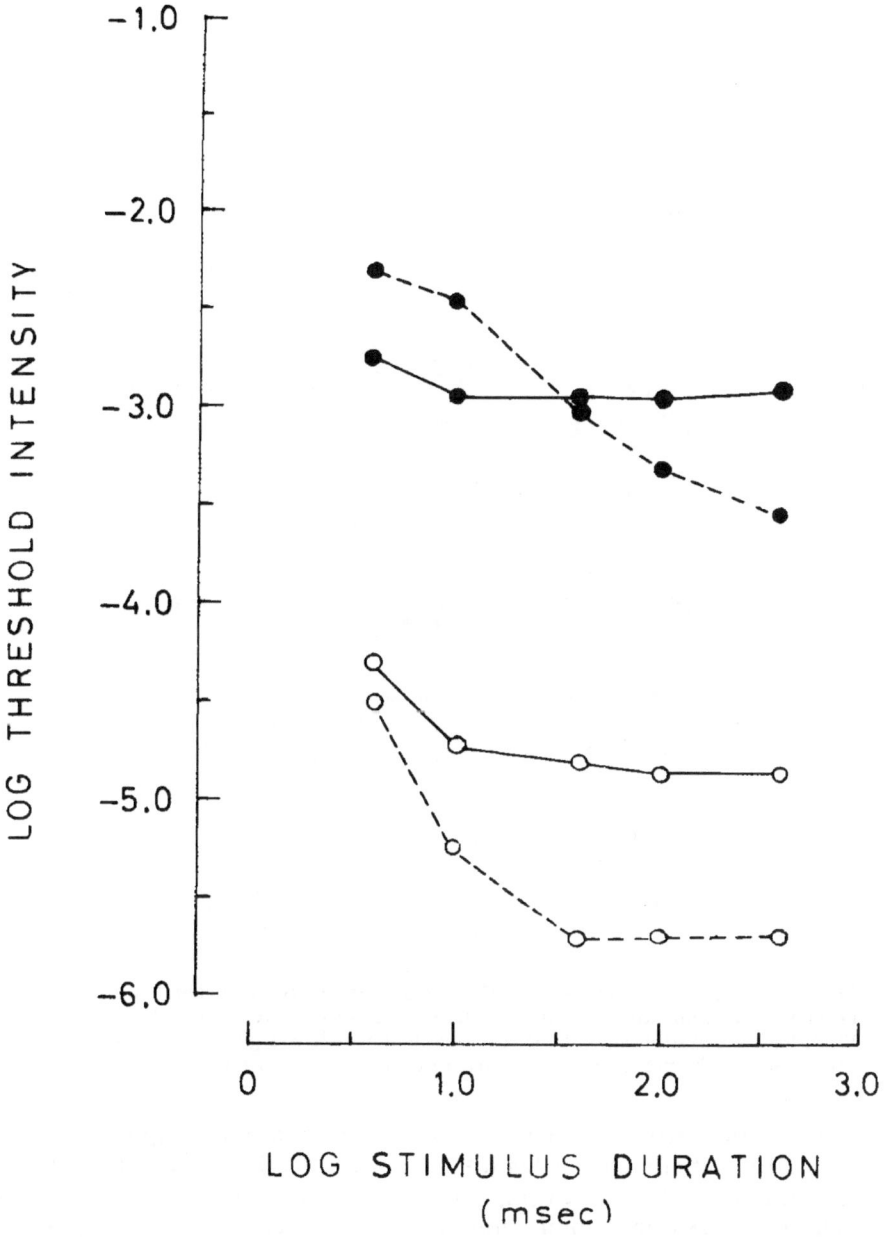

Fig. 2. Comparison between the electric threshold curve of the b-wave and the oscil-latory potentials in relation to duration of stimulus. Threshold criterion was 33 uV for the a- and b-wave and 2.5 a.u. (arbitrary units) for the oscillatory potentials. Average of three subjects. Black circles: oscillatory potentials. Open circles: b-wave. Continuous line: strong light adaptation by stimuli given at an interval of 15 sec. Dashed line: weak light adaptation by stimuli given at an interval of 2 min.

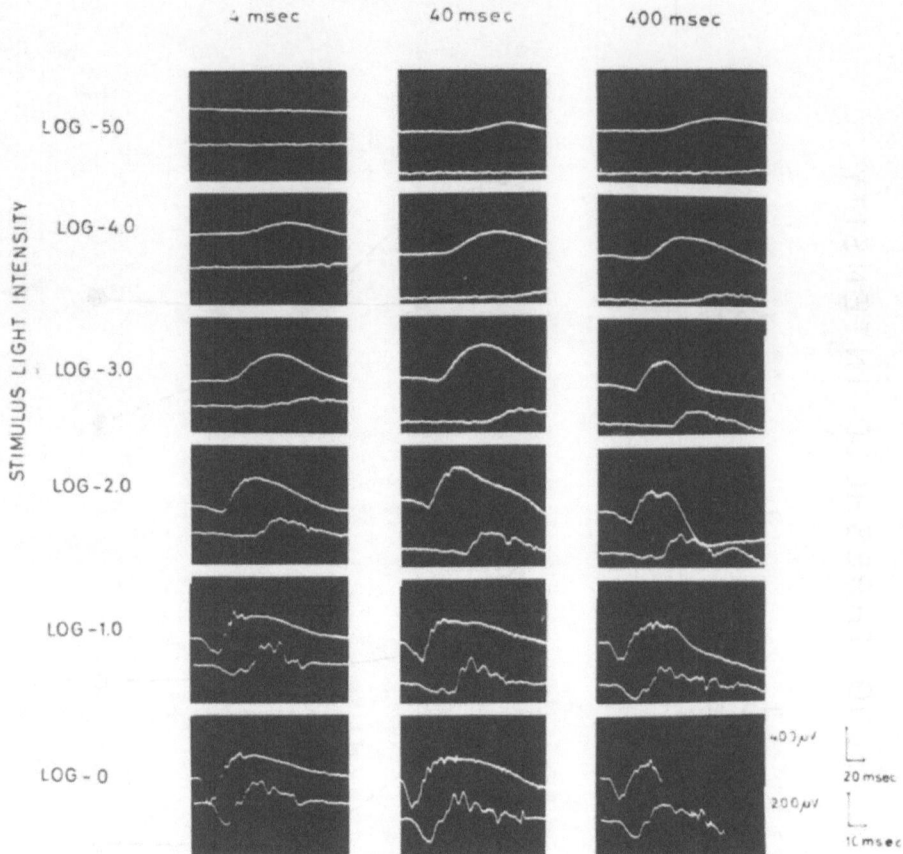

Fig. 3. Threshold and relation to stimulus light intensity of the amplitude of the slow (a- and b-wave) and the oscillatory potentials for three different durations of stimulus. Weak light adaptation caused by stimulus light which was given at 2 min intervals. In other respects the procedure was similar to that described in Fig. 1.

When the second procedure was performed a b-wave appeared in response to light stimulus of $\log I_S = -4.3$ when the shortest duration of light stimulus (4 msec) was used (Fig. 3). A b-wave was induced by light stimulus of $\log I_S = -5.3$ when stimulus duration was 40 msec or more. In response to light stimulus of $\log I_S = -2.3$ and 4 msec duration an a-wave appeared. When duration increased to 40 msec or longer an a-wave was recorded in response to $\log I_S = -3.3$. The oscillatory potentials were elicited by stimulus light of $\log I_S = -2.0$ and 4 msec duration. When longer duration (40 msec) was used the oscillations appeared in response to light stimulus of $\log I_S = -3.0$. Using 400 msec duration they were recorded in response to $\log I_S = -3.3$.

346

Evidently, the threshold of the slow (a- and b-wave) as well as oscillatory potentials changed as the stimulus duration increased. The slow potentials revealed a temporal summation up to 40 msec, whereas the oscillatory potentials were integrated up to the longest duration (400 msec) used (Fig. 2). In summary, the threshold of the oscillatory potentials was deter-

In summary, the threshold of the oscillatory potentials was determined by intensity of stimulus light alone when short intervals between stimuli were used. When longer intervals were used and weak light adaptation by stimuli was induced, the threshold was dependent of intensity as well as duration of stimulus i.e, temporal summation existed over a range of at least 2 log units. Thus, temporal summation of the oscillations varied with retinal light adaptation caused by stimuli. The rapid oscillations behaved differently to that of the slow potentials (a- and b-wave).

REFERENCES

ALGVERE, P., L. WACHTMEISTER & S. WESTBECK On the oscillatory potentials of the human electroretinogram in light and dark adaptation. 1. Thresholds and relation to stimulus intensity on adaptations short flashes of light. A Fourier analysis. *Acta ophthalmologica* 50: *737-759* (1972).

ALPERN, M. & J. FARIS Luminance-Duration Relationship in the Electric Response of the Human Retina. *J. Opt. Soc. Am.* 46: *845-850* (1956).

JOHNSON, P.E. & N.R. BARTLETT Effect of Stimulus Duration on Electrical Responses of the Human Retina. *J. Opt. Soc. Am.* 46: *167-170* (1056).

VAN LITH, G.H.M. Simultane bestimmung der elektroretinographischen und senso rischen Reizschwelle. *Vision Res.* 6: *185-197* (1966).

WACHTMEISTER, L. Luminosity functions of the oscillatory potentials of the human electroretinogram. *Acta opthalmologica* (Kbh) 52, *353-366* (1974).

WIRTH, A. La durata dello stimolo como mezzi di separazione delle componenti fotopica e scotopica dell' electroretinogramma. *Arch. Sci. Biol.* 40, *163-170* (1956).

SENSORY AND ELECTROCORTICAL DETERMINATION OF THE AREA-LUMINANCE RELATIONSHIP IN RESPONSE TO INTERMITTENT LIGHT STIMULATION IN MAN

V. GAVRIYSKY & W. HERBOLZHEIMER

(Frankfurt/Main-Bad Nauheim, FRG)

According to FERRY (1892) and PORTER (1902) the critical flicker frequency (cff) is linearly related to the logarithm of the stimulus amplitude of the flickering light. Furthermore, there is a relation between the critical flicker frequency and the logarithm of area stimulated (GRANIT & HARPER, 1930). Since then many authors have reinvestigated the influence of area on the critical flicker frequency (HECHT & SMITH, 1936; HYLKEMA, 1942; LANDIS, 1954). However, we have failed to find measurements on the relation between the area stimulated and the critical flicker threshold (cft), i.e. the luminance necessary for the impression of fusion in response to intermittent light stimuli of constant frequency. Such a procedure is desirable for several reasons. First, to replace the measurement of the critical frequency where fusion occurs by the measurement of luminance at the fusion point in response to a constant stimulus frequency within the photopic range ($\geq$ 30 cps). Secondly, to adapt the psychophysical measurement of the critical flicker frequency to the electrical recording techniques of the visual system such as the electroretinogram (ERG) or the visually evoked cortical potential (VECP) where the determination of the absolute threshold or the critical flicker frequency is less precise than the determination of luminance at a given response amplitude.

The following experiments describe the relation between the size of retinal area stimulated and the luminance necessary for a constant response (critical flicker threshold in psychophysical measurement, amplitude of a fixed size in the VECP) during intermittent photic stimulation in man.

METHODS

(1) *Sensory measurement.* Subjects were a 23 year old female and a 22 year old male, both in good health. Presenting of the light stimulus was made by a Tübingen projection perimeter (Oculus/Dudenhofen) with hemispheral illumination of stepwise variable luminance of the adaptation field and the test stimulus. Interruption of the test stimulus for intermittent light was performed by a motor-driven sectored disk providing light stimuli of equal light and dark period. Constancy of the stimulus frequency of 30 cps (in some experiments 40 cps were used) was controlled by a frequency counter (Wandel & Goltermann/Reutlingen) and readjusted if necessary.

The subject observed a steady adaptation field upon which flickering light stimuli of different field diameters ranging from 7 to 116 minutes were superimposed. The test stimulus was either foveally presented (central measurements) or at various angles of eccentricity ranging from 20° to 60° in the horizontal meridian of the temporal retina. During the measurement the subject looked with one eye at the fixation point of 10' diameter; the other eye was covered with a black eye-patch. Fixation was controlled by means of a telescope in the position of the blind spot.

Mydriaticum Roche and Neosynephrine 2.5% were used for dilatation of the pupil.

Measurement was made by determining the luminance at the flicker fusion point by inserting neutral (Schott NG) filters in steps of 0.1 optical density. The critical flicker threshold was determined by the up- and down-method deviating randomly twice from the rule. The luminance of the surround was kept constant at about 12 cd/m². The luminance of the test stimulus (maximum value about 1200 cd/m²) and the adaptation field were measured with a SEI exposure photometer (Salford Electrical Instruments). (2) *Electrocortical measurement.* A xenon was employed at the source for both the flickering light and for the background illumination. The luminance of the test beam was varied by inserting neutral density absorption filters. The background illumination was kept constant at 2000 td. Interference band filters served to obtain flickering lights of 630 nm and background illumination of 467 nm. Flicker was produced by rotating sectored disks in place of the shutter providing equal light and dark periods.

The subject fixed through the dilated pupil of his left eye in Maxwellian view (central fixation) a steady circular adaptation field of 18° upon which the flickering light of various size (24' to 12°) was concentrically superimposed. A hair-cross served for fixation. The right eye was covered with a black eye-patch.

The potentials were led off by a gold-disk electrode placed about 3 cm above the inion (monopolar recording). They were amplified and fed into a Tektronix 502 A oscilloscope which was connected to a Biomac Computer. Negativity of the recording electrode is indicated by downward, positivity by upward deflection of the potential recorded.

Measurements began with the determination of the sensory and the VECP threshold. Thereafter, the radiant power of the flickering beam was increased in steps of 0.3 to 0.45 log units. At each level to VECP was recorded (n = 256) and displayed on an X-Y recorder.

RESULTS

(1) *Sensory determination.* The luminance at the threshold criterion chosen, i.e. the fusion point in response to the flickering light of constant frequency (critical flicker threshold, cft) decreases as the retinal area increases. For small fields, i.e. less than 44 min of arc, the decrease of stimulus luminance roughly corresponds to the increase of the retinal area; for larger fields, i.e. up to a stimulus diameter of 116 min of arc, the decrease of luminance is less than the increase of area stimulated (Fig. 1A). Generally, the different slopes of the area-luminance relationship are more clearly seen

350

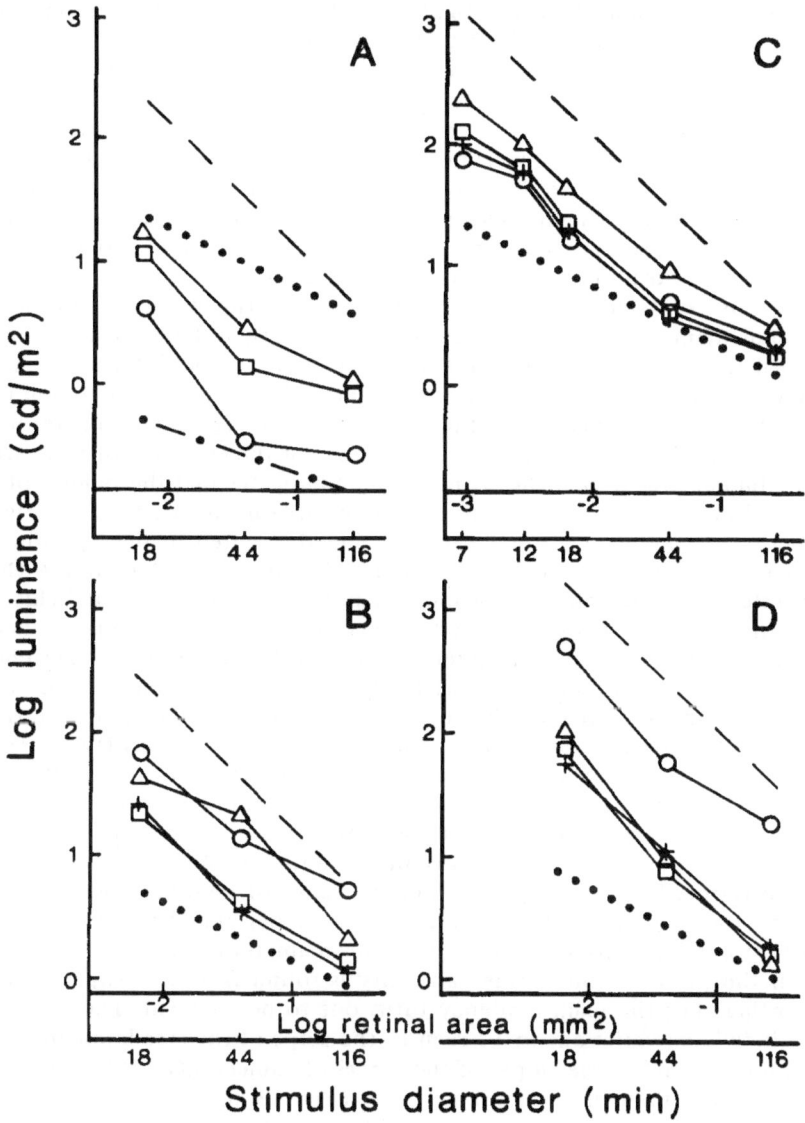

Fig. 1. Graphs showing the relation of log luminance (cd/m²) of the test stimulus at the flicker fusion point (sensory determination) in response to intermittent light of constant frequency (ordinate) and log retinal area (mm²) stimulated (abscissa). On the second abscissa the diameter of the test light (in min of arc) is indicated. A and C – subject S.G., B and D – subject A.M. Stimulus frequency A and B – 30 cps, C and D – 40 cps. Foveal fixation. Central stimulation – circles, eccentric stimulation 20° – crosses, 30° – squares, 60° – triangles. Background luminance 12 cd/m² (A); 8.6 cd/m² (B); 13.6 cd/m² (C); 10.8 cd/m² (D). Graph C includes stimulus diameters of 7 and 12 min of arc. Ricco's law (I · A = constant) – dashed line; Piper's law (I · √A = constant) – dotted line; Pieron's law (I · ∛A = constant) – dashed-dotted line.

in the center (circles) than with stimulation of the peripheral retinal field (crosses − 20°, squares −30°, triangles − 60°).

Fig. 1B illustrates an experiment in another subject. The different slopes with smaller and larger test fields at central and peripheral (20°, 30°) stimulation are not as impressive as in A. There is an exception of the curve at 60° where the slope deviates from the course at stimulus diameter of 44 min of arc which may be ascribed to the eccentric stimulation that sometimes turned out to be difficult. Occasionally it occurs that the slopes for smaller and larger peripheral test fields are nearly equal resulting in a roughly linear course of the area-luminance relationship (cf. also fig. 1D).

Because of technical reasons the present experiments were confined to stimulus diameters up to 2° (116 min of arc). In their determinations of the critical frequency of flicker (cff) GRANIT & HARPER (1930) used larger stimulus fields (up to 6°). With central and 10° peripheral stimulation they observed a further increase of the cff in areas for a stimulus diameter up to 6°. With still larger stimulus fields, the course of the curve relating the cff to the stimulus area became horizontal, which indicates that the validity of the Granit-Harper law is confined to a stimulus area up to 6°. In their original experiments the cff was approximately linearly related to the logarithm of area between 21 min and 6° of stimulus diameter. GRANIT & HARPER suggested that the relationship did not hold at smaller stimulus fields and that the complete curve would be S-shaped. We recognize a similar tendency in Fig. 1C at the stimulus diameter of 7 min of arc (except at 60° peripheral stimulation). According to GRANIT & HARPER, the linear relation between cff and log area would be an approximation referring to the rising branch of the curve or perhaps only to its upper part. BROWN (1945) examined the validity of the Granit-Harper law between 25° and 90° retinal location for a stimulus diameter between 23.4 min of arc and 13.6° under the conditions imposed by the Talbot level surround, which matches the brightness at fusion of the intermittent stimulus. Under these conditions the Granit-Harper law was confirmed but the range of its validity was found to exceed the stimulus diameter limit of 6°. At peripheral location 50°, the relation was found to hold up to a stimulus diameter of 13.6°.

In the present study some variability is found from one experiment to the other, but the main tendency turns out to be constant. There are also interindividual variations to be seen in the slope of the area-luminance relationship; generally, the slopes of the curves of subject S.G. (Fig. 1A and C) are more flat than those of subject A.M. (Fig. 1B and D). Accordingly, we can say that the effect of the size of the stimulated area is less in subject S.G. than in subject A.M.

(2) *Electrocortical determination.* As compared to the high threshold of the electrical response of the eye (electroretinogram) where the determination of the area-luminance relationship is complicated by the presence of stray light, the relation between the VECP and the sensory threshold is much more favourable (HUBER & ADACHI, 1971). Nevertheless, the use of strong adaptation fields to suppress the rod activity is advisable (HENKES & VAN LITH, 1969). While in previous studies at low repetition rates of the light stimulus, fields as small as 24 min of arc have been used (RIETVELD et al., 1965; ARMINGTON, 1968; DE VOE et al., 1968) the smallest field

diameter presently used to evoke measureable flicker responses at 30 cps in the VECP is 48 min of arc. Clear-cut responses are seen at a field diameter of 2° (Fig. 2). It is seen that at larger fields the amplitude of the VECP wavelets increases. The shape of the wavelets is similar to destroyed sinusoids, and at 6° field diameter the wavelets become double-positive at stronger radiant power. Up to a field diameter of 10°(in some subjects up to 6°) the amplitude of the wavelets increases.

Accordingly, a smaller radiant power is necessary for a VECP of constant amplitude when the retinal area increases. This is shown in Fig. 3 where an almost linear relation is seen between log radiant power of the stimulus and log area stimulated up to a filed size of 6°. The slope of the curve is more than what is predicted by Ricco's law ($I \cdot A$ = constant, indicated by dashed line). Instead it is close to the relation $I \cdot A^{3/2}$ = constant (line interrupted by crosses).

Different to the above data obtained with the 30 cps flicker VECP are the results of sensory threshold measurements at the fusion point obtained in the same experiments (Fig. 3, filled symbols). Within the range of areas tested, hardly any effect of area is seen, the slope of the area-luminance curve is more flat than Piper's law ($I \cdot \sqrt{A}$ = constant, indicated by dotted line) and approaches Pieron's law ($I \cdot \sqrt[3]{A}$ = constant, indicated by dashed-dotted line).

With a repetition rate of 2.3 cps ADACHI & KELLERMANN (1973)

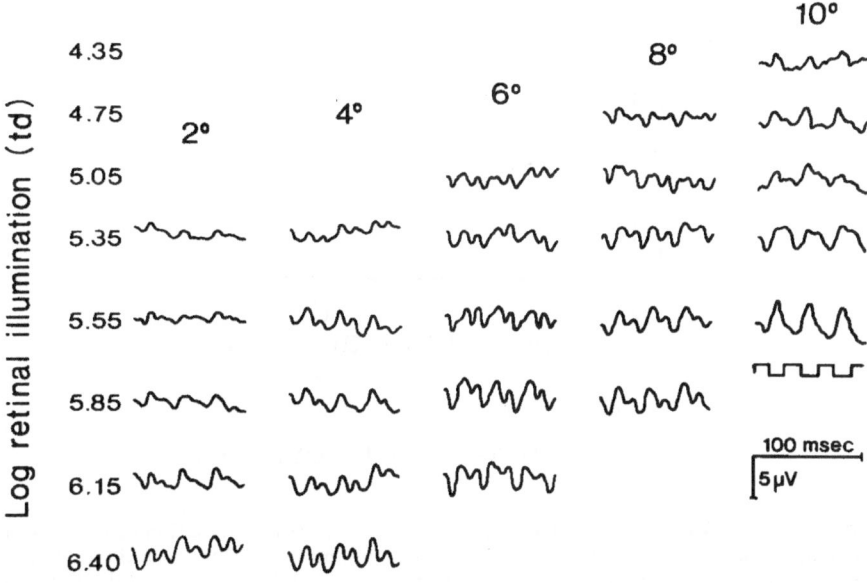

Fig. 2. Averaged (n = 256) VECPs in response to intermittent light stimuli (λ = 630 nm central fixation) of 32 cps, concentrically superimposed upon an adaptation field (λ = 467 nm) of 2000 td. Diameter of test field – horizontal columns; test light illumination (log td) – vertical columns. Light pulse, amplitude and time calibration as indicated. Subject G.S.

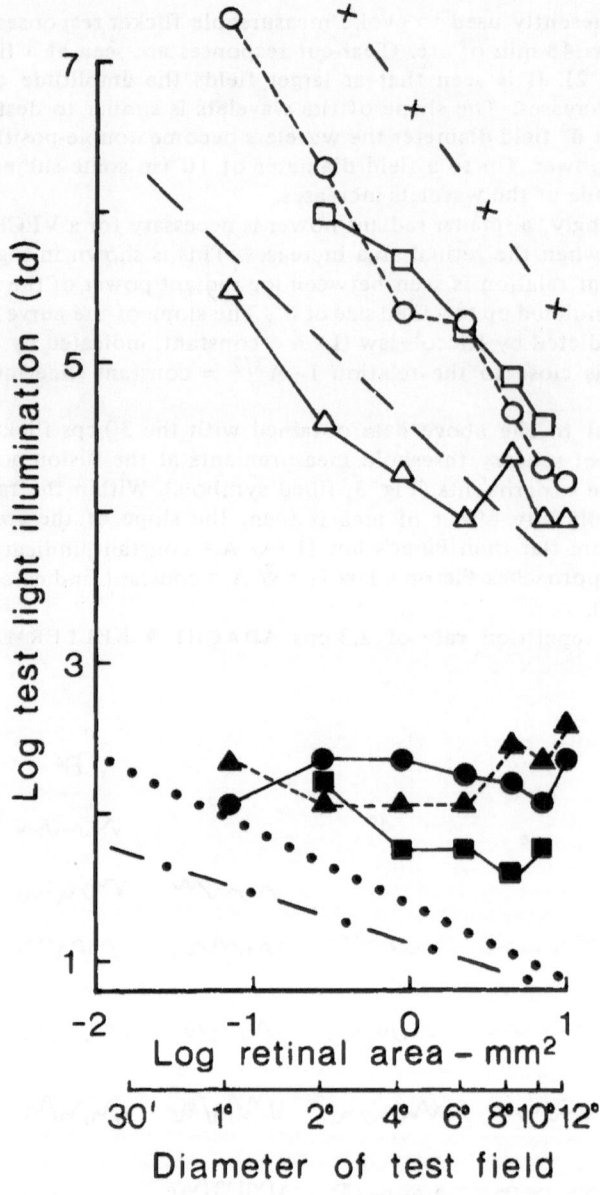

Fig. 3. Graph showing the relation between log test light illumination of intermittent stimuli of 30 cps, necessary for VECPs of constant amplitude (log td, ordinate) and log retinal area stimulated (abscissa). The test light (λ = 630 nm, central fixation) was concentrically superimposed by background illumination (467 nm) of 2000 td. Circles – criterion amplitude 1.5 μV, subject B.M.; triangles – criterion amplitude 1.5 μV, subject V.G.; squares – criterion amplitude 2.0 μV, subject G.S. Filled symbols – data of sensory threshold measurements obtained from the same subjects. The dashed line denotes Ricco's law (I · A = constant), the dotted line Piper's law (I · √A = constant), the dashed-dotted line (Pieron's law (I · ∛A = constant).

studied the area-luminance relationship in the *scotopic* VECP. Using latency as the criterion and a stimulus duration of 0.1 sec the data obtained were similar to those of the present investigation. However, the sensory data obtained by these authors were different. The slope of the area-luminance relation of the sensory threshold was similar to the VECP findings, whereas in the present photopic conditions it was flat.

DISCUSSION

The present study describes the relationship between the luminance necessary for a given critical flicker frequency and the stimulated retinal area superimposed to a photopic background. The results are compared with the likewise determined luminances required for a given height of response obtained with the VECP. In the sensory series the slope of the critical flicker threshold area approximates Ricco's law at small stimulus fields ($< 1°$ field diameter) and Piper's law (in some experiments Pieron's law) at larger fields (up to $2°$ field diameter). At still larger fields (up to $6°$ diameter) the slope decreases and approaches Pieron's law. With the VECP as index the slope of the curve between 1 and $6°$ is more than what is predicted by Ricco's law.

Assuming a direct relationship between stimulus luminance and critical flicker frequency (Ferry-Porter law) as well as between critical frequency and area (Granit-Harper law) a similar relation can be expected between area and stimulus luminance of a flickering light of constant frequency. The present experiments show such a relation under photopic conditions up to about 6 to $10°$ in the VECP and up to $1°$ in the sensory determinations. Why is the range so much different for the two sets of measurement where the reciprocity law of Granit and Harper holds? (1) There are inhomogeneities within the field tested, and the minimum field size where VECP recordings were made is much larger than for the sensory measurements. (2) The contribution of stray light which is considerably more in the VECP recordings than in the sensory series. (3) In the VECP measurements the criterion was a given height of response about half between the threshold and the maximum response in the VECP.

It is well known that the course of the curve describing the VECP amplitude versus luminance is S-shaped and that at threshold near luminances there is a linear relation between the luminance and the height of response, whereas at higher luminances there is a linear relation between the logarithm of luminance and the height of response. Such an effect could be of major importance for the different range of validity for the VECP and the sensory series where the reciprocity law holds. Light scatter could provide the extension of the validity of the reciprocity law in the VECP series in the direction of bigger areas stimulated. While such an effect could be present in the dark adapted VECP measurements of ADACHI & KELLERMANN (1973) and in the electroretinographic measures of VAN LITH (1966), this is less so in the present photopic measurements where the light signals were superimposed to a bright surround and the frequency of intermittent stimulation is in the photopic range.

The present results support the conclusion that the parafovea significantly contributes to the photopic VECP. Therefore, we share REGAN's (1972) conclusion that the relative effectiveness of central foveal stimulation for evoking cortical potentials extremely stressed by RIETVELD et al. (1965), ARMINGTON (1968) and DE VOE et al. (1968) is fairly exaggerated.

SUMMARY

The area-luminance relationship in response to intermittent light stimuli of constant frequency (30 and 40 cps) is determined in man by measuring the luminance at the flicker fusion threshold (psychophysical measurements) and for a flicker response amplitude of constant height (measurements of the visually evoked cortical potential).

In the sensory measurement the slope of the critical flicker threshold versus area approximates Ricco's law at small stimulus fields($< 1°$ field diameter) and Piper's law at larger fields (up to $2°$ field diameter). At still larger fields (up to $6°$ diameter) the slope approaches Pieron's law.

With the VECP amplitude the slope of the curve between $1°$ and $6°$ is more than what is predicted by Ricco's law. The results support the conclusion that the parafoveal region of the retina significantly contributes to the photopic VECP.

REFERENCES

ADACHI-USAMI, E. & KELLERMANN, F.-J. Spatial summation of retinal excitation as obtained by the scotopic VECP and the sensory threshold. *Ophthal. Res.* 5, *308-316* (1973)
ARMINGTON, J.C. The electroretinogram, the visual evoked potential and the area-luminance relation. *Vision Res.* 8, *263-276* (1968).
BROWN, H.C. The relation of flicker to stimulus area in peripheral vision. *Arch. Psychol.* 298, New York, 1945
FERRY, E.L. Peristence of vision. *Amer. J. Sci.* 44, *192* (1892)
GRANIT, R. & HARPER, P. Comparative studies on the peripheral and central retina. *Amer. J. Physiol.* 95, *211-228* (1930).
HECHT, S. & SMITH, E.L. Intermittent stimulation by light. VI. Area and the relation between critical frequency and intensity. *J. gen. Physiol.* 19, *979-989* (1936).
HENKES, H.E. & VAN LITH, G.H.M. Evaluation and clinical application of macular responses in ERG and VER. *J. Chiba Med. Soc.* 45, *489-502* (1969)
HYLKEMA, B.S. Examination of the visual field by determining the fusion frequency. *Acta Ophthal.* 20, *181* (1942).
LANDIS, C. Determinants of the critical flicker-fusion threshold. *Physiol. Reviews*, 34, *259-286* (1954).
VAN LITH, G.H.M. Simultane Bestimmung der elektroretinographischen und sensorischen Reizschwelle. *Vision Res.* 6, *185-197* (1966).
PORTER, T.C. Contributions to the study of flicker. Part II. *Proc. Roy. Soc.*, 70, *313* (1902).
REGAN, D. EPs in Psychology, Sensory Physiology and Clinical Medicine. London, Chapman and Hall, Ltd., 1972.
RIETVELD, E.J. W.E. TORDOIR & J.W. DUFFY Contribution of fovea and parafovea to the VER. *Acta Psysiol. Phyrm. Neerl.*, 13, *330-339* (1965).
DE VOE, R.G., H. RIPPS & H.G. VAUGHAN Cortical responses to stimulation of the human fovea. *Vision Res.* 8, *135-147* (1968).

OCULAR DIPOLE MOMENT (ODM) – VARIATION EXCITED BY PHOTOFLASH[1]

R. TÄUMER, N. ROHDE, J. HENNIG & L. WOLFF

(Freiburg, West Germany)

Via skin electrodes it is possible to record eye movements. This method (electronystagmography, electrooculography) is due to the rotation of the electrical dipole of the eye in relation to the fixed electrodes. If the person moves the eyes with a constant amplitude the variation of the amount of the dipole can be measured indirectly. The recorded amplitude of a 40 deg eye-movement will vary like the ocular dipole moment (ODM). With this method we can investigate the slow potential changes of the retina. If the eyes move frequently a resolution in time of about 1 sec is possible. We demonstrated two components of the ODM-variation (TÄUMER et al., 1974):
1. a sinus of 26 min cycle-time (main oscillation). This main oscillation is much more damped at the lower levels of the ODM (Fig. 1)

COMPONENTS OF THE ODM - VARIATION

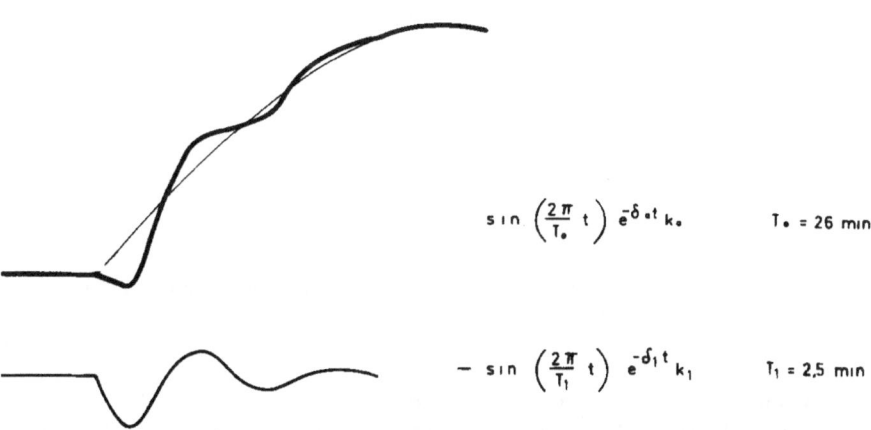

$$\sin\left(\frac{2\pi}{T_0} t\right) e^{-\delta_0 \cdot t} k_0 \qquad T_0 = 26 \text{ min}$$

$$- \sin\left(\frac{2\pi}{T_1} t\right) e^{-\delta_1 t} k_1 \qquad T_1 = 2{,}5 \text{ min}$$

Fig. 1. The two components of the variation of the electrical ocular dipole moment (ODM)
Main oscillation with a cycle-time of 26 min
Fast oscillation with a cycle-time of 2.5 min

1. Supported by the Deutsche Forschungsgemeinschaft SFB 70.

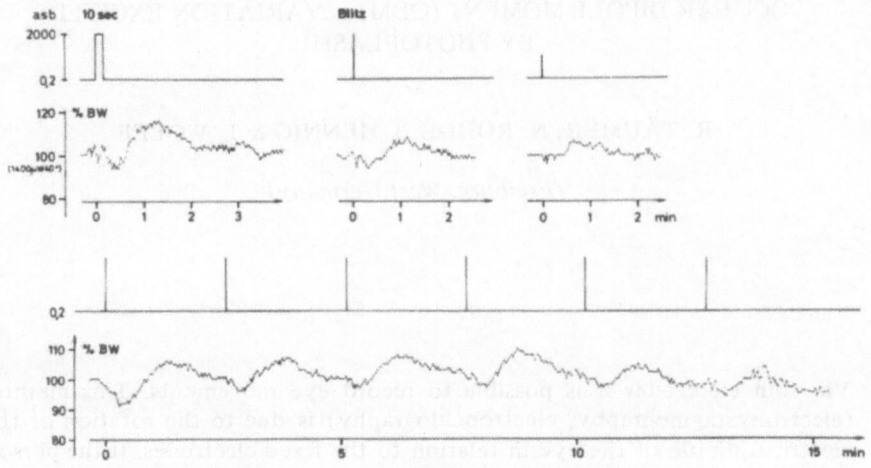

Fig. 2. Response of the ODM to a luminance step of 4 log units and 10 sec duration. Elicitation of the fast ODM-wave by photoflashes of large and small light-exposure. Steady oscillation of the fast wave by stimulation with repeated flashes

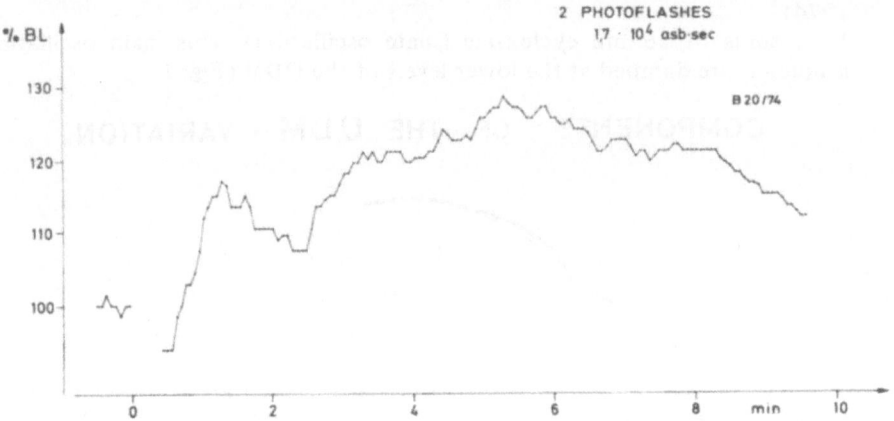

Fig. 3. Response of the ODM to large photoflash with the main oscillation and the superpositioned fast waves

2. a sinus of 2.5 min cycle-time (fast oscillation).

Especially short light pulses elicite the fast oscillation (HENNIG et al., 1974). The upper part of Fig. 2 (left) shows this in an experiment with a luminance step of 4 log units amplitude and a duration of 10 sec. The fast oscillation appears with an amplitude of 21% BL (percent basis level). Also with very short luminance steps, like photoflashes, the fast oscillation can be evoked. That is shown in the upper part of Fig. 2 (right) with a large and a small flash. A repetition of the flashes at each 2.5 min forces the ODM to a steady oscillation with an amplitude larger than 10% BL.

If the flash is large enough also the main oscillation will be stimulated. On the response of Fig. 3 the clearly detectable fast wave is superpositioned to the main oscillation. Here we used two photoflashes separated by 1 sec with an lightexposure of 1.7×10^4 asb x sec.

The photoflashes were performed by a xenon-filled discharge tube. This tube was fixed at the edge of the perimeter and flashes inside it. The intensity-characteristic in time of the 20 asb x sec-flash is drawn in Fig. 4. The peak intensity is reached in a very short time (range: μsec) and decreases 3 log units in about o.1 msec. The peak-intensity for flashes with different light-exposure is always the same. The technical realisation of the different light-exposures of the used flashes is managed by changing the slope on the decreasing part of the intensity-characteristic. So for instance the largest flash has the same intensity-characteristic, but on the time-scale the 0.5 msec must be changed to 50 msec.

The effect of the flashes is roughly proportional to the logarithm of the light-exposure (Fig. 5). Increasing light-exposure causes an increase of the amplitude of the fast wave. In the upper curve the ongoing main oscillation is noticable. The beginning part of the curves is quite unsure. The reason is the spasm of the periocular muscles connected with large luminance increase. It seems that this muscle-contraction changes the electrical resistance of the tissue and causes this large increase of the amplitude for the 40 deg eye movements during a period of about 15 sec.

Now we looked for the effect of repeated flashes. We stimulated with 300 flashes within 30 sec following a long adaptation to a luminance of 0.2 asb. The flashes had a light-exposure of 20 asb sec. Two cycles of the fast wave are detectable (Fig. 6). The first amplitude takes the value of about 30% BL.

In an other experiment (Fig. 7) we adapted the person to complete darkness. During the experiments only the small fixation lights (yellow light emmiting diodes) illuminated the perimeter. Every 2 min there begins a

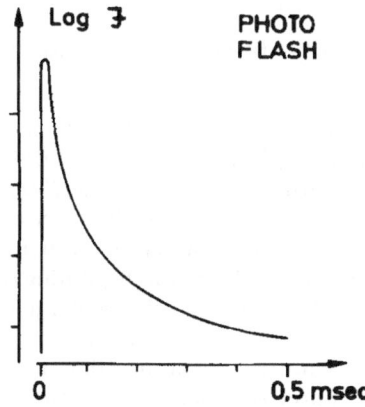

Fig. 4. Intensity-characteristic of the 20 asb sec-flash

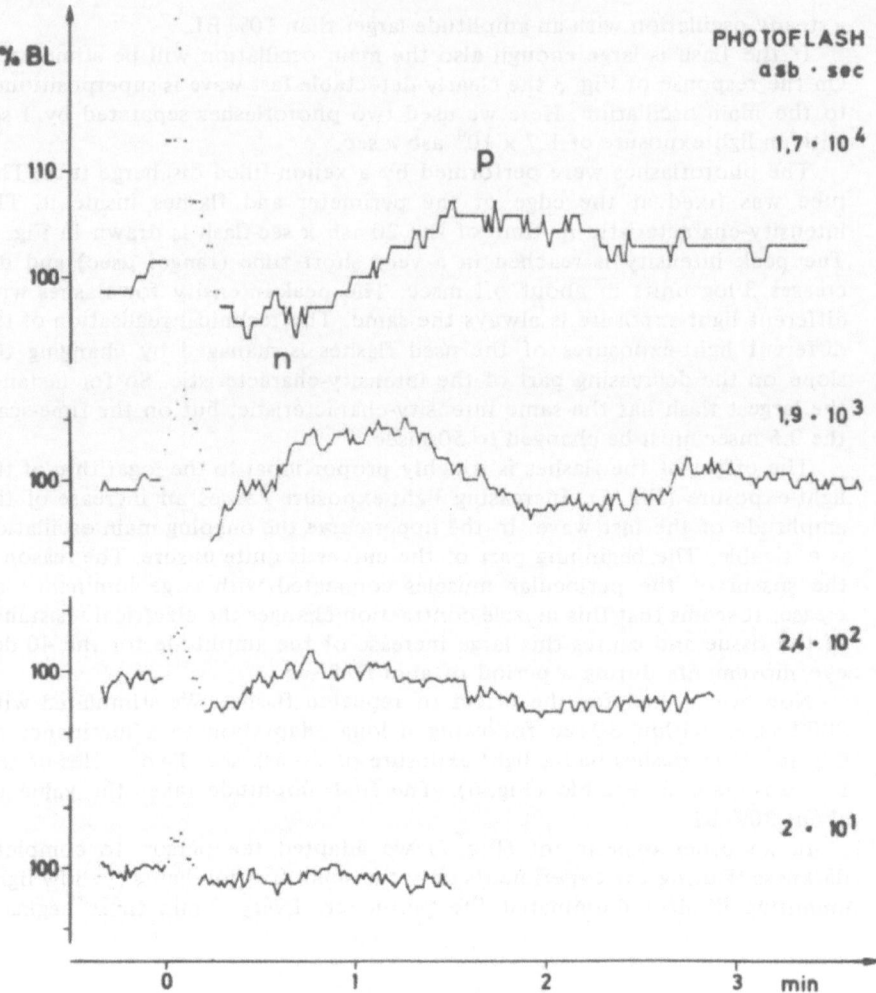

Fig. 5. Response of the ODM to flashes of different light-exposure

flash-period of 30 sec. Again the muscle-disturbance occurs at the beginning of each flash-period. The amplitude of the fast ODM-wave increases with the number of the flashes. With 0.4 cps (12 flashes/30 sec) the fast wave has an amplitude of 16.8% BL; with 20 cps (600/30 sec) about 26.3% BL. These are mean values of the 8 stimulation periods. Furthermore the amplitude of the fast wave increases slightly from the beginning of the experiment to the end. The upper curves show an underlying main oscillation. In Fig. 8 the amplitude of the fast wave is drawn in relation to the logarithm of the number of flashes. It is not sure whether the amplitude of the fast ODM-wave depends linearly upon the logarithm of the flash-number. Perhaps in the region between 1 and 10 cps a saturation occurs. This fact will be object of further experiments.

The experiment of Fig. 9 with an other person supports our belief. Between 6 and 60 flashes/30 sec we get a strong increase (6 to 24% BL). But from 60 to 600 flashes the amplitude changes only slightly (24 to 27% BL).

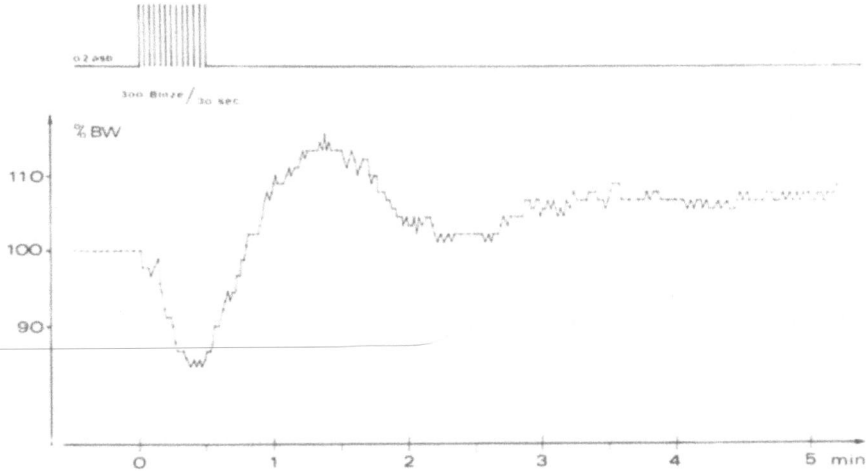

Fig. 6. Excitation of the fast wave by 300 flashes applied during 30 sec.

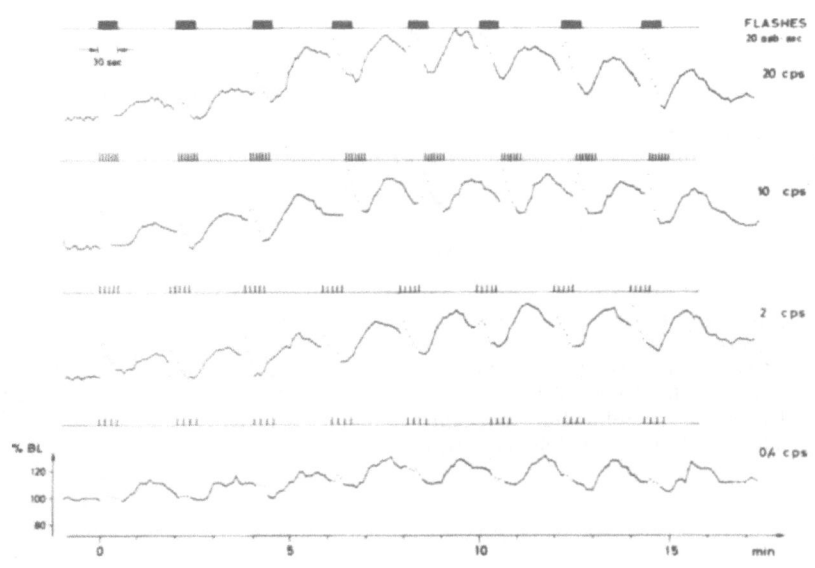

Fig. 7. Stimulation of the ODM with repeated flash-periods of 30 sec. The used flash-frequency during the flash-periods is drawn on the right. Experiment with the same person

361

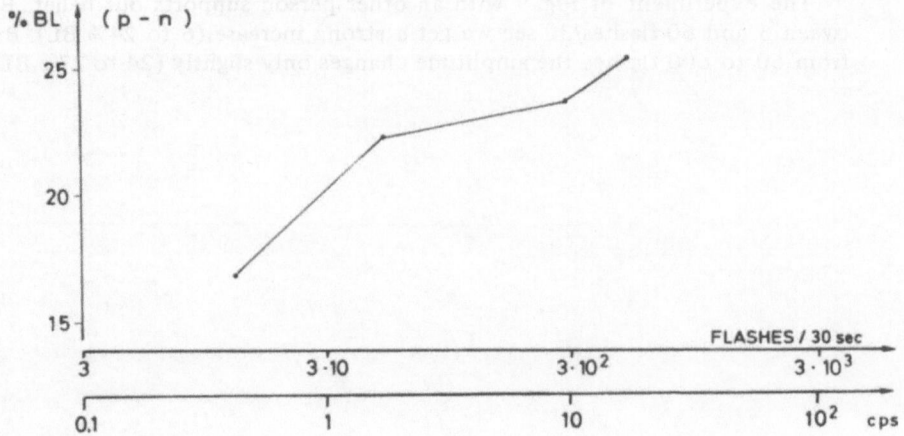

Fig. 8. The amplitude of the fast wave of Fig. 7 in relation to the flash-frequency

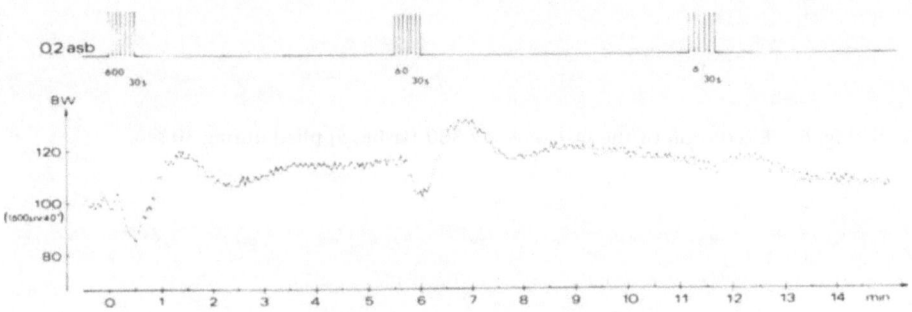

Fig. 9. Variation of the amplitude of the fast wave with the number of flashes delivered during the stimulation interval of 30 sec.

REFERENCES

TÄUMER, R., HENNIG, J. & PERNICE, D. The Ocular Dipole – a Damped Oscillator Stimulated by the Speed of Change in Illumination. *Vision Res.* Vol. 14. (1974).

HENNIG, J., TÄUMER, R. & PERNICE, D. Die Änderung des elektrischen Dipolmoments des menschlichen Auges (ODM) bei kurzen und mittellangen Hell- und Dunkelreizen (Sekunden- und Minuten-Bereich). Berichte von der 72. Zusammenkunft der Deutschen Ophthalmologischen Gesellschaft. Heidelberg 1973,

THE SLOW DARK OSCILLATION OF THE OCULAR DIPOLE MOMENT (ODM) - DEPENDENCE UPON THE AMPLITUDE OF THE STEP TO DARKNESS*

R. TÄUMER, N. ROHDE & R. HAUBACH

(Freiburg, West Germany)

Whereas the light step response of the electrical ocular dipole moment (ODM) had been investigated intensively (KRIS, 1958; KOLDER, 1959; TÄUMER et al. 1974) the dark oscillation had found small interst, since ARDEN (1962) stated an independence of the dark step reponse from the amplitude of the step to darkness. In this study we will deal with the dark response to steps of a large range of amplitudes.

In Fig. 1 our apparatus is shown. A perimeter hemisphere is illuminated by a halogen lamp of 1000 watt. The intensity of the luminance is changed by a shutter which is controlled by a function generator. The amout of the ODM is recorded indirectly by the electrooculogram in dc.-coupling.

Following a step decrease in luminance a damped oscillation of the ODM occurs which lasts with several cycles more than 2 hours. On this response to a step of 3 log units (Fig. 2) the first minimum with a value of

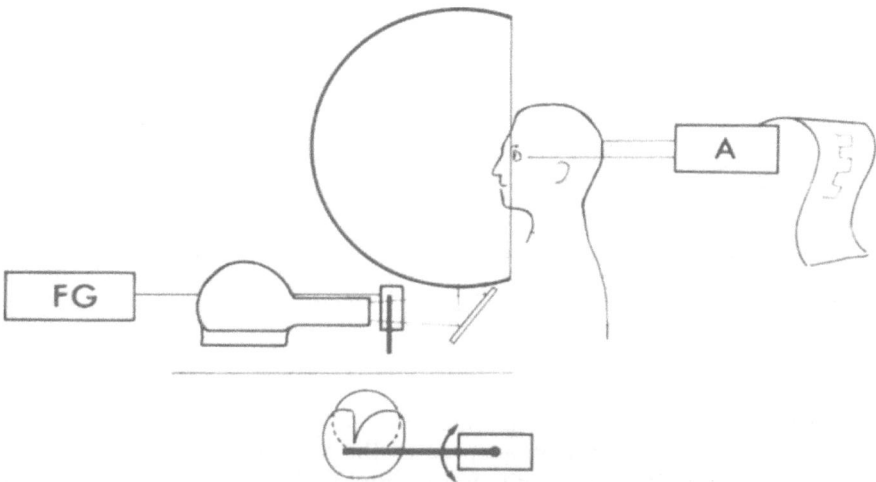

Fig. 1. Experimental equipment. The perimeter hemisphere is illuminated by a 1000 watt halogen lamp. The luminance is changed by a shutter which is driven by a function generator. The eye movements of 40 deg are recorded in dc-coupling via skin-electrodes

* Supported by the Deutsche Forschungsgemeinschaft SFB 70

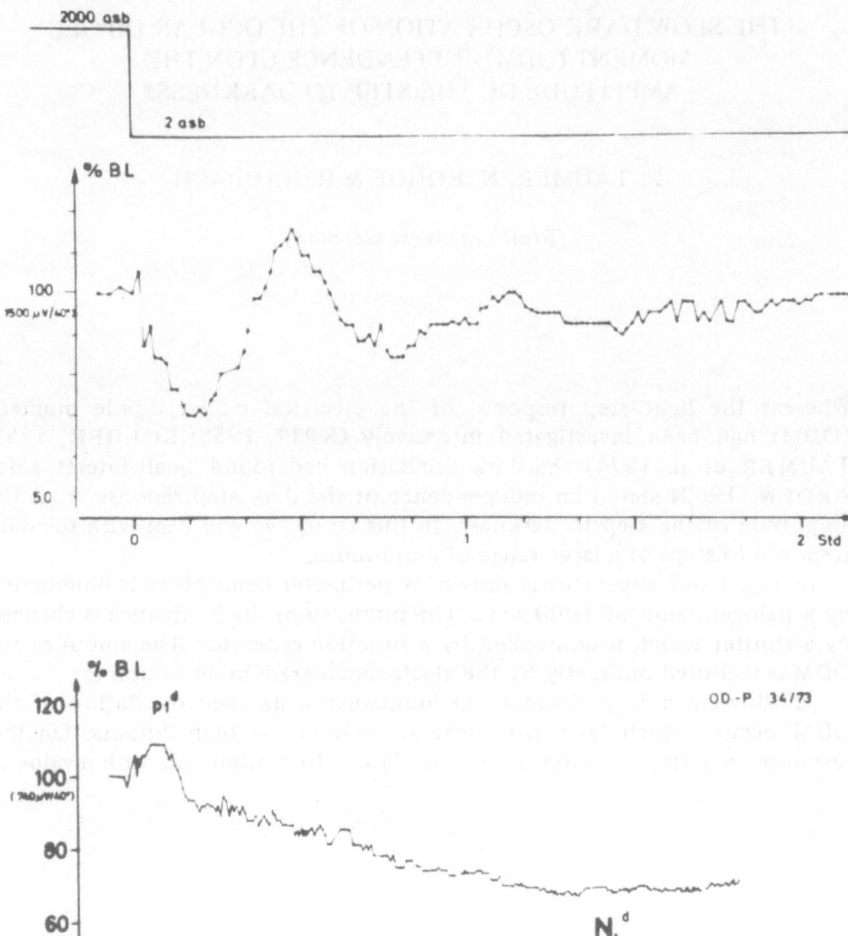

Fig. 2a. The ocular dipole response to a 3 log unit step to darkness with a damped oscillation of 3 cycles; b. Beginning part of a 4 log unit step response with better resolution in time. The first elevation (p₁ᵈ) comes from the superpositioned fast oscillation.

70% BL is reached after 10 min. Each point of the curve is the mean value of 10 eye movements of 40 deg done by the person after each minute. Before each experiment the person adapted to the first luminance level for about 1 hour. In this time any oscillation excited by luminance variations before the experiment would have vanished. A steady Basis Level (BL) is reached. Then we measure all values of the ODM in percent of this BL (% BL). In the curve of Fig. 2 we can distinguish 3 cycles of the dark damped oscillation. If the person carries out eye movements each second the beginning of the dark response can be investigated more precisely (Fig. 2b). On this response to a

364

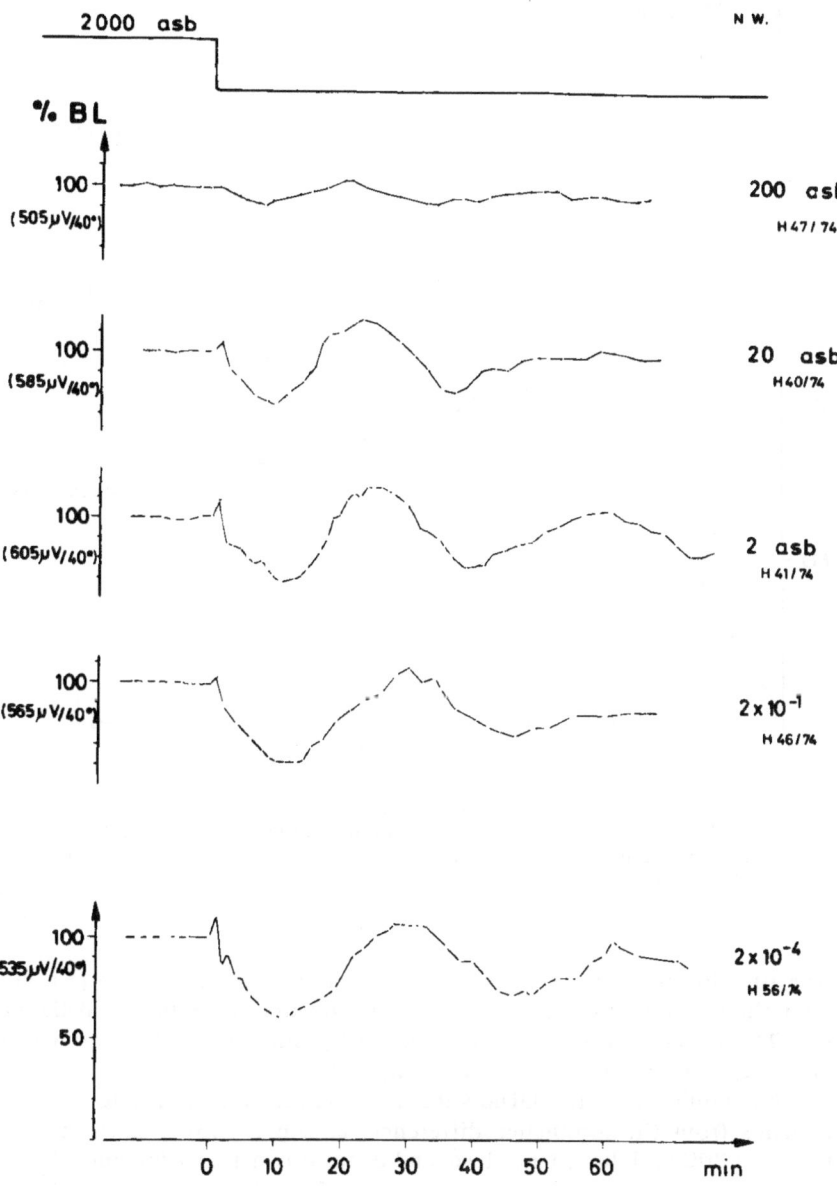

Fig. 3. Responses of the ODM to dark steps of different amplitude (1, 2, 3, 4 and 7 log units). All curves from one person. 1 hour adaptation at 2000 asb before the dark step.

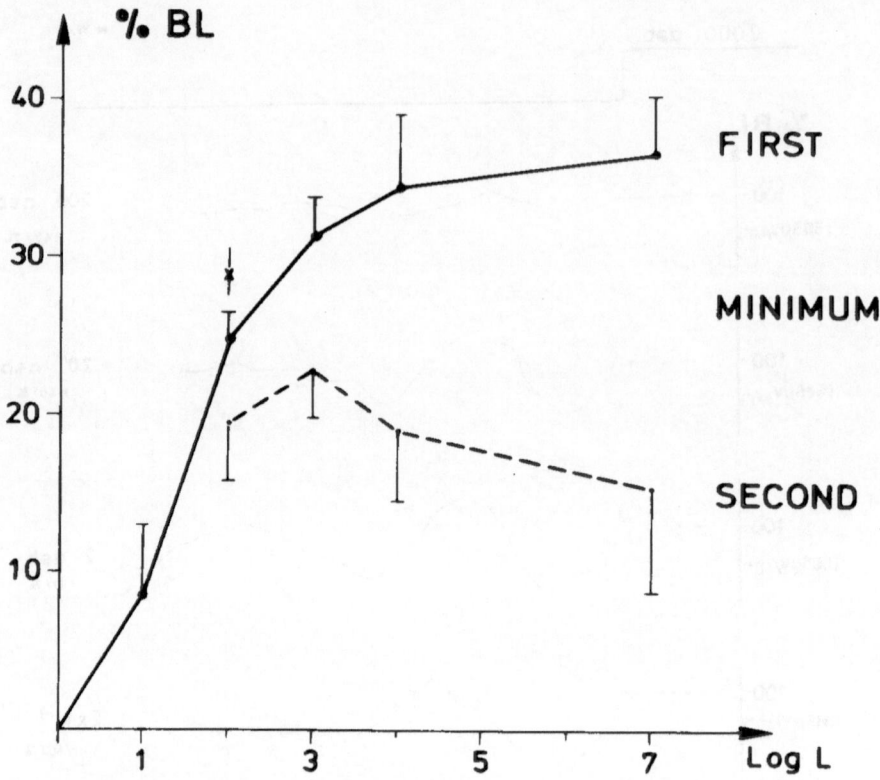

Fig. 4. Dependence of the first minimum and the second minimum upon the step amplitude. Each point is the mean value of 6 experiments of the one person. The vertical lines represents the standard deviation. The cross shows the value from experiments with an adaptation to 20 asb.

step of 4 log units we find the first minimum after 12 min ($N_1{}^d$). 40 sec after the step a first elevation to + 10% BL occurs. It disappears at the 80 th sec. This superpositioned fast wave upon the main oscillation we have studied in an earlier paper (HENNIG et al., 1974).

The amplitude of the ODM's main oscillation in response to a dark step depends from the luminance difference, as Fig. 3 shows. Each step starts from the 2000 asb luminance level and drops down 1 to 7 log units. The end levels are shown on the right side of Fig. 3. Especially between the first and second curve there is a large amplitude-difference. But also the other curves encreases with larger step amplitude. In the same way the cycle time becomes longer with larger steps.

The relation between the value of the first minimum and the step amplitude is shown in Fig. 4. During the first 3 log units the value of the minimum increases largely (about 11% BL per log unit). Between 3 and 7 log units only a small increasing occurs. This fact gives the explanation, why KOLDER (1959) found no amplitude variation of the dark oscillation. He always has used steps to complete darkness. That means he has large steps, for instance effective 8 or 9 log units. These large steps he varied in amplitude by 0.7 or 1.7 log units. So he could get only a small variation of the amplitude, because the system is still saturated.

The second minimum increases with the log units up to 3 log units. With larger steps the second minimum becomes more inconstant and decreases in value.

With the cross we show in Fig. 4 a step response from a beginning level of 20 asb to 0.2 asb (2 log units). This response is significantly larger than the responses with the 2000 asb beginning level. Such an experiment shows Fig. 5. We see a larger amplitude and a longer cycle time of the response to the second step of 2 log units.

Fig. 6 demonstrates the dependence of the first minimum time and the first cycle time (time from the first minimum to the second one) upon the step-amplitude. Again the times increase with the step-amplitude. Whereas the cycle time increases steadily up to 7 log units the curve of the first minimum flats above 4 log units. The point of the step beginning at 20 asb lies again above the other curve.

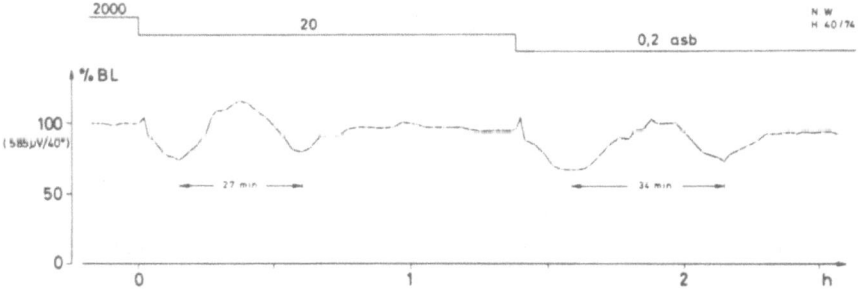

Fig. 5. Original record of an experiment with 2 log units steps. At the first adaptation to 2000 asb; at the second to 20 asb.

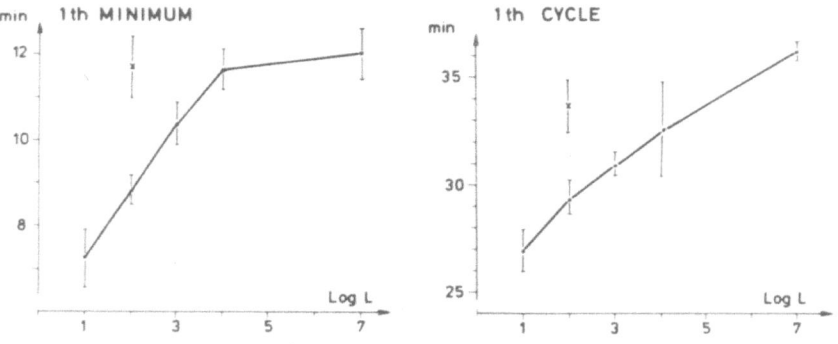

Fig. 6. Relation between the time of the first minimum and the first cycle (time from the first minimum to the second one) and the step amplitude.

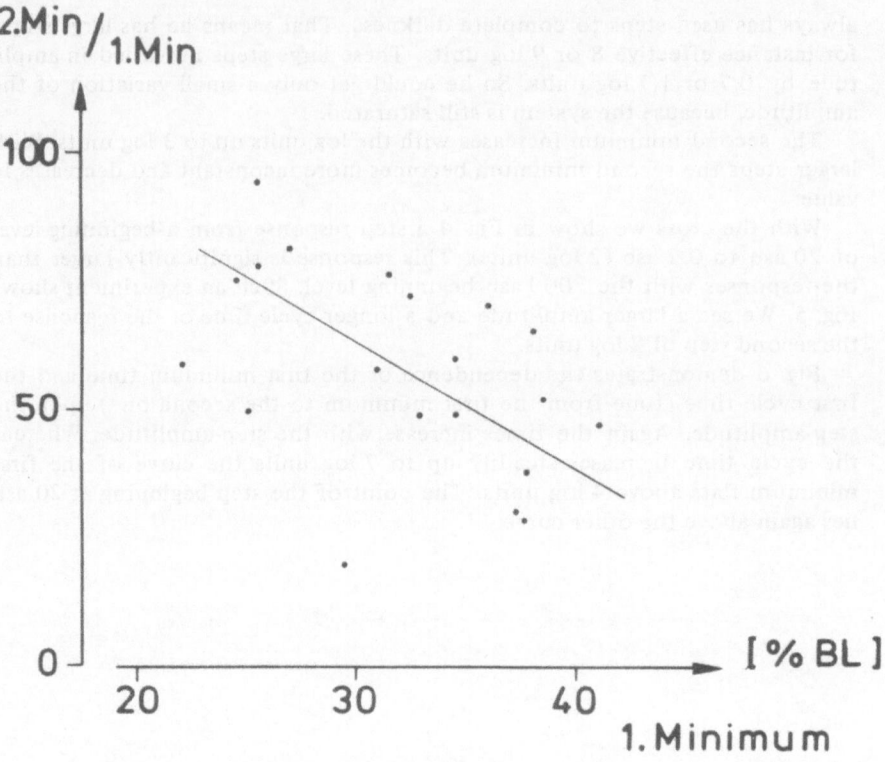

Fig. 7. Dependence of the second minimum (given in percentage of the first minimum) upon the value of the first minimum. With a larger first minimum the second one becomes smaller compared with the first minimum.

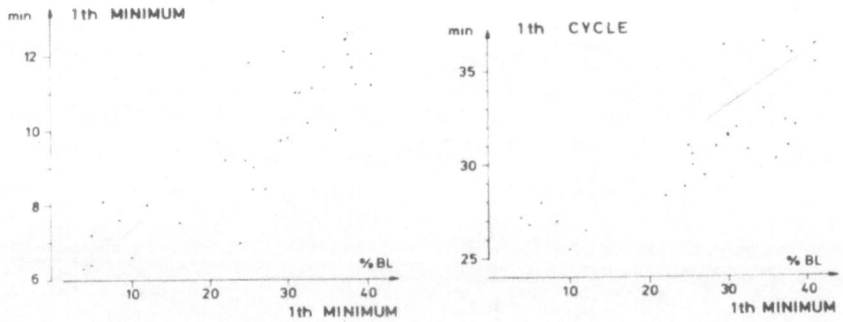

Fig. 8. The first minimum time and the first cycle time in relation to the value of the first minimum.

In our opinion the explanation for this behaviour of the values and the times of the extrema is the higher damping of the oscillating system in the lower levels of the ODM. The decrement (2th minimum/ 1th minimum) is a gauge for this damping. Fig. 6 shows that the second minimum (as percentage of the first) becomes smaller with the larger values of the first minimum. The oscillating process loses more and more energy as deeper it dives into the smaller levels of the ODM-amount. The same fact may be responsible for the variation of the times of the extremes. The first minimum takes more time to develop with larger values (Fig. 8). In the same way the cycle time (first minimum to second minimum) becomes larger. The process oscillates slowlier through levels with larger damping.

REFERENCES

ARDEN, G.B. & KELSEY, J.H. Changes produced by light in the standing potential of the human eye. *J. Physiol.* 161, *189-204* (1962).

HENNIG, J., TÄUMER, R. & PERNICE, D. The fast ocular dipole oscillation 11th ISCERG-Symposium. Bad Nauheim (1973), 424-430. Documenta ophthalmologica-Proceedings series

KOLDER, H. Spontane und experimentelle Anderungen des Bestand-Potentials des menschlichen Auges. *Pflügers Arch. ges. Physiol.* 268, *258-272* (1959)

KRIS, CH. Corneo-fundal potential during light and dark adaptation. *Nature* 182, *1027-1028* (1958).

TÄUMER, R., HENNIG, J. & PERNICE, D. The ocular dipole — a damped oscillator stimulated by the speed of change in illumination. *Vision Res.* Vol. 14, (1974).

ELECTROPHYSIOLOGICAL AND PSYCHOPHYSICAL EXAMINATIONS OF A FAMILY WITH PROGRESSIVE CONE DYSTROPHY*

EDGAR AUERBACH & BERNARD KRIPKE

(Jerusalem, Israel)

This presentation is the continuation of a study of 39 congenital achromats with autosomal recessive inheritance (AUERBACH & MERIN, 1974; AUERBACH & KRIPKE, 1974). In addition to these subjects, we had the opportunity to examine nine members of a family, the G-Family, of which the five adults suffered from achromatopsia, typical in most respects, but who claimed to have had color vision when they were younger, and that their visual acuity gradually decreased over the years. Of the youngest generation, four of the five children of the two afflicted adults were examined (Fig. 1). The fifth child, we were told, is healthy. There is no consanguinity in this pedigree. In short, we seemed to deal with a family with progressive cone dystrophy with autosomal dominant inheritance.

Progressive cone dysfunction has been described by several groups of investigators (FRANÇOIS et al., 1956; STEINMETZ et al., 1956; SLOAN & BROWN, 1962; GOODMAN et al., 1963; GOODMAN et al., 1964/1966). The most recent studies on autosomal dominant inheritance of this condition are those of BERSON, GOURAS & GUNKEL (1968), KRILL & DEUTMAN (1972) and AUERBACH & KRIPKE (1970) presented at a society meeting.

The same ERG findings described in the recent study (AUERBACH & MERIN, 1974) of the congenital achromats characterize in its extreme form the recordings of the five adult members of the G-Family (Fig. 2). There is

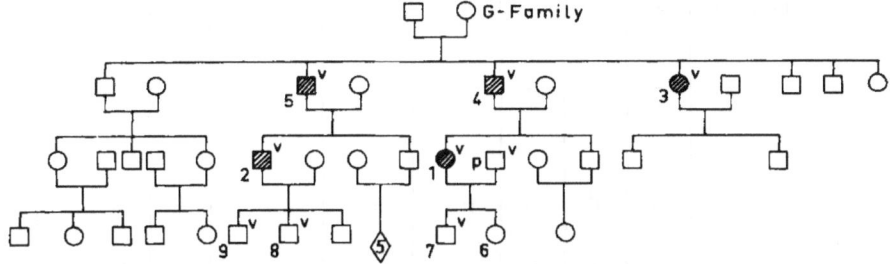

Fig. 1. Pedigree of the G-family. V: examined; Shaded symbols: patients 1 to 5 who are afflicted by progressive cone dystrophy. P: severely protanopic subject.

* Supported by Stiftung Volkswagenwerk under contract number 11 1538.

371

Table 1

No.	born	sex	Nystagmus	Photophobia	corrected visual acuity R	L	refraction R	L	Ishihara	scotopic line	ERG light	ERG dark	EOG
1	1942	f.	(+)	+	2/60	2/60	−6.0○1.0	−6.0e1.0	none	+	extinct	scotopic	
2	1928	m.	(+)	+	6/18	6/18	−2.25	−1.75	none	+	extinct	scotopic	
3	1900	f.	−	+	2mFC	2mFC	−12.0○1.0	−10.00	none	+	extinct	scotopic	
4	1906	m.	−	+	low	low	−11.0 telescopic for reading	−10.00−2.0 telescopic for reading	8,14, 15,16	+	extinct	scotopic	
5	1900	m.	−	+	low	low	−11.0○3.0 telescopic for reading	−12.0○3.0 telescopic for reading	none	+	extinct	scotopic	
6	1968	f.	+	−	6/60	6/9	−2.75−1.75	c.−1.50	normal	−	+ all components present; 0.4. subnormal: o.d.		
7	1964	m.	−	−	6/12p.	6/12p.	−3.75	−4.75	normal	−	+	normal	
8	1962	m.	−	−	6/36	6/18	−2.75○1.0	c.+0.50	all, except 9, 13	−	0	0	235%
9	1959	m.	−	−	?	?	?	?	normal	−	0	0	0

no response in the light. In the dark, the ERG is of typical scotopic nature, being characterized by a shallow negative wave of long extension along the time axis and a slow positive wave whose amplitude gradually increases during dark adaptation.

Of the four children examined (patients 6 to 9), three appeared absolutely normal according to color vision tests or, in patient 7, to eletroretinography (Table 1). The fifth child was too young to be examined. In one of the four children (patient 8) a slight disturbance of color vision was found (two mistakes in the Ishihara test) which is so little that it is unclassifiable as yet and may well later turn out not to be true. At least three of the four children are myopic. The ERG was normal in one of the two children tested. In the other child (patient 6), the ERG in the squinting eye was moderately subnormal and its vision could not be improved with glasses. However, this may be due to pathology other than cone dystrophy since the photopic components were present in the ERG. In view of the evidence

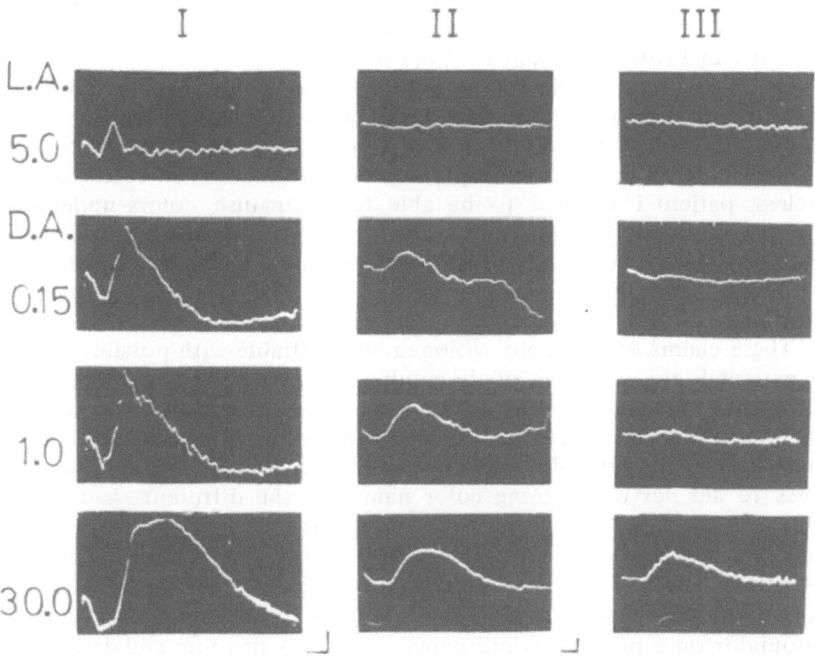

Fig. 2. The ERG of a normal subject (I), of a congenital achromat (II) and of an achromat due to progressive cone dystrophy (III), recorded after 5 minutes (5.0), in light adaptation (L.A.) and in dark adaptation (D.A.) after 15 seconds (0.15), one minute (1.0) and 30 minutes (30.0). The pattern of the ERG in both kinds of achromatopsia is generally identical. In contrast to the normal case, in the achromat the ERG is missing during light adaptation. In the dark the negative wave (downward) is shallow and of long extension since the large photopic negative wave and the fast, photopic positive component of the normal ERG are absent in the extreme form of achromatopsia. The positive wave is the slow scotopic component of gentle slope. Note that the ERGs in column III are very subnormal. Calibrations below each column: 20 msec. 100 μV.

presented below, that achromatopsia in the G-Family is progressive, it will be necessary to re-examine these children periodically.

All the achromatic adults in the G-Family (patients 1 to 5) are myopic with corrections ranging from two diopters to more than ten diopters (Table 1). In all but patient 2 the myopia has been increasing which is substantiated by former prescriptions for corrective lenses. The same four patients also reported a marked decrease in visual acuity in adulthood. Patient 1 told us that she could read the blackboard in school without difficulty and that at the age of 22 her visual acuity began to deteriorate rapidly. Her aunt, patient 3, was a seamstress in her youth, and her father and uncle (patients 4 and 5) also engaged in occupations requiring reasonably good visual acuity. In 1968, however, when we examined them the first time, patients 3, 4 and 5 could read only with telescopic glasses at a distance of about 10 cm. In patients 1, 2 and 3 we were able to verify the presence of small central scotomata. Patient 2, an engineer, was probably exceptional in that his corrected visual acuity of around 6/18 did change only slightly during the last 28 years. However, this may not mean too much since the three older patients claimed to have seen quite well until about the age of patient 2 in 1968 (he died in 1970) (Table 1).

In tables 1 and 2 all the five adults showed some macular involvement and no foveal reflexes were found. Otherwise, the findings from the ERG and color vision tests were typical of achromats in the five affected adults. The Farnsworth panel D-15 displayed the scotopic line in each case. Nonetheless, patient 1 claimed to be able to distinguish colors under certain conditions. Her father, uncle and aunt independently informed us that they had been able to see colors until middle age, when they had gradually lost the ability. Patient 2 denied having had color vision except perhaps in his early youth before the age of 12.

These claims of lost color vision are unverifiable with possible exception of patient 1, the youngest of the adults, who has still (in 1974) some color vision and appears to be at an advanced stage of transition to total color blindness. This was proved on a subsequent visit in 1968 when patient 1 said that she had thought over our explanation to have learned to use external clues to aid her in assigning color names to the different shades of grey which we first supposed she saw. She said that she found it unconvincing since she was sure she could distinguish colors. In fact, she claimed that sometimes she had to correct the color naming of her husband, a severe protanope. We showed her a spot of light of about 1 cm^2, cast by a monochromator on a piece of white paper in a dimly lit room and demonstrated to her that she saw only changes in intensity as the wavelengths changed. She then, however, demonstrated to us that she could name correctly the colors of such subjects as curtains, clothing, signs, pieces of colored filter glass and books which latter, however, had to be removed from the shelf and viewed at a distance of 15 to 20 cm. After this performance, we began to doubt our interpretation that she had been using external clues. We, therefore, tested her with our psychophysical apparatus. She sat in a lightless cell from which she observed, without a fixation point, a patch of ground glass, subtending 1° at her eye and which was illuminated by a monochromator. The intensity of the light could be varied by means of

No.	Color Vision & Visual Acuity	Fundus	
1	sees still *color* under favorable conditions. *visual acuity:* according to her began to deteriorate rapidly from 1963	*1968:* no foveal reflexes in O.U., slight glittering around foveae. *1972:* slight degenerative macular changes. *1974:* macular degeneration O.U. & choroidal atrophy, maculae invaded by blood vessels.	small central scotoma (1-2 letters missing) ,, larger central scotoma	latent strabismus and nystagmus when tired
2	*color vision* perhaps until 10 years. *visual acuity:* according to patient did not deteriorate since childhood	normal	very small central scotoma O.D. if at all	latent nystagmus when trying to fix at reading and when tired
3	*color vision* until approximately age of 30	normal, perhaps slight macular changes	small central scotoma	slight latent strabismus
4	*color vision* until age of 30	staphyloma posticum O.U. marked choroidal atrophy especially in macular areas. moderate pallor papillae	sees the test light as not exactly round, central scotoma?	eccentric fixation above fovea
5	*color vision* until age of 40 *visual acuity:* good until age of 40	normal except for slight macular changes	central scotoma?	small latent nystagmus small latent strabismus
6	*color vision* normal at age of 4	fine pigmentary changes in right macular, otherwise normal	no scotoma	posterior synechiae O.D. strabismus? parafoveal eccentric fixation O.D.
7	*color vision* normal at age of 10	*1972:* foveal reflexes O.U. very weak foveal reflex O.S otherwise normal. *1974:* fundus normal	no scotoma	no strabismus
8	*color vision* practically normal at age of 6	normal	no scotoma	no strabismus, small eccentric fixation in O.D. about 3° of fovea nasally
9	*color vision* normal	normal	no scotoma	no strabismus

Table 3 Color naming of monochromatic lights by patient 1

Wavelength (nm)	Color name 1968	Color name 1972
400	blue	no color
420	blue	,,
440	blue	,,
460	blue	,,
480	green	,,
500	green	,,
520	green	,,
540	green	green?
560	green or yellow green	no color
570	yellow-green or yellow	,,
580	yellow	,,
590	yellow or orange	,,
600	orange or red	,,
620	red	,,
650	red	,,
700	red	,,

calibrated neutral density wedges. She was asked to name the colors of spectral light of wavelenghts ranging from 400 nm to 700 nm in steps of 20 nm or less, presented in random order. She named each color correctly in three separate tests performed by two different experimeters (Table 3). However, she could see the color only at intensities about 2 log units above the normal photopic threshold. At lower intensities her sensation was achromatic. We repeated the Ishihara and Farnsworth D-15 tests illuminated by a Macbeth daylight lamp allowing her to hold the test objects at a convenient distance and to observe them through a powerful magnifying glass. She was unable to read the numerals in the Ishihara plates although she correctly named the color of the background. On the Farnsworth D-15 she found she could see and name correctly the colors of some of the disks but only if she held them so close that the magnified image of a disk filled her visual field in Maxwellian view. However, her first arrangement in 1968 was unsatisfactory and almost completely disordered. Two years later, in 1970, the arrangement was surprisingly different in that it indicated the scotopic line (Fig. 3A). The experimenter now removed the disks 14 and 15 and instructed her to arrange again the remainder. When she was then asked to replace disks 14 and 15, after finishing her new arrangement, the result was almost normal (Fig. 3B). When she was re-examined two years later, in 1972, a better approximation of the scotopic line was obtained and this time removal of buttons 14 and 15 did not give a result (Fig. 3C). The last test was performed in 1974 (Fig. 3D), and now the arrangement follows the scotopic line. She is still able, as mentioned, to name the color of objects, such as books, correctly if she holds them close to her eyes, although with more difficulty than in 1972.

In the face of the evidence that patient 1 seems to have trichromatic color vision under very favorable conditions and that it deteriorated within

376

six years, we now accept the reports of her father, uncle and aunt that they had seen colors in their youth up to middle age. This assumption was strengthened by a repetition of the test with monochromatic spectral lights with patient 1, four years after the first time (in 1972). In contrast to the earlier examination, this time she was unable to name any spectral color at all, even at highest intensities available, except for 540 nm which appeared to her greenish, but only at highest intensity available which is about 4 log units above the normal photopic threshold. Already 550 nm appeared colorless (Table 3).

We have made psychophysical dark adaptation tests with the five affected adults. It is obvious that these curves are far less reliable than those from normal observers because of the patients' photophobia and their difficulties to fixate. Nonetheless all of these patients were intelligent and co-operative so that we were able to obtain fairly reproducible results. Fig. 4 shows dark adaptation curves measured at 500 nm which we obtained from patient 1, patient 5, her uncle, and patient 3, her aunt. The results from her father, patient 4, were not reliable. Three sets of these data practically fit the same curve; the data from patients 1 and 5 measured 6° above the fovea and the data from patient 3 measured at central fixation. The data from

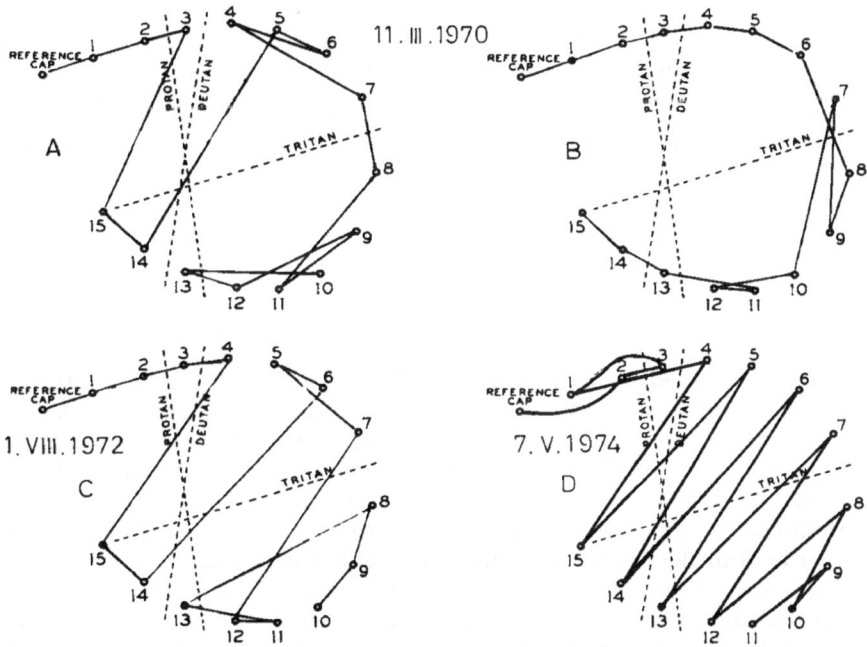

Fig. 3.   Results of Farnsworth panel D-15 test from patient 1. A: in 1970 the transversal lines indicate the 'scotopic line'. B: the buttons 14 and 15 were removed prior to the retest; the subject was then asked to rearrange the other buttons and thereafter to put 14 and 15 in place. An almost faultless result was achieved though slow and with difficulties. C: two years later the direction of the 'scotopic line' is more typical; this time removal of buttons 14 and 15 did not work as it did two years before. D: another two years later yields a possibly extreme form of the 'scotopic line'

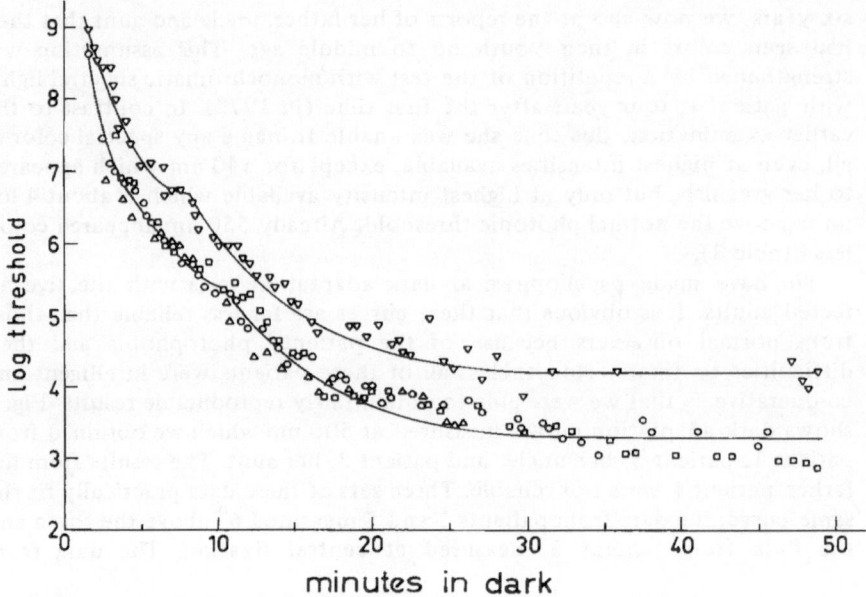

minutes in dark

Fig. 4. Psychophysical dark adaptation curves of patients 1, 3 and 5 after one minute of white light adaptation. The test light of 500 nm subtends 1°. At central fixation: patient 3 (circles) and patient 5 (triangles, base up). Fixation 6° above fovea: patient 1 (squares) and patient 5 (triangles, base down). Fixation in all experiments between two small lights each of 0.2° subtense, equal brightness and separated by 1.7° of arc or more. Note that the data of patients 3 and 5 at central fixation and of patient 1 at fixation 6° above fovea practically fit one curve, while the other curve of patient 5 would also fit the same curve were it not 1 log unit higher. The curves drawn through the data after the 'kink' represent the scotopic branch of the standard dark adaptation curve (see text).

patient 5, measured at central fixation, fit almost exactly the other three curves, but the threshold is elevated by nearly 1 log unit. In these curves there is perhaps just a hint of the kink between 11 to 12 minutes after the end of the light adaptation which divides a possible photopic branch from the scotopic. There is, however, no good fit to the scotopic branch of our standard dark adaptation curve published in our former paper (AUERBACH & KRIPKE, 1974) as seen by the line drawn in the figure. Also the final thresholds of the peripheral data are up to half a log unit higher than the upper limit of the normal absolute threshold of our standard curve.

When we made dark adaptation measurements on patient 1 closer to, and at the fixation point the picture changed entirely. For comparison, the data from patient 1 of measurements 6° above the fovea are transferred from Fig. 4 and appear as curve A in Fig. 5 together with curve B obtained under the same conditions except that the measurements were made 4° above the fixation point. Curve B shows a clear plateau during the photopic phase, and the part below the break is similar to the corresponding branch of curve A. Curves like curve B at 4° above the fovea were obtained from this patient for eight wavelengths.

378

Measurements of dark adaptation at central fixation were carried out with patient 1 at six wavelengths and displayed a second plateau during the normally photopic phase. Three of these curves are illustrated in Fig 5: one practically complete curve (C) together with two incomplete curves (D and E). All showed two early plateaux before the curve measured at 480 nm drops to a final third plateau. There is good reason to assume from the data that the curves measured at the other wavelengths also descend to a third plateau, had we followed them long enough. This is ascertained by a few isolated measurements about 35 minutes after discontinuation of light adaptation, which showed thresholds nearly three log units lower than the second plateau. Not only the two early plateaux but also the third plateau is surprising since we measured at central fixation. To verify these measurements, they were repeated and essentially the same result was obtained although the thresholds of the plateaux showed variations.

To identify the receptors responsible for the early plateaux and that late in the dark, we tried to plot the spectral sensitivity of the data from central fixation and from fixation 4° above the test light. However, the results from

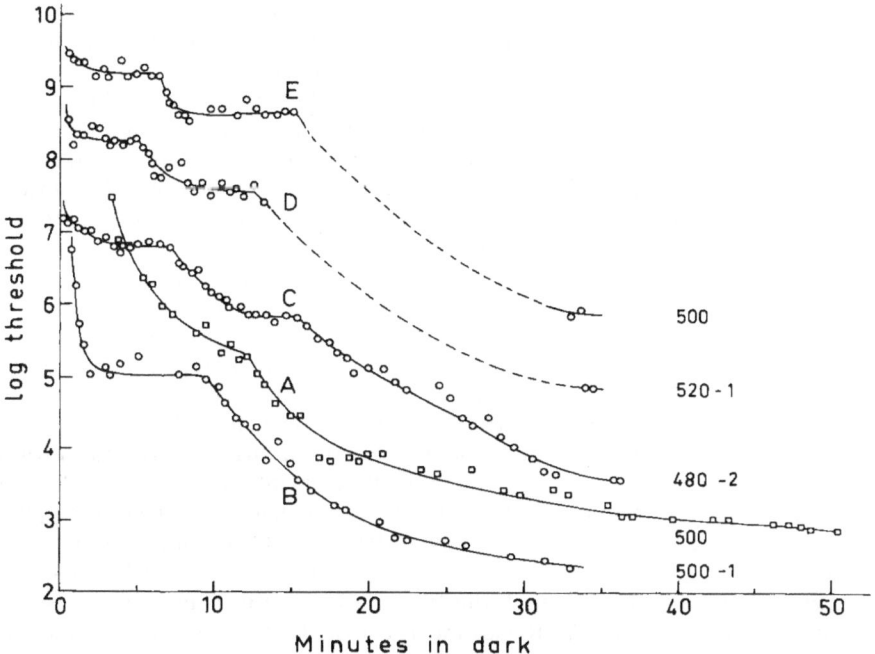

Fig. 5. Dark adaptation curves of patient 1 at three retinal locations, each after a one-minute light adaptation. Test light subtends 1°. Wavelengths are indicated at the curves. In order to illustrate the curves separately in the graph, some are shifted upward (+) or downward (-) from the measured data which is indicated behind the wavelengths. A: is the curve from subject 1 in Fig. 4, with 500 nm, measured 6° above the fovea. B: at 500 nm, measured 4° above fovea and moved 1 log unit below the measured data (-1). C, D and E: test lights of 480 nm, 520 nm and 500 nm all at central fixation. Note the two plateaux during the first 15 minutes of dark adaptation before the curve falls to the final scotopic plateau.

the plateaux measured at central fixation, such as shown in curves C, D and E of Fig. 5, though essentially reproducible, did not fit any reasonable curve. Due to her central small scotoma, the subject probably did not maintain accurate fixation, although the fixation was held between two points of light subtending 1.7° and centered on the 1° test patch.

The spectral sensitivity reflected by the high plateaux could, however, be determined from the series of dark adaptation curves measured 4° above the fovea, such as Fig. 5B. The curve drawn through the data is the reciprocal of the 1951 CIE scotopic curve (WYSZECKI & STILES, 1967) translated upwards to give the best fit, which is reasonable from 520 nm to 580 nm of the measured data (Fig. 6). The sharp departure of the data from the CIE curve in the range of 480 nm to 520 nm is shown in the inset (circles). The other symbols in the inset refer to similar data from patient 2 and will be explained below. This experiment was repeated with patient 1 four years later (in 1972), and the data showed a reasonably good fit to the earlier ones (Fig. 6, squares).

We also tested her spectral sensitivity against a white background illumination which in normal subjects sufficed to saturate the rods. Fig. 7 shows both the data obtained from subject 1, despite her photophobia, and an average curve from eight normal observers with the same background illumination all with central fixation and a test light subtending 2°. Her curve remarkably differs from the one obtained with the normal subjects in that it essentially displays a maximum at around 500 nm with a possible indication of another maximum at 440 nm. Except for the latter maximum, this is in contrast to the normal photopic sensitivity curve obtained under identical conditions, which exhibits three maxima: one at about 440 nm, the second at 540 nm and the third at 610 nm. Moreover, the threshold of the scotopic peak at 500 nm is about 1 log unit higher than the lowest photopic threshold from the normal observers at 540 nm. Also the peak at 440 nm is less sensitive by 0.7 log units than that in the normal observers. In other words, the reverse of the normal condition appears to occur here. The apparently scotopic function of subject 1 appears to be less sensitive than the photopic function of normal observers. It is, however, very doubtful whether the 'scotopic' curve obtained from patient 1 under conditions of rod saturation can be due to rods. It may be possible that essentially cones filled with rhodopsin are responsible and that also the π_1 mechanism of Stiles may play a role, i.e. cones which may contain cyanolabe. The latter may then point to a remnant of color vision as the π_1 cone monochromat's dichromacy at relatively low luminances, which the two color vision tests used were insufficiently sensitive to detect. Regarding the essentially scotopic character of the sensitivity curve, even granted that, due to the then small central scotoma of patient 1, her central fixation was probably not completely accurate but only reasonably so, the rods should be saturated under the experimental conditions as seen in the color normal subjects. Therefore, even with inaccurate fixation, no scotopic curve should be obtained. On the other hand, it is much easier to fixate with background illumination than in the dark. When we tried the same test in 1974, we were unsuccessful since her macular degeneration has alarmingly increased during these last two years.

A three-branched curve from a 500 nm test light was also obtained from

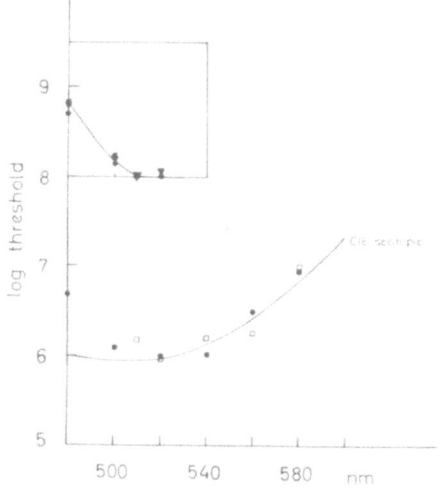

Fig. 6. The log threshold of the first plateau from dark adaptation curves of patient 1 measured 4° above the fovea as a function of wavelength. Test light subtends 1°. Circles: measurements in 1968, squares: measurements under the same conditions in 1972. The curve fitted to the data is the 1951 CIE scotopic sensitivity curve translated vertically to give the best fit. The inset with the same abscissa shows the departure of the data from the CIE scotopic curve at wavelengths below 520 nm (circles). The other symbols (triangles, and circles with slanting line) are taken from similar departures of data from patient 2 (see Fig. 10).

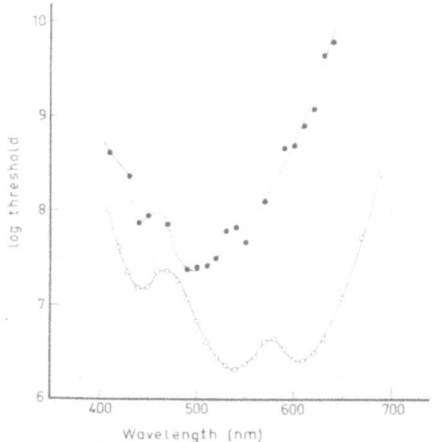

Fig. 7. Spectral sensitivity curves from measurements at white background illumination sufficient to saturate the rods, measured at central fixation and a 2° subtense of the test light. The upper curve was obtained from patient 1 and each point represents the average of at least five readings. The lower threepeaked curve is averaged from eight normal observers and each point represents the average of eight times five readings. While in the normal observers the threshold was determined by increasing the intensity of the test light until it was just seen, the reverse procedure was necessary in patient 1 in whom an essentially scotopic curve with a maximum at about 500 nm was obtained. Another possible maximum at 440 nm is indicated by an intermittent line.

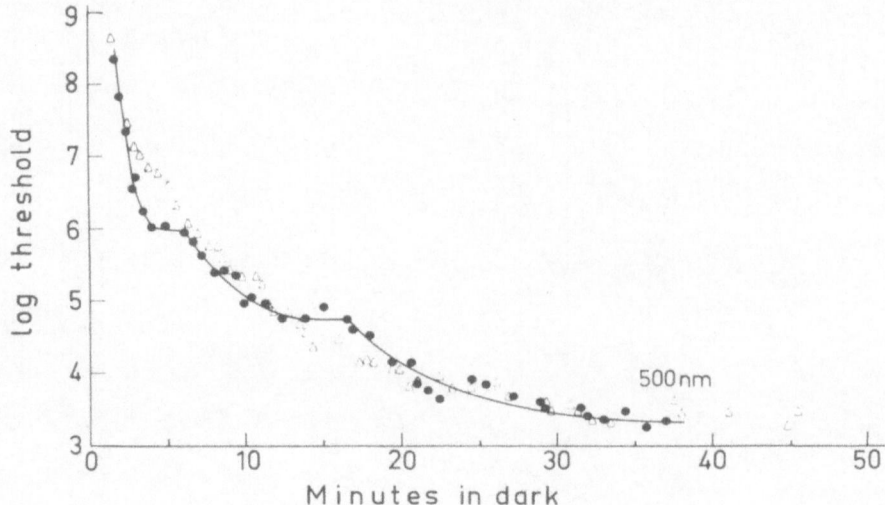

Fig. 8. Two dark adaptation curves of patient 3 measured 6° above the fovea (rings) and at central fixation (triangles) following a one-minute white light adaptation. The test light of 500 nm subtends 1°. Note the difference between the two curves: the two higher plateaux obtained at 6° above fovea seem smoothed out in the curve at central fixation except for some irregularities. The points of the latter were not connected, but the curve falls to the same absolute threshold as the peripheral one.

patient 3, measured 6° above the fovea (Fig. 8). The curve displays one early plateau onr irregularity at around 5 minutes. A second one between 12 and 16 minutes in the dark although apparently well delineated and repro-duced in another test, appears to us questionable. The curve falls then to a final scotopic plateau after about 32 minutes in the dark which is about 0.3 log units above the upper limit of the range of the absolute threshold od our standard dark adaptation curve. When we measured her dark adaptation at central fixation, the decline of the curve was quite different (Fig. 8). The threshold was steadily falling to the same low scotopic threshold obtained in the periphery showing only two humps. This subject was also completely color-blind but claims to have seen colors until the age of approximately thirty. Her central scotoma seems to be very small and could not be mea-sured. She says that sometimes one or two letters seem to be missing. We were, however, unable to measure her dark adaptation with test lights of other wavelengths. We succeeded to determine only the scotopic sensitivity at 6° above fovea and obtained a quite reliable curve with a maximum around 520 nm.

Patient 2 was a subject with relatively good visual acuity and concentra-tion on the task. The data, a series of curves from test lights of different wavelengths measured at central fixation (Fig. 9), were repeated to check on their reliability. The retests confirmed the presence of different early irregu-larities, but varied in threshold. The branches may shift to the left or the right if there are variations in the initial level of light adaptation from curve to curve as expected from an untrained photophobic observer. These curves have several branches, especially the curve measured with test light of 500 nm, the lowest plateau of the latter being more than half a log unit above the upper limit of the standard curve. Various plateaux during the photopic phase of dark adaptation were obtained in subjects with normal color vision and in dichromats and shown to reflect the different rates of adaptation of different kinds of cones (AUERBACH, 1958/60; AUER-BACH & WALD, 1954, 1955). Multibranched curves were found also in congenital achromats (AUERBACH & KRIPKE, 1974). These displayed up to three plateaux during the normally photopic phase of dark adaptation and a scotopic plateau, all exhibiting spectral sensitivities at 500 nm. This may then be assumed to be the case also with our present data. In other

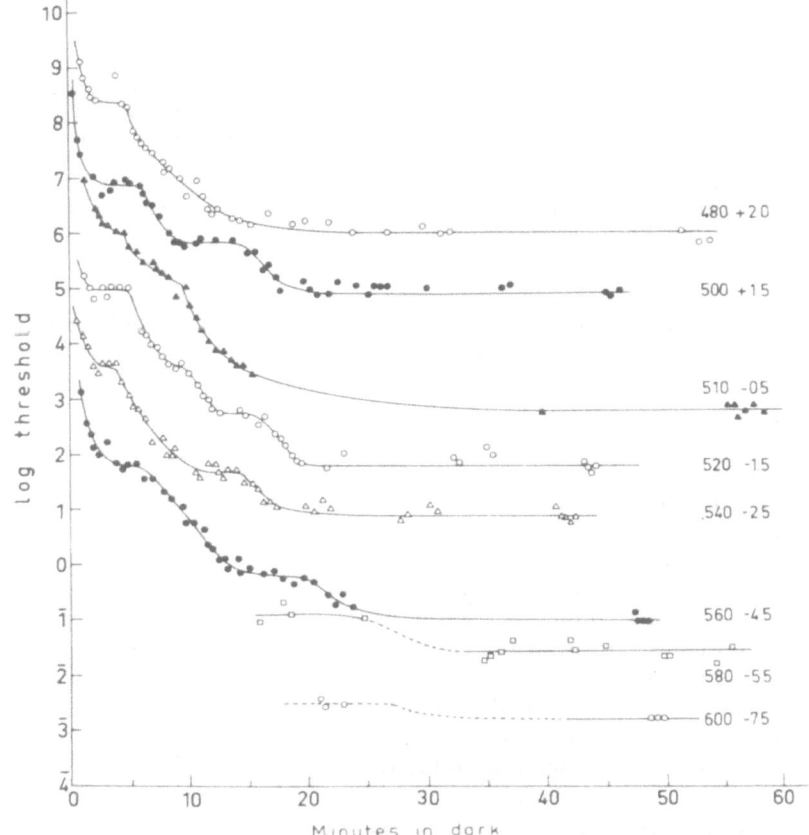

Fig. 9. A set of dark adaptation curves of patient 2 measured at central fixation following a one-minute white light adaptation. The test light of 1° was between two fixation points each subtending 0.2° and separated from each other by 2°. The wavelengths are indicated at each curve. The curves are displaced vertically by the indicated amounts behind the wavelengths to separate them from each other. The values for the incomplete curves of 580 nm and 600 nm were obtained by interspersing these readings between those of other wavelengths.

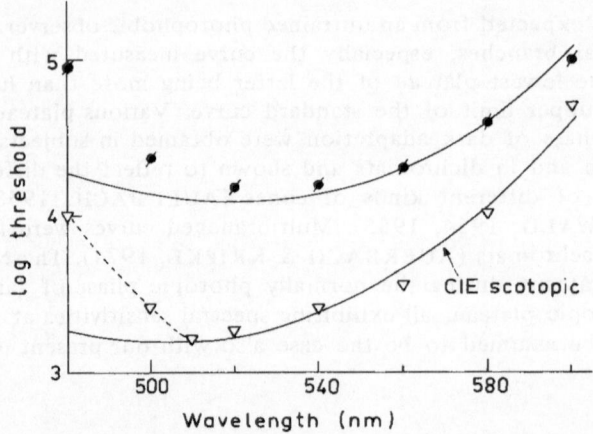

Fig. 10. The thresholds of the two lowest plateaux of dark adaptation curves in patient 2 obtained at central fixation as a function of wavelength. The lowest curve is the 1951 CIE scotopic curve translated vertically to give the best fit to the data. The curve above it is the average sensitivity curve of five achromats studied by ALPERN, FALLS & LEE (1960) also translated vertically to give the best fit. Regarding the earlier plateaux in the dark adaptation curves of Fig. 9, see text. The data below 520 nm from both curves are plotted in the inset of Fig. 6.

words, the branches of each of the curves in Figs. 5 and 9 should reflect the varying sensitivity to the different wavelengths. We did not, however, succeed in demonstrating this phenomenon with the plateaux at high thresholds in the patients studied here.

The lowest two plateaux obtained in the measurements with patient 2 were generally clearly delineated in most of the curves in Fig. 9.

The points for the lowest plateau and the one above were plotted as a function of wavelength (Fig. 10). The curve fitted through the lower set of points at the different wavelengths is once more an approximation to the 1951 CIE scotopic curve although measured at foveal fixation. Similar to Fig. 6 of subject 1, the fit is good down to 510 nm. Then there is a sharp departure of the data from the CIE curve in the short wavelengths, which is inserted with the appropriate symbols in the inset of Fig. 6. The curve fitted through the next higher set of points was taken from ALPERN, FALLS & LEE (1960). It represents the mean spectral sensitivity of their five achromats measured at the fixation point. It was translated vertically to fit our data. There is also a good fit down to 520 nm. Also here a departure from the spectral curve was found for the wavelengths below 520 nm, which is indicated by the appropriate symbol in the inset of Fig. 6; it is remarkable how closely the three departures shown there fit the same curve. However, the irregularities and plateaux at higher thresholds mostly do not permit a reliable assessment or extrapolation and are, therefore, not inserted into the graph of Fig. 10.

As to the close fit of the three departures shown in the inset of Fig. 6 in the spectral range below 520 nm. The sensitivity of patient 1 measured 4°

above the fovea and that of her cousin, patient 2, of the lowest plateau measured at the fovea, departs from the CIE scotopic curve in practically exactly the same way. The departure does not fit the absorption spectrum of the macular pigment nor of the lens. Tentatively, we may hypothesize that it shows the presence of some light-absorbing material not present in normal observers which screens the receptors of these patients. The sensitivity of the second-to-lowest plateau of patient 2 is not that of rhodopsin (Fig. 10). However, above 520 nm it nearly fits the average sensitivity, as mentioned, of the five achromats reported by ALPERN, FALLS & LEE (1960), who show that the departure from the sensitivity of rhodopsin can be accounted for by the absorption of the yellow macular pigment (WALD, 1964). Below 510 nm, the sensitivity of this plateau departs from that of rhodopsin screened by macular pigment. The departure (inset of Fig. 6) is the same as the one of the sensitivity of the same patient's lowest plateau from the CIE scotopic curve. This is consistent with the hypothesis of an abnormal screening substance in these two patients. BLACKWELL & BLACKWELL (1961) also observed a shift in spectral sensitivity with increasing dark adaptation from the sensitivity of rhodopsin screened by macular pigment to that of rhodopsin, and took this as evidence that their subject used increasingly eccentric fixation as he became more dark-adapted. This may be the explanation of the shift in sensitivity of patient 2.

Vision in all the adult subjects was scotopic, even with central fixation or its near approximation, a fact which is expected in achromats. Likewise, in progressive cone dystrophy at the final stage of achromatopsia, as in congenital achromatopsia, there were special retinal loci with either one or more high-threshold plateaux in the normally photopic phase of dark adaptation implying cone function, but always, even in the fovea, displaying the low-threshold scotopic plateau as well. We were able to trace down the photopic function in one case in the periphery only, in others in the fovea and close by. There were loci in which almost monophasic dark adaptation curves were obtained. However, some of the 'photopic' plateaux, no matter whether in the periphery or the fovea, displayed the scotopic function, although not as regular by far as found in congenital achromats reported in another study. In the present cases, some of the 'photopic' plateaux did not provide any meaningful spectral sensitivity. It should be emphasized that the ERG was typically scotopic in all cases.

Special importance we attribute to the experiment performed under constant background illumination. Despite rod saturation, an essentially scotopic sensitivity curve was obtained at central fixation which was of even higher threshold than the corresponding photopic sensitivity curve of normal subjects. It should be mentioned that this subject is the only one among the five adults who still possesses some trichromatic color vision under special favorable conditions (which, however, over the years gradually fades away) although this is reflected neither by the color vision tests nor the ERG, let alone the spectral sensitivity curves obtained. These observations, together with the multibranched dark adaptation curves, may be due to extensive damage of retinal elements on the one hand, and, as mentioned, to abnormal cones containing rhodopsin on the other hand. The fact that she still sees colors under special conditions is probably due to spared islands of normal cones, which cover, however, so small a retinal area that they are not brought out by the tests performed and which we were permitted to perform. In ordinary surroundings, she is still (in 1974) able to recognize colors only when the colored objects occupy a relatively large portion of her visual field activating the normal cone islands spared by the dystrophy. She could identify, as described, the color of a book held in her hands, but not of books two meters away on a shelf. It is, however, not size alone which is the determining factor. The test light which she correctly identified in our psychophysical apparatus is quite small, and she was still in 1968 successful even when we used a still smaller light. A light of approximately the same size reflected from a piece of paper in dimly lit surroundings gave rise only to achromatic sensations. The change in the shape of her psychophysical dark adaptation curve in Fig. 5 suggests the location of the island, i.e. that part of her retina which can distinguish colors and which seems confined to a small area around her fixation point, where the dark adaptation curve shows the presence of one class and of two classes of rapidly adapting receptors. We may also suppose that the neutral mechanisms in her retina which mediate color contrast are very disturbed. In contrast vision, disturbances may account for, or participate in her deteriorating visual acuity. This may be so up to 1972 when the macular changes were only little but not any more in 1974 when she had a marked macular degeneration.

The adult members of the G-family seem to show the same symptoms as the patients of dominantly inherited 'progressive cone degeneration' described by BERSON, GOURAS & GUNKEL (1968). In both families, there is progressive loss of color vision becoming marked in adulthood, accompanied by deteriorating visual acuity and high myopia; the ERG is typical of achromatopsia.

To conclude, the facts that we obtain scotopic thresholds at retinal loci where normally there should not be any, and that there are retinal elements with fast kinetics and high thresholds as normally found only in cones but lacking photopic spectral sensitivity, may point to rods at retinal loci where there are normally none and to cones containing rhodopsin. However, the problem is inexplicable to the authors how cones, which have functioned normally earlier in the life of these achromats, could have acquired in their outer segments such fundamental changes in the membranes of their invaginations and outer membrane which contain the visual pigment to account for the phenomena. It seems to argue against this hypothesis, and points to a machanism completely different from that found in congenital achromats. We may come closer to an explanation by regular follow-up examinations of the still color-normal children of the afflicted parents of the second generation of the G-family. We may add, whatever hypothesis is advanced for typical achromatopsia need not also account for the dominantly inherited disease of the G-family, which is evidently of a different genotype.

SUMMARY

Five adults and four children belonging to three generations of a family with progressive cone dystrophy were examined electrophysiologically and psychophysically. All were myopic and photophobic. Four of the five adults were total achromats but claimed to have seen color in their youth. The fifth adult, the youngest of the group, still displayed some traces of color vision when examined six years ago, but lost even these during the following four years. In all five achromats the scotopic line was found. All children have normal color vision, but three are myopic.

The ERGs in the adults tested and recording during dark adaptation were characteristic of achromatopsia. The psychophysical dark adaptation tests in two of the five adults displayed multiple plateaux at certain retinal areas (up to three or perhaps four) similar to findings in congenital achromats reported before (*Doc. Ophthal.* 1974). Foveal sensitivity curves obtained from these achromats were of scotopic nature.

REFERENCES

ALPERN, M.; FALLS, H.F. & LEE, G.B. The enigma of typical total monochromacy. *Am. J. Ophthal.* 50: Pt. II, *997-1011* (1960).

AUERBACH, E. Violet receptor. In Mechanisms of Colour Discrim. Proc. Int'l. Symp. Paris 1958, pp. *177-182*, Pergamon Press, 1960.

AUERBACH, E. & KRIPKE, B. Some studies of rod monochromatism: a dominant pedigree. *EEG & Clin. Neurophysiol.* 28: 643 (1970)

AUERBACH, E. & KRIPKE, B. Achromatopsia with amblyopia. II. A psychophysical study of 3 cases. *Doc. Ophthal.* 37-1: *119-144* (1974).

AUERBACH, E. & MERIN, S. Achromatopsia with amblyopia. I. A Clinical and electroretinographical study of 39 cases. *Doc. Ophthal.*, 37: *79-117* (1974).

AUERBACH, E. & WALD, G. Identification of a violet receptor in human color vision. *Science*, 10: *401-405* (1954).

AUERBACH, E. & WALD, G. The participation of different types of cones in human light and dark adaptation. *Am. J. Ophthal.* 39: Pt. II. *24-40* (1955).

BERSON, E.L.; GOURAS, P.; & GUNKEL, R.D. Progressive cone degeneration, dominantly inherited. *Arch. Ophthal.* 80: *77-83* (1968).

BLACKWELL, H.R. & BLACKWELL, O.M. Rod and cone mechanisms in typical and atypical congenital achromatopsia. *Vision Res.* 1: *62-107* (1961).

FRANÇOIS, J.; VERRIEST, G.; DEROUCK, A.; & HUMBLET, M. Dégénérescense maculaire juvénile avec atteinte prédominante de la vision photopique. *Ophthalmologica* 31: *393-402*, (1956).

GOODMAN, G.; RIPPS, H.; & SIEGEL, I.M. Cone Dysfunction Syndromes, *Arch. Ophthal.* 70: *214-231* (1963).

GOODMAN, G.; RIPPS, H.; & SIEGEL, I.M. Progressive cone degeneration In H.M. BURIAN & J.H. JACOBSON (ed.): Clinical Electroretinography. Proc. 3rd Int'l Symp. in 1964, Pergamon Press, 1966, pp. 363-372.

KRILL, A.E. & DEUTMAN, A.F. Dominant macular degenerations. The cone dystrophies. *Am. J. Ophthal.* 73: *352-369* (1972).

SLOAN, L.L. & BROWN, D.J. Progressive retinal degeneration with selective involvement of the cone mechanism. *Amer. J. Ophthal.* 54: *629-641* (1962).

STEINMETZ, R.D.; OGLE, K.N.; & RUCKER, C.W. Some physiologic considerations of hereditary macular degeneration. *Amer. J. Ophthal.* 42: *304-317* (1956).

WALD, G. The receptors of human color vision. *Science* 145: *1007-1017* (1964)

WYSZECKI, G. & STILES, W.S. Color Science: concepts and methods, quantitative data and formulas. John Wiley & Sons, Inc., New York, 1967.

VISUAL EVOKED RESPONSE AND ANTIMALARIAL DRUGS:
Clinical and pathophysiological data

J. PATY, L. CORCELLE & J.M.A. FAURE

(Bordeaux, France)

The retinal toxicity of synthetic antimalarial drugs is well knownn. Among many tests for the early detection of toxicity is the electroretinogram. Fluorescence stimulation increases the specificity of detection of the drug in the retina (ALFIERI & SOLE 1966).

We were led to investigate the use of the VER in these circumstances from both practical and theoretical considerations with particular reference to three factors:

— The detection of specific 'perifovealopathy' (according to Haches' denomination) (HACHE, TURUT & DUFOUR 1971) would be more evident because of the preferential cortical amplification of macular inputs.

— Many drugs have the same visual toxicity and the same quinonic nucleus as the antimalarial drugs but not their specific fluorescence.

— There may be other sites at which antimalarial drugs exert a toxic effect, although less frequently than in the retina. For instance, optic neuritis, neuromyopathy or brain disorders (CAMBIER, MASSON, BERKMAN & DAIROU 1972, GRENIER, ROLLAND, KIFFER & MAUPAS 1973, LATERRE, STEVENS, GOFFIN & VERLGHE 1973, LYLE & SCHMIDT 1962).

The ERG and the VER were recorded in patients on long term treatment with antimalarial drugs. They were also studied in rabbits after experimental intoxication so that the toxic mechanism may be determined and further VER methods developed.

METHODS

A) In Man

Eighteen patients (14 females, 4 males) were examined. They were on long term treatment with quinoline derivatives for chronic disease (rheumatoid arthritis or systemic lupus erythematosis. Three had prophylactic antimalarial treatment only. Nine patients were aged about 50, six about 20 and there were three children less than 5.

The VER was recorded monopolarly comparatively right and left 2 cms. above the inion with an Alvar retinograph amplifier. An SAIP ART 1 000 averager was used to average 50 or 100 sweeps. The ERG was recorded at the same time.

The examination was carried out as for dynamic electroretinography with white, red and blue stimuli before and during dark adaptation. This usual method in our laboratory gives parameters of modulation and further the best identification of characteristic components and culmination times. (Using CIGÁNEK notation) (CORCELLE, MABON, ROZIER, VINCENT, BENSCH & FAURE 1969)

B) In animals

Rabbits were acutely or chronically intoxicated with chloroquine sulphate. Electrodes were stereotactically implanted along the visual pathway, being stainless steel macroelectrodes for deep levels and silver at cortical levels. Records were time-switched after acute intoxication and taken 24 hours after the last injection in chronic intoxication. The ERG and VER were recorded (using MOPEV II) on atropinised awake animals under five conditions: red or white flash, light or dark adaptated, or with electrical stimulation of the optic nerve.

The rabbit was chosen as an experimental animal as there have been previous studies on antimalarial drug retinopathy and on the visual functions of this animal (BABEL, & ENGLERT 1969, DALE & PARKHILL 1965, FRANCOIS & MAUGDAL 1964, MONNIER, FAURE, ROZIER & BENSCH 1971, RAMSEY, BLOODWORTH & ENGERMAN 1970, VAN HOF & COLLEWIJ 1971)

RESULTS

A) In man

Correlation of the VER and ERG results with clinical tests shows four levels of involvement (fig. 1).

0 level: (2 cases) with a normal VER and no ERG or clinical abnormality. These patients were on low dosage (100 mg/day of chloroquine sulphate) for malaria prophylaxis.

Ist level: (7 cases) the clinical tests are normal and the ERG is normal with a fusion frequency over 50 c/s. The VER shows the following abnormalities:
— the amplitude is higher than usual with red and white stimuli.
— the negative IIIrd wave shape seems to be increased and takes a triphasic aspect.
— the culmination times may be delayed, not above 75ms. (normal 60 ± 5 ms with our stimulation parameters)

IInd level: (4 cases) these patients have a supranormal ERG with no clinical signs. The critical fusion frequency may be higher than normal (70-80 cs in two cases). The VER shows marked changes:
— there is an increase with the red stimulus compared with white or blue.
— the culmination time of the negative IIIrd wave is delayed more than 80 ms (80-100 ms).
— the IIIrd wave is very abnormal with a large polyphasic shape.

IIIrd level: (4 cases) There are ERG defects in the photopic components (the b-wave has a blunted aspect, the red response is of low voltage and the fusion frequency is lower than 30 c/s). Three of the patients have clinical defects.

The VER shows three features in our three patients:

— selective modification related to the stimulus wavelength and a marked decrease of the III-IV wave amplitudes (more marked with a blue stimulus than with a red one).

— delaying of the IIIrd wave culmination time more than 80 ms.

— low voltage of the IIIrd wave, detected only with the red stimulus, with polyphasic shape.

By our methods the VER shows changes as the ERG changes progress but the VER is affected earlier with antimalarial drug impregnation. These changes enhance the value of the less marked electroretinographic signs such as supranormality which is very difficult to assess.

The VER seems to have a prognostic value. With some patients followed for a long time during treatment electrophysiological signs have progressed through levels as shown in table I.

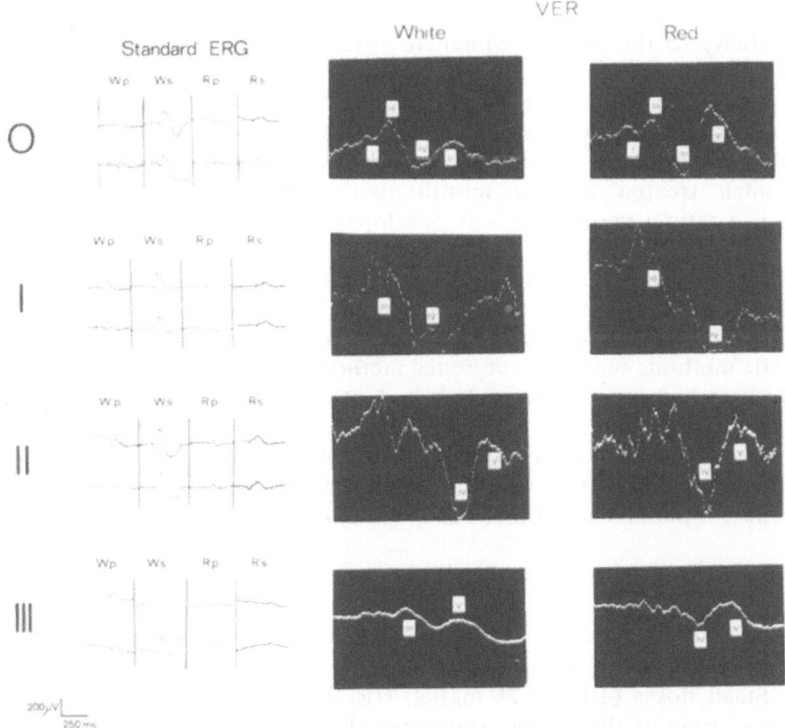

Fig. 1. Antimalarial drugs in Man. Comparative VER and ERG records. O. Normal; I. VER impregnation with normal ERG; II. Retinal impregnation with supranormal ERG; III. Retinal damage, with clinical signs, photopic defects of ERG and following VER's signs (note persistence of polyphasism of IIIrd wave of VER).

TABLE I

	Ophtalmological signs	E.R.G.	V.E.R.	Comment
0	–	Normal	normal	normal
I	–	Normal	Red increased Short delayed Polyphasic IIIrd wave	VER impregnation
II	–	Supranormal	Red increased Delayed (more than 20 ms) Polyphasic III rd wave	Retinal impregnation
III	+	Photopic defect	Decreased more with blue stim. Delayed Early polyphasism.	Retinal toxicity
NS	+	abnormal	No polyphasism.	Non Specific

Specificity of the changes which are different from those in other pathological circumstances are illustrated by the following cases. In the first case it was possible to identify an optic neuritis due to antimalarial drugs. There was a selective decrease of the VER associated with a polyphasic shape of the earlier components. The ERG was normal. In the second case, a 60 years old woman treated for six months with synthetic antimalarial drugs (S.A.D.), a retinal vascular defect developed with ERG abnormalities but with no VER abnormality. The antimalarial treatment was continued and after a further six months visual acuity was recovered. The clinical value of the VER method may therefore be presumed but other clinical studies are still necessary. We could benefit by adding the VER method to other early diagnostic methods such as fluoresence methods.

. Three mechanisms for the nature and site of the action of SAD on the VER may be suggested:

– there is a central expression of the retinal modification.
– there is a conduction defect at the optic nerve level
– there is parallelism of brain and retinal toxic accumulation.

B) In the Rabbit

1) *Photic evoked response.* Chloroquine sulphate injections induce VER changes all along the visual pathway.

A) Small doses (10 and 20 mg/kg) (fig. 2) produce a slight increase of conduction time of the evoked responses at the level of the optic nerve and the geniculate body. At a cortical level the earlier components (t1 wave with a culmination time of 22.2 ± 0.75 ms which is regarded as a presynaptic component) have the same decrease (about 2 ms). On the other hand the later components of the primary complex of the VER are delayed only at cortical levels with mean doses of 20 mg/kg. (t3 wave, culminating normally

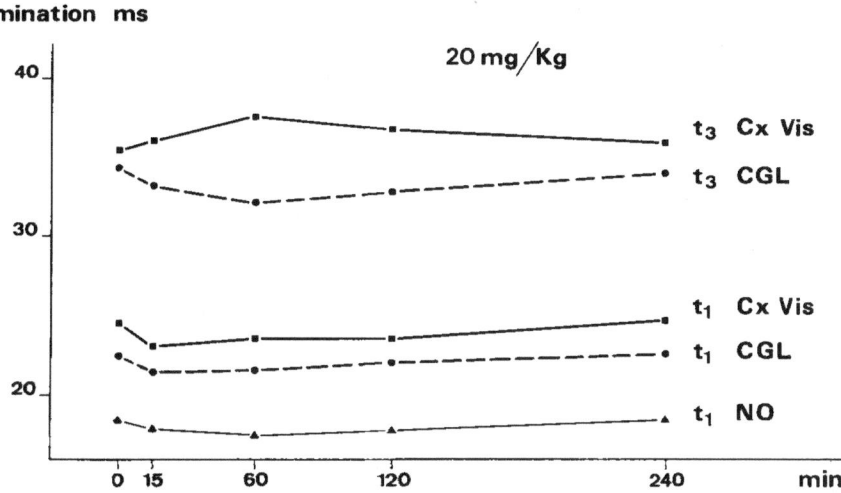

Fig. 2. Acute chloroquine intoxication in rabbit. Decreasing of VER's lateness at a subcortical level of earlier component (t₁ presynaptic), increasing of late component (t₃ postsynaptic) at a cortical level.

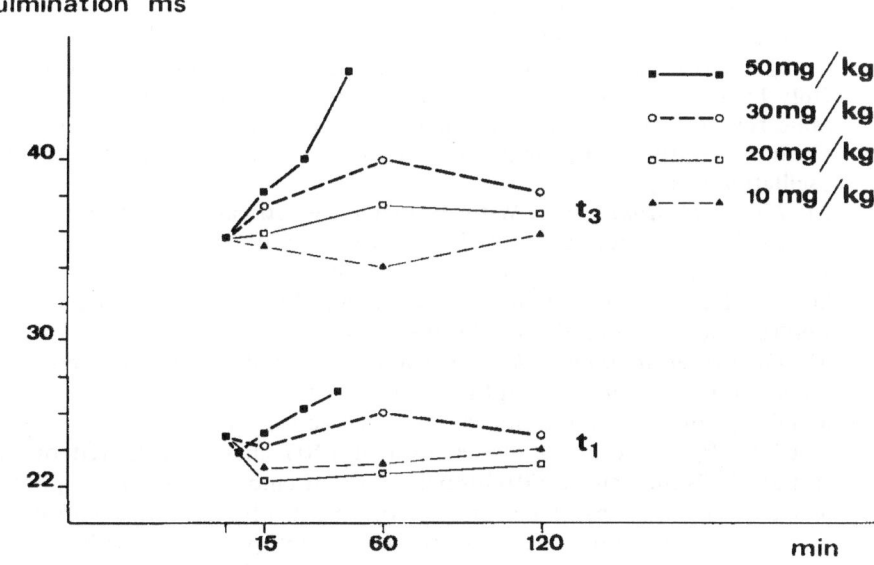

Fig. 3. Evolution of culmination times of early and late components of primary complex of cortical responses after various chloroquine doses injection (rabbit).

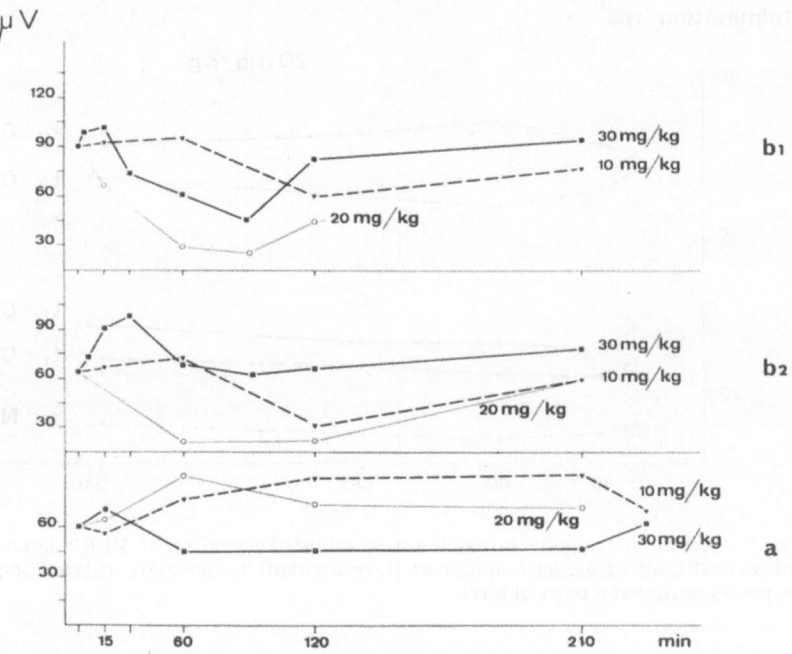

Fig. 4. Evolution of ERG after chloroquine injection: note differential action upon b1 and b2 wave with 30 mg/kg (white stimulation).

at 34.8 ms ± 1.46, is 3 ms. delayed), but not at subcortical level. This delay involves an increase of synaptic time.

B) Increasing doses of chloroquine increase the cortex delay (fig. 3). Only high doses (30 mg/kg) generated delay at a subcortical level and at the same time affected earlier (presynaptic) components of the visual response. *Qualitatively* the post-primary response is also increased with changes in the oscillation's shape.

2) *Electrical Stimulation.* With optic nerve electrical stimulation it is possible to shunt the retinal level. In this case modifications of response were seen at cortical level but not at subcortical level, after acute of chronic intoxication. This method demonstrates that there is a direct brain action as well as a modification of retinal transmission.

3) *Electro-retinographic changes.* Chloroquine induces first an increase and second a decrease in the amplitude of the ERG, mainly the *b* wave (fig. 4). Mainly qualitative alterations can be observed following drug doses. As indicated by fig. 5 there is a dissociation of ERG changes with red or white stimuli. This indicates a differential action of chloroquine on the photopic and scotopic systems and a drug involvement with the photopic/scotopic interaction. With moderate doses there is a scotopic defect, with increasing red ERG the photopic system seems protected. This may be due to the reduced vasoconstictive reaction of retinal vessels (MEIER-RUGE 1969) with higher doses. Thus with the highest lethal dose (50 mg/kg) an increase

394

of the scotopic components is observed before death. So it may be assumed that there are functional interactions at a retinal level which may alter the electro-retinogram without retinal alteration.

4) *Comparison between acute and chronic intoxication.* With the chronic procedure all levels obtained with the various drug doses were found. With the ERG there is found first an increase and then a decrease in voltage. With evoked potentials there is a cortical delay and then a subcortical delay. These changes were the same during chronic and acute intoxication and they indicate cumulative drug effects, not only at a retinal but also at a cortical level. The main difference is that with chronic intoxication there are more marked changes in the pattern of the VER.

5) *Controls of drug accumulation* at brain level were finally done chemically with PROUTY method (ALFIERI & SOLE 1966). We find comparable quantities in the brain as in the kidney or the liver (about 1 μg/g of tissue).

CONCLUSIONS

Studies of the experimental and clinical VER indicates pathophysiological sites and action of synthetic antimalarial drugs which are of interest in neuropharmacology and neurotoxicology.

1) With SAD accumulation there are not only retinal but cerebral effects. This would accord with clinical data (such as anti-epileptic effects) and chemical data (relating to the affinity of these drugs with macromolecular compounds) (REINERT & RUTTY 1969, RUBIN, MANSOUR, ZVAIFLER & BERMSTEIN 1965).

2) There is evidence of a neural action. The antimalarial drugs increase

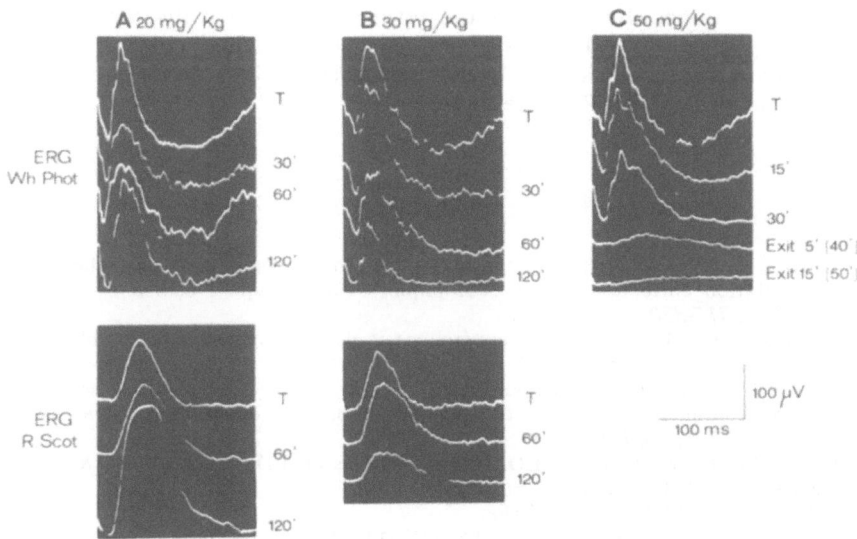

Fig. 5. Retinographic changes after chloroquine injection showing dissociation between photopic and scotopic responses.

395

synaptic delay. This effect occurs at retinal level and also at cortical levels. With a more sensitive test it could be that an abnormality at cortical level could be the first indication of toxic impregnation.

3) The VER could be a good method for the detection of an organic lesion of the retina. Moreover it adds to the value of retinographic changes. It seems likely that a simultaneous VER and fluorescence examination in a longitudinal study would allow confirmation and precision of diagnosis.

4) Theoretical considerations are considered by relating comparative data in man and the rabbit.

Antimalarial accumulation at a cortical level can alter the earlier components of the VER in man as in the rabbit. The prominent cortical function in man explains the marked increase of VER sensitivity. Therefore on the basis of our experiments we assume that the earlier components of the VER are first generated at a cortical level.

ACKNOWLEDGMENTS

We particularly thank G. Labayle and R. Miguelez for their technical aid.

SUMMARY

A method of visual evoked response (V.E.R.) is proposed for the early diagnosis of visual complications of antimalarial drugs.

Eighteen patients were examined: VER changes related to drug accumulation and visual toxicity are observed earlier than with the classical ERG.

Other experimental studies using the VER and ERG were carried out in rabbits in acute and chronic intoxication. Cerebral accumulation and synaptic effects of the drug were detected.

As functional alterations of the retina may modify the ERG it seems necessary to add the VER to diagnose an organic lesion.

Clinical applications and theoretical considerations about the morphological analysis of the VER are discussed.

REFERENCES

ALFIERI R. & SOLE P. Quelques aspects electrorétinographiques des phénomènes d'inhibition entre les système scotopiques et photopiques. *C.R. Soc. Biol. Paris* 1966, 2, *317-320*.

BABEL J. & ENGLERT U. Etude expérimentale de la rétinopathie par la chloroquine *Bull. Mem. Soc. Franc. Ophtal.* 1969, 82, *491-505*.

CAMBIER J., MASSON M., BERKMAN N. & DAIROU R. Neuropathie sensitive et névrite optique après absorption prolongée de chloroidoquinone. *Nouv. Presse Med.*, 1972, 1, 30, *1991-92*.

CORCELLE L., MABON A., ROZIER J., VINCENT J.D., BENSCH Cl. & FAURE JMA. Potentiels évoqués rétiniens corticaux chez l'enfant amblyope strabique. *Arch. Opht.* 1969, 29, 3, *187-192*.

DALE A.J.D., PARKHILL E.M. & LAYTON D.D. 'Studies on chloroguine retinopathy in rabbits'. *J.A.M.A.* 1965, 193, *241-243*.

FRANÇOIS J. & MAUGDAL M.C. Experimental chloroquine retinopathy. *Ophtalmologica (BASEL)* 1964, 148, 6, *442-452*

GRENIER B., ROLLAND J.C., KIFFER A. & MAUPAS Ph. Myélorédiculonevrites subaiguës et chloroiodoquinoléine. *Nouvelle Presse Med.* 1973, 2, n° 16, *1076.*

HACHE J.C., TURUT P. & DUFOUR D. Etude des lésions maculaires par antipaludéens de synthèse. *Lille Med.* 1971, 16, 1, *217.*

LATERRE E.C., STEVENS A., GOFFIN L. & VERLGHE. Myélopathie subaiguë (SMON) après absorption d'hydroxyquinoléines. *Nouvelle Presse Med.* 1973, 2, n° 38, *2550.*

LYLE D.J. & SCHMIDT I.G. The selective effects of drugs upon nuclei of the oculogyric system *Amer. J. Opht.* 1962, 54, n°4, *706-716.*

MEIER-RUGE W. Drug induced retinopathy. In FRANÇOIS J.: 'Occupational and medicative hazard in Ophtalmology'. Congr. Europ. Soc. Opht. Amsterdam 1968. Karger édit. (Basel) 1969, *561-573.*

MONNIER M., FAURE J.M.A., ROZIER J. & BENSCH Cl.- Variations des activités évoquées d'origine rétinienne selon la stimulation chromatique et la période de l'année chez le lapin. Journ. of Neuro-visc. Relations, 1971, suppl. X, *204-219*

PATY J. Potentiels évoqués visuels et électrorétinographie au cours des traitements par antipaludéens de synthèse chez l'Homme et l'Animal. Medical Doctoral Thesis Bordeaux 1972, n° 266 (136 pp,261 Ref.)

PROUTY R.W. & KURODA K. Spectrophotometric determination and distribution of chloroquine in human tissues. *J. Lab. Clin. Med.* 1958, 52, *477-480*

RAMPON S;, ROUHER F., ALFIERI R., SOLE P., BUSSIERE J.L. & SAUVEZIE B. Surveillance ophtalmologique des malades traités par antipaludèens de synthèse: mise en évidence électrorétinigraphique de l'imprégnation rétininienne toxique. *Rev. Rhum.* 1970, 3, *233-235*

RAMSEY M.S., BLOODWORTH J.M.B. & ENGERMAN R.L. Chloroquine retinopathy in the rabbit. *Canad. J. Opthal.* 1970, 5, 3, *273*

REINERT H. RUTTY D.A. Mechanisms of chroroquine and phenothiazine retinopathies *Toxicol. Appl. Pharmacol.* 1969, 14, *635-636.*

RUBIN M., MANSOURA.M., ZVAIFLERN.J. & BERMSTEIN H. Binding of chloroquine to melanine granules *Invest. Ophtal.*, 1965, 4, 2, *236.*

VAN HOF M.W. & COLLEWIJ H. Vision in rabbit. *Documenta Ophtamologica* 1971, vol.30, *361* pp.

COMPARATIVE ELECTROPHYSIOLOGICAL OBSERVATIONS OF INTRAOCULAR TUMOURS AND RETINAL DETACHMENTS

ANNA BOHÁR & ÁGNES FARKAS

(Budapest, Hungary)

The first surveys published on clinical electroretinography reported that intraocular tumours influence the bioelectrical retinal activity. It was stated that small tumours, not exceeding one or two papil diameters, may increase this activity. Supernormal potentials could even be indicative of this. A reduction however, more or less proportional to the extension of the tumour, is more typical. This responds better to the expectations of both the electrophysiologist and the clinician. It confirms the diagnosis, but has in itself no diagnostic value. The electrophysiological results in retinal detachment are in several respects identical with those observed in intraocular tumours. In retinal detachment the bio-electrical activity may have prognostic value, but in tumours it does not. In patients, observed in our Institute due to retinal detachment or intraocular melanoblastoma, we noted some remarkable phenomena during the electro-retinographical (ERG) and

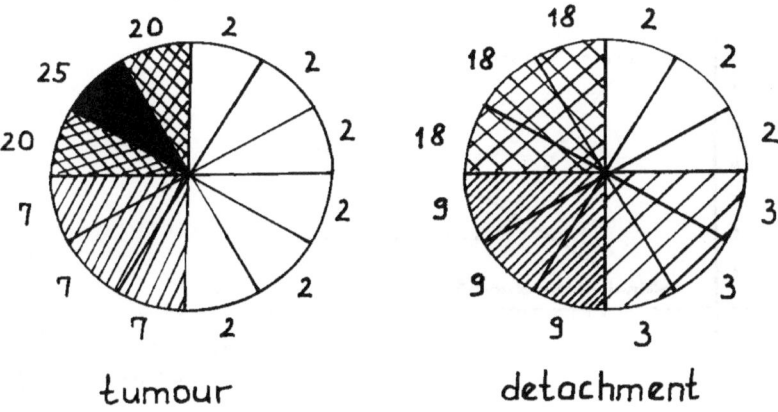

Fig. 1.

electroculographical (EOG) examinations. In the following, we propose to evaluate them briefly.

As an appropriate starting-point, we compared the electrophysiological data available of 25 histologically verified melanoblastic eyes with those of retinal detachments.

Fig. 1 illustrates schematically the extension of intraocular melanoblastoma and retinal detachments as found clinically. In the sectors of corresponding size, the deepening of the tint is proportional to the incidence of the process. It may be noted that in our material the retinal detachments are more extensive than the circumscribed tumours.

We follow the international procedure, considering the ERG amplitude of the healthy eye as 100 per cent. In comparison to this a 30 per cent reduction in the response of the affected eye is qualified as pathological.

Fig. 2 represents an actual recording. The reduction in ERG amplitude of the upper recording amounting to 80-100 per cent occurred in a proportion of 1:6 (Fig. 3).

We observed melanoblastoma of small extension significantly in more cases than retinal detachments of the same extent. In the latter ophthalmoscopical and electrophysiological findings show a certain parallelism, particularly in recent processes. Circumscribed tumours of small extension in-

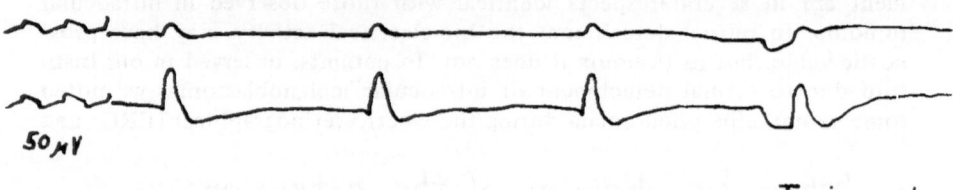

50 µV

Tu. ioc. o.d.

Fig. 2.

Reduction of ERG - amplitude by 80- 100%

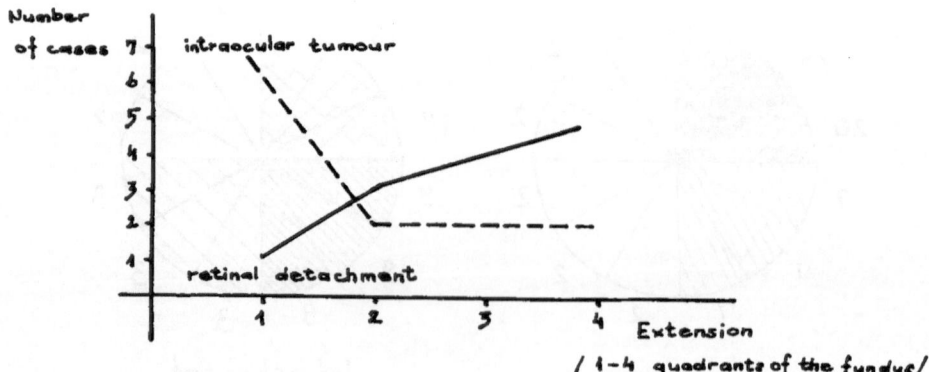

Fig. 3.

fluence the bioelectric activity of the entire retina to a higher degree as one would expect. This is shown in Fig. 4 representing the ERG results of 8 melanoblastomas and 8 retinal detachments, both extending over one-quarter of the fundus. It is obvious that a melanoblastoma reduces the bioelectric activity of the retina more than a retinal detachment, although the latter is a real retinal disease while the former will only reduce the first two retinal neurons indirectly.

The EOG primarily gives information about the function of the pigment epithelium. In cases of retinal detachment and intraocular melanoblastoma, there are basic potential changes, indicative of accelerated or retarded photochemical processes, which are generally identical. This was investigated in our material using Arden's quotient.

Fig. 5 represents an actual recording. Arden's quotient is the ratio between the highest value of the standing potential during light adaptation and the lowest value during dark-adaptation. The normal value of this quotient

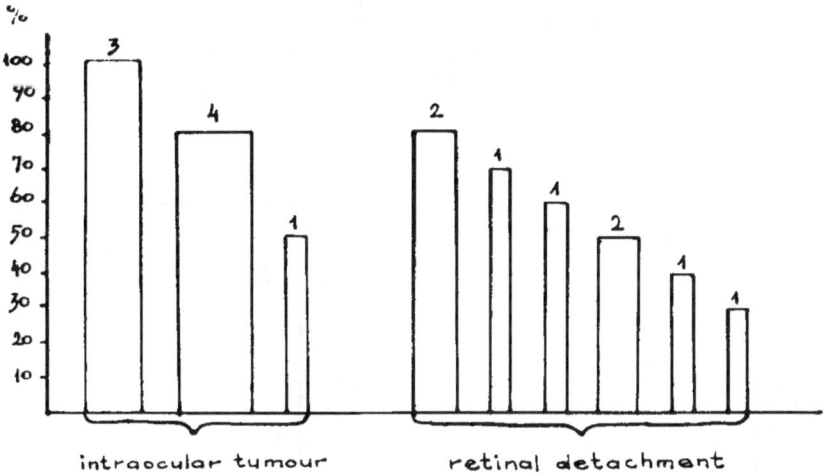

Fig. 4.

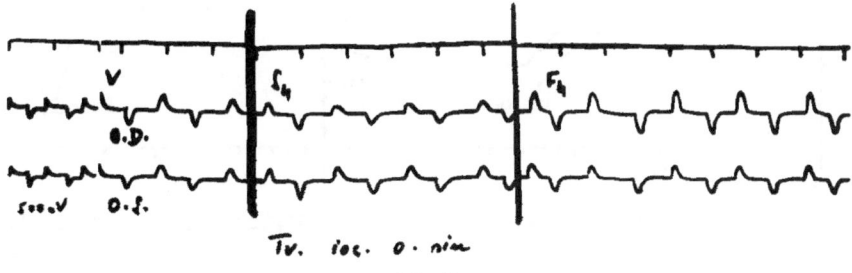

Fig. 5.

is approximately 2.0, which can be observed in the right eye of Figure 5. In the eye with the melanoblastoma the standing potential does not change; Arden's quotient is 1.0.

In Fig. 6 Arden's quotient of the two groups is drawn in comparison with a healthy group. The graph indicates that tumours have a much stronger blocking effect of the bioelectrical activity as compared to the

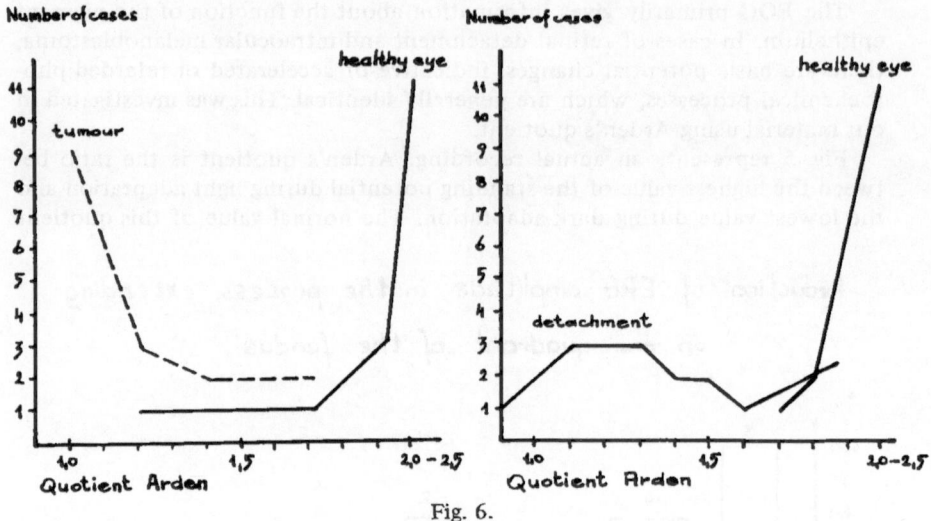

Fig. 6.

Conditions of the EOG basic potential in the affected and healthy eye

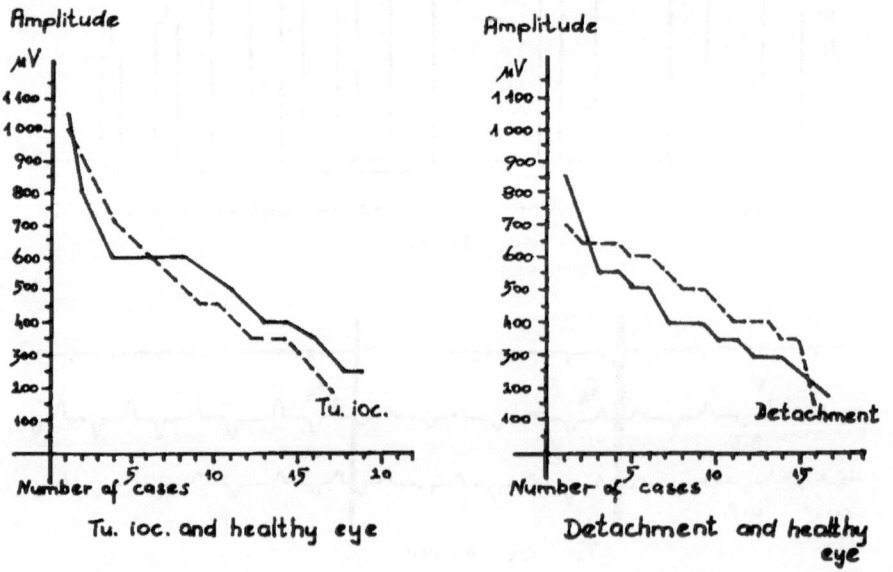

Fig. 7.

detachments. The standing potential itself tends to increase in the detachment and decrease in the tumours.

SUMMARY

Both the ERG and the EOG appear to be more damaged in cases of intraocular melanoblastomas than in recent retinal detachments, if in both groups the visible extension of the abnormality is about the same. The difference may assist in establishing the diagnosis.

LITERATURE

ALGVERE, P.: Clinical studies on the oscillatory potentials of the human electroretinogram with special reference to the scotopic-b wave. *Acta Ophthal.*, 46, *993*, (1968).

FRANÇOIS, J. & ROUCK, A.: L'électroretinographie dans la myopie et les décollements myopigenes de la rétine. *Bull. Soc. Belge Ophthal.* 107, (1954).

FRANÇOIS, J. et al: Study of retinal electrical activity in cases of choroidalmalignant melanomata treated by light coagulation. *Ann. Ocul.* 199, *1049*, (1966).

KARPE, G.: The basis of clinical electroretinography. Acta Ophthal. Suppl. 24, (1945).

KARPE, G. & RENDAHL, J.: The clinical electroretinogram. VI. The electroretinogram in detachment of retina. *Acta Ophthal.* 30, *303-316*, (1952).

RENDAHL, J.: Advances in electrophysiology and pathology of the visual system. Thieme, Leipzig, 319, 1968.

STRAUB, W.: Das Elektroretinogramm. Klin. Mbl. Augenheilk. Beiheft, 36, (1961).

SUNDMARK, E.: The electroretinogram and malignant intraocular tumours. *Acta Ophthal.* 36, *57*, (1958).

THE MACULAR FUNCTION IN THE ERG

G.H.M. VAN LITH

(Rotterdam, the Netherlands)

For patients, as well as ophthalmologists, macular function plays a very important role in total retinal function. Measure of the visual acuity, central sensivity and colour vision are the usual methods of testing the macular function. They fail, however, in small children, in the state of unconsciousness, in the presence of media opacities and sometimes in elderly people. Furthermore, these methods are not objective. It is logical, therefore, that clinicians have always been especially interested in determining macular function by means of electrophysiological methods. We will recapitulate on what can be done nowadays, what the failings are and what may be expected in the near future. Since I was asked to report about the macular function in the ERG, the EOG and VEP will not systematically be dealt with. Concerning the VEP, more data can be found in the paper of OGUCHI et al. (1975) in this issue.

Concerning the macular function in the electroretinogram (ERG), many data are rather old fashioned. In the early beginning of applying the ERG for clinical purposes, it was already established that the ordinary ERG, registered without special amplification methods, was merely a function test of the entire retina. Even after local stimulation, the ERG did not reflect the activity of the stimulated area, but that of a much larger region, stimulated by stray light (ASHER, 1951). The reason for this was that a real local response was too small to be visualized amidst the noise level. Later on, improvement of the signal to noise ratio having been achieved by means of averagers and lock-in amplifiers (PADMOS & van NORREN, 1972), the registration of local responses, including those of the macula or fovea, became possible (ARDEN & BAUKES, 1966). First of all, we want to discuss what can be deduced about the macular function from the global ERG (G-ERG), i.e. an ERG, with total or almost total retinal stimulation. After that, the so-called macular-ERG (M-ERG) or foveal-ERG (F-ERG) will be debated. In this report we will limit ourselves to the ERGs, derived from the cone system, since with the term macular function usually the cone function is meant. ERGs of the cone system can be obtained either by using a high adaptative illumination, suppressing the rod system, or with a high flicker rate over 20 cps. We use the first method, both for the G-ERG and for the M-ERG, since for the latter a high adaptive illumination is also needed to prevent stray light responses.

In the presence of media opacities, local illumination of the retina cannot be achieved without having stray light. Therefore, since only G-ERGs are obtained in this situation, it is most important to know whether it is possible to predict the existence of a macular degeneration from the global electrical responses. The contribution of the macula to a G-ERG is rather small, since the macula is only a small part of the retina. Although its receptor density is the highest of the retina, the absolute number of receptors which it contains, is low as compared to the total number of receptors of the entire retina. This can best be illustrated by furnishing some data of POLYAK, quoted from DEUTMAN's book concerning the foveal dystrophies (DEUTMAN, 1971).

The term macula is mostly used in clinical terminology, such as in senile macular degenerations and macular oedema, indicating that usually the pathological process covers more than the fovea only. Anatomically, the macula represents that part of the retina which contains the yellow pigment. This area is not sharply demarcated. According to POLYAK, it amounts to about 16° visual angle, i.e. somewhat smaller than the retinal area, which lies between the temporal branches of the central retinal artery. For clinical purposes, the latter is often described as the posterior pole. The number of cones within the real macular area would only be 650.000, which is approximately 10% of the total number of cones, the latter being 7 million.

The question arises, as to whether a total loss of macular function, thus a 10% loss of the receptor system, can be found with the aid of a G-ERG. Actually, we should be able to find a loss less than 10%, since it may often occur that macular degenerations do not attack all the receptors within the affected area. Furthermore, macular degenerations are often limited to the fovea, and the fovea, bordered by the foveal margin reflex, encompasses a 5° visual angle. This area contains a 100.000 cones, which is only 1.5% of all cones. Since biological variations are far greater than this percentage, it may hardly be expected, that a local foveal abnormality can be detected by means of a G-ERG. Going back to a theoretical 10% function loss caused by a macular disease, it has to be looked into, whether such a loss can produce a significant reduction of the ERG.

Generally, the ERG is considered to be a summation potential of the entire retina. An argument in favour of this hypothesis is, that with local stimulation under photopic conditions, the height of the ERG seems to correlate with the number of receptors stimulated (VAN LITH & HENKES, 1970). It is not certain, however, that the correlation found for the macular area, holds true for the rest of the retina. This problem of the relative contribution of the various parts of the retina to the ERG, registered with a contactlens, has not yet been investigated enough. BRINDLEY & WEST-HEIMER (1965) did some basic work in this field. Assuming that the ERG is a summation potential, we have to consider what a 10% loss in amplitude may signify in relation to the ERG variability. In most reports, including that of PETERSON, 1968, the interindividual variability of the normal ERG is 20% or more. Per individual, the variability should still be about 10%. The same percentage may be found when the right and left eye are compared. In respect to these data, a 10% receptor loss will by no means be significant. Hence, theoretically it should be impossible to detect a macular disturbance by means of G-ERG.

If we diminish the stimulus field from a total one to a local macular one, an abnormal electrical response of the macula will not longer be hidden in the mass response of the entire retina. In order to obtain a local ERG stray light responses have to be avoided with a strong background illumination which, if it also suppresses the rod system, will reveal a local cone response, (VAN LITH & HENKES, 1968). Furthermore, averaging techniques are a prerequisite, since local responses are too small to be registered with an ordinary amplifier. The unsolved problem of the fixation limits the value of a M-ERG greatly. Since the height of a M-ERG depends on the cone density in the stimulated area, the amplitude will not only be decreased by a pathological process, but also by an improper fixation of the stimulus spot (VAN LITH, 1971). This means that a normal M-ERG will indicate a normal macula, while a lowered M-ERG does not say very much. In this aspect more may be expected from the registration of the VEPs, which reflect for the greater part the macular area, especially if patterned stimulation is used. Clinical data of these methods, however, are scarce. Coming to some clinical results, the senile macular degenerations and the juvenile foveal dystrophies will be a separately dealt with, since ERG results are quite different in both groups.

SENILE MACULAR DEGENERATIONS

In the books of JAYLE et al. (1965) and FRANCOIS et al (1974) it is reported that electrophysiological examination in senile macular degenerations may reveal normal or subnormal responses. That the ERG may be normal is not astonishing, but how can subnormal responses be explained? Since actual local macular abnormalities, such as traumatic or inflammatory scars do not reveal lowered ERGs (JACOBSON, 1961), it is most probable that low ERGs in senile macular degenerations are not caused by the ophthalmoscopically visible macular abnormality only. Involvement of the retina outside the macula must also have contributed to a decrease in the responses. The finding that scotopic ERG, as well as the oscillatory potentials (PERDRIEL, 1969) are often lowered, supports this view. Another indication for a more generalized retinal disturbance is obtained, if the alterations in the photopic b-wave after total retinal and local macular stimulation are compared. From a $10°$ stimulus field, often covering the degenerated area, we obtain under our stimulus conditions a response of about $10 \mu V$, being approximately 10% of the global response, which is normally $100-150 \mu V$. Decrease or even absence of the macular response can by no means explain the decrease in the G-ERG, which we often see. Furthermore, the decrease in the G-ERG does often not correlate with the macular alterations. Some examples may clear this up. The ERGs of figure 1 are made with total retinal stimulation, using a ball-stimulator (VAN LITH et al. 1973). A bright blue background is used to suppress rod activity. White light flashes are given in a frequency of 4 per second. The lower limit of our normal range amounts to $100 \mu V$.

The first patient had a disciform macular degeneration of the left eye. Visual acuity of this eye was 1/300. In the other eye, only small pigment alterations were found in the fovea. Visual acuity of this eye was rather

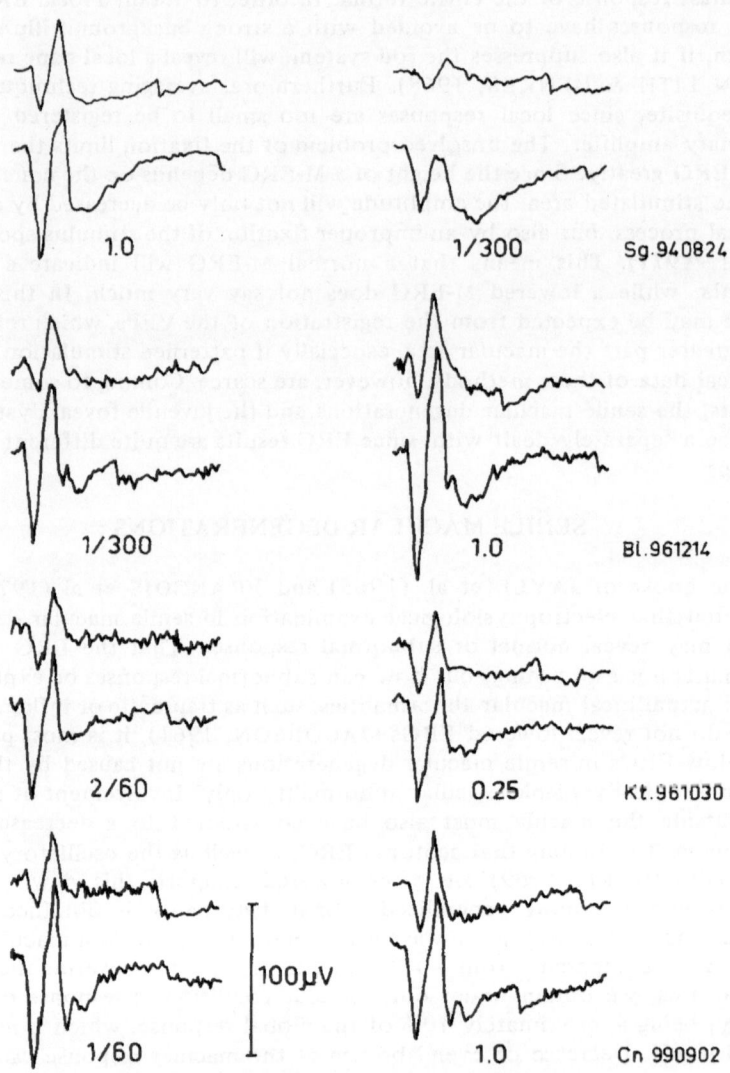

OD   OS

1.0   1/300   Sg.940824

1/300   1.0   Bl.961214

2/60   0.25   Kt.961030

100μV

1/60   1.0   Cn 990902

Fig. 1. ERGs of the cone system with total retinal illumination. Upper recording: 0.1 J, lower recording: 1 J. Time basis 250 msec.

good. The low responses of the left eye were obvious, the right eye having much better responses.

The second patient also had a disciform macular degeneration with a visual acuity of 1/300, but of the right eye. In this patient, too, the unaffected eye showed small pigment alterations. The affected eye again had lower responses than the unaffected eye. Comparing, however, the ERGs of the first and second patient it appeared that the responses of the bad eye of the second patient were as high as those of the good eye of the first patient. It cannot be demonstrated more clearly that there is no correlation.

The third patient had an atrophic macular degeneration of both eyes. Although the maculae seemed to be about the same ophthalmoscopically, the visual acuity of the right eye was 2/60, that of the left eye 0.25. The ERGs, on the contrary, were of the same height, reflecting the appearance better than the visual acuity. This is understandable, since on one hand the photopic ERG, if it is a summation potential, reflects the total number of functioning and stimulated cones, while on the other hand the visual acuity reflects the highest density of functioning cones in the macular area. This may result in some connection between the ERG and the visual acuity, but not in a real correlation. The discrepancy between visual acuity and ophthalmoscopic appearance in this patient is difficult to explain on the basis of a local abnormality. A visual acuity of 0.25, which can be obtained in a normal eye at 10° eccentricity, could indicate a destruction within a 20° area. Following this idea, a visual acuity of 2/60 would point to a damaged area of 80°. Ophthalmoscopically, this area was only 10°. If we assume that also outside this 10° area retinal tissue is out of function, the ERGs should be much lower. A similar problem was encountered with the last patient of this group. This patient had a colloidal macular degeneration of the right eye. Visual acuity of this eye was 1/60, that of the other eye 1.0. In this patient the responses of the right eye were even higher than those of the other eye. It may be doubted, however, whether this low visual acuity was caused by the degeneration only. An amblyopia cannot be excluded.

From all our data, of which these recordings are only some examples, we can deduce that, considered as a whole, senile macular degenerations often have lowered photopic responses, reflecting very probably a lowered activity of the entire posterior pole. Therefore, per individual, a low global photopic response may indicate in elderly people the existence of macular alterations. A normal response, on the other hand, does not exclude a macular disease.

Of the same group of patients, shown in Figure 1, the M-ERGs are represented in Figure 2. A normal response is seen only in the left eye of the second patient. All the others are clearly lowered, the left eye of the first patient is even too low to be registered. In this respect, the results are better than those obtained after total retinal stimulation, in which most responses are rather good. There is even some tendency for the M-ERG to be lower as visual acuity decreases. A clear correlation, however, is lacking, if we look at the results of the left eye of the second and fourth patient. Evidently, a 10° area is still too large to be compared with visual acuity, the latter being determined by far less than even a 1° area.

CHLOROQUINE RETINOPATHY

In early chloroquine retinopathy the ERG is generally normal. In advanced cases, which we never see anymore, especially the scotopic ERG may be lowered according to the known abnormalities in the retinal periphery. The bull's eye itself is very probably too small an alteration, to cause ERG

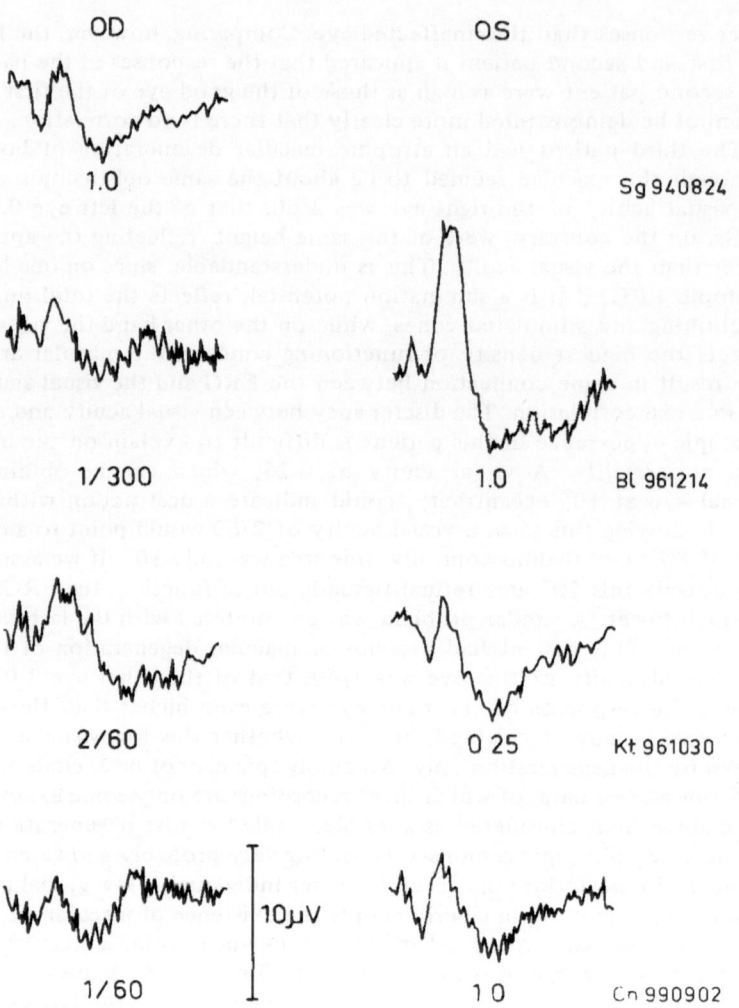

OD   OS

1.0   Sg 940824

1/300   1.0   Bl 961214

2/60   0 25   Kt 961030

1/60   10μV   1 0   Cn 990902

Fig. 2. ERGs of the cone system with a 10° macular stimulation of 0.1 J. Time basis 250 msec.

alterations. A lowered photopic ERG, therefore, will indicate an extensive abnormality in the posterior pole. In our opinion, lowered scotopic or photopic ERGs are rather late symptoms, the EOG being more reliable. Of 1333 chloroquine controls, we performed in Rotterdam over the last 4 years, 31% of the EOGs were lowered. Of the cases, in which the EOG was abnormal, less than 20% showed an abnormal scotopic or photopic ERG.

JUVENILE FOVEAL DYSTROPHIES

Of the juvenile foveal dystrophies the most common are the dominantly inherited vitelliform dystrophy and the recessively inherited Stargardt's

410

disease. An X-linked inheritance is seen in the juvenile foveal dystrophy, combined with retinoschisis. The cone-rod dystrophies which begin often as a foveal dystrophy may have different modes of inheritance. Ophthalmoscopically, the cone-rod dystrophy may resemble the bull's eye of the chloroqoine retinopathy; electrophysiologically, however, both diseases are quite different from one another. We have already observed that the chloroquine retinopathy may have a reduced EOG, while the scotopic and photopic ERG are normal or only a slightly lowered. In the cone-rod dystrophy, on the contrary, the reduction of the photopic ERG is the most striking symptom. Although the EOG is usually reduced, a totally absent lightrise is only seen in very late stages. Figure 3 represents the typical electro-ophthalmological results. The scotopic ERG is at the lower limit of the normal range, while the photopic ERG is clearly reduced, its amplitude being only 25 μV, i.e. 25% of the normal value. The EOG is lowered, but a lightrise is

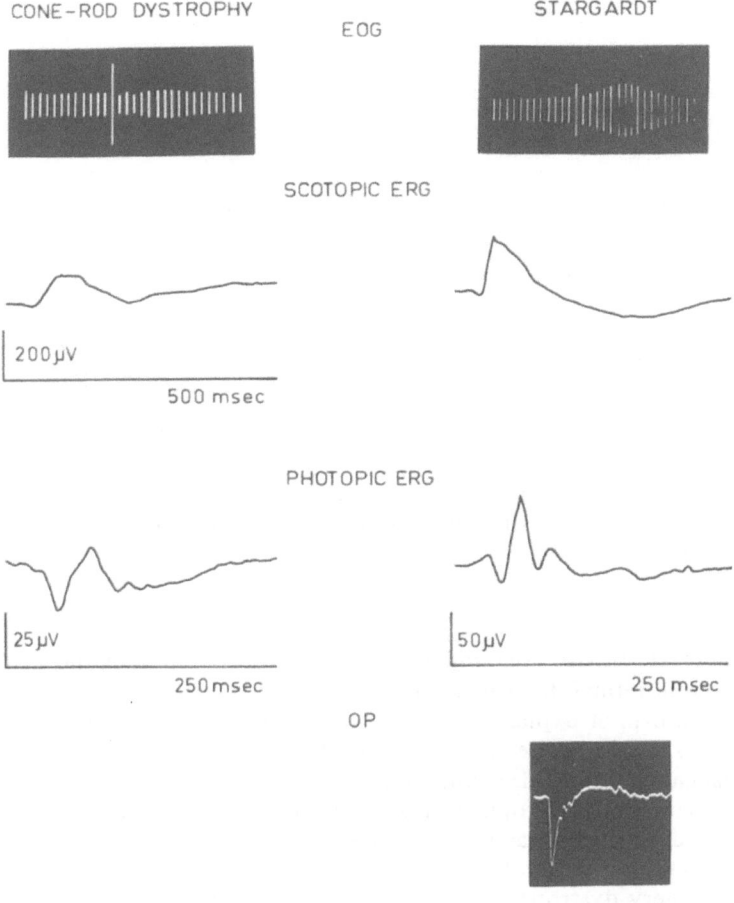

Fig. 3. EOG, ERG, and OP in the cone-rod dystrophy (left) and Stargardt's disease (right).

411

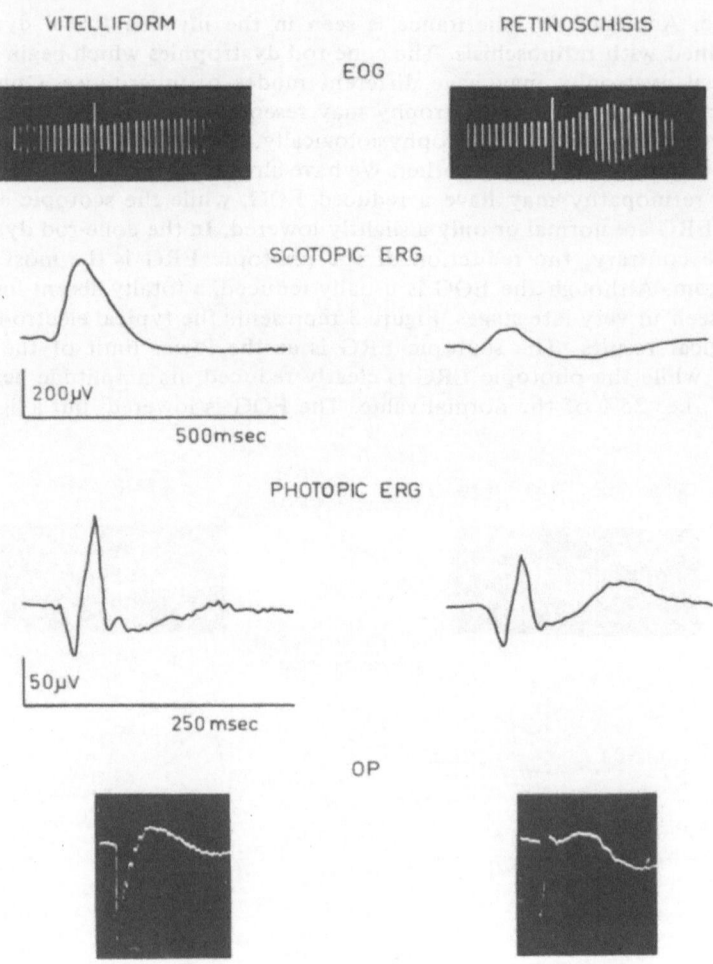

VITELLIFORM   RETINOSCHISIS

EOG

SCOTOPIC ERG

| 200µV

500msec

PHOTOPIC ERG

| 50µV

250 msec

OP

Fig. 4. EOG, ERG and OP in the vitelliform dystrophy (left) and the cystoïd foveal dystrophy (right).

still present. In the cone-rod dystrophy, it is evident that the ERG better reflects the retinal disturbance than the ophthalmoscope. The local macular alteration cannot explain the strong reduction of the G-ERG. On the other hand, psychophysical examination and the progress of the disease prove the general character of this disturbance.

The cone-rod dystrophies may also have the configuration of an atrophic macular degeneration and as such resemble Stargardt's disease. In the latter, round yellowish white flecks often surround the zone of atrophy. Even in the periphery dystrophic areas may be present. Electrophysiologically, Stargardt's disease reveals responses which are much less disturbed than those found in the cone-rod dystrophy. The disturbances are more like those in the chloroquine retinopathy. EOG and ERG are often normal. If the abnormalities in the posterior pole are rather extensive, then a lowered photopic ERG may be expected. An involvement of the retinal periphery will be expressed in an abnormal EOG and an abnormal scotopic ERG. The case, shown in figure 3, has a somewhat lowered photopic ERG, while EOG and scotopic ERG are normal.

The alterations in response found in the vitelliform dystrophy are almost pathognomonic. This dystrophy is well-known by its lesions in the fovea. Among others, FRANCOIS et al. (1967) and DEUTMAN (1969) described the absence or strongly reduced lightrise in the EOG in the presence of a normal ERG. The abnormal EOG points to a diffuse disturbance of the pigment epithelium. The normal ERG suggests a normal neuro-epithelium. Quite the reverse can be found in the X-linked cystoid foveal dystrophy which is often combined with a retinoschisis (Figure 4). The normal EOG, combined with the normal a-wave or receptor/potential, indicates a normal pigment epithelium and receptor system. The low scotopic and photopic b-waves, and the absent OPs point to a disturbance in the superficial retinal layers. These alterations in the ERG resemble those seen in retinal circulatory disturbances. It is rather strange that the ERG-abnormalities are not in accordance with the extent of the schisis. THALER, HEILIG & SLEZAK 1973, even found that independent of the existence of a retinoschisis, the

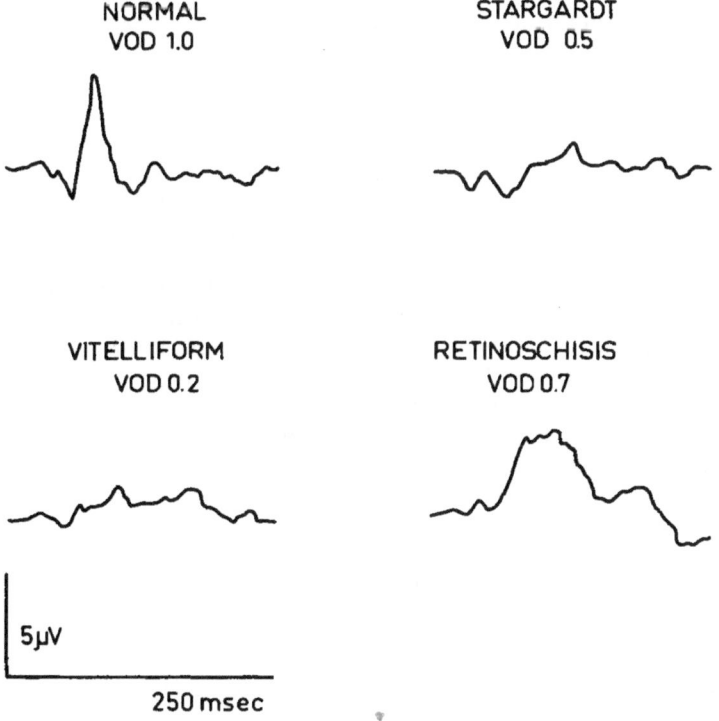

Fig. 5. 8° Macular ERGs of a normal and 3 types of juvenile foveal dystrophies.

413

b-waves are lowered. This is also our own experience. The patient whose recordings are shown in figure 4 had actually no retinoschisis. In this aspect, juvenile retinoschisis differs from retinal detachment.

Surveying these 4 juvenile foveal dystrophies, it appears that in Stargardt's disease, the electrical responses correspond very well with the fundus alterations. In the other three dystrophies: the cone-rod, the vitelliform and the retinoschisis, this is by no means the case. The macular alteration must only be part of the disease, electro-ophthalmology providing us with a much better insight as to the real retinal disturbances, but at the same time lacking this information of the macular function.

We have already discussed the problems of the M-ERG. We will only shortly discuss the data we obtained in the juvenile foveal dystrophies (figure 5). The cone-rod dystrophy is not included. Its macular responses do not differ essentially from those in Stargardt's disease and the vitelliform dystrophy. The macular ERGs are lowered in all 3 cases. Furthermore, the degree of reduction reflects more or less the degree of the foveal disturbance. Correlation with the visual acuity, however, could not be established. · These results therefore do not differ substantially from those in the senile macular degenerations. A very typical finding is the broad response, which we always find in the juvenile retinoschisis (VAN LITH & DEUTMAN, 1975). This is not seen in the global responses. The finding of the broadened photopic M-ERG is not pathognomonic for the retinoschisis. Macular oedema from other causes, such as circulatory disturbances, disciform macular degenerations and traumatic oedemas may produce the same type of response.

SUMMARY

A loss of function of the macula can not alter a G-ERG (global ERG) significantly, despite its high cone density, since it contains only 10% of the total number of cones. Both in senile macular degenerations and in juvenile foveal dystrophies the alterations in the G-ERG point to a more general disturbance of the retina as can be seen ophthalmoscopically. In media opacities a low global photopic ERG often indicates in elderly people a macular degeneration while a normal response does not exclude a macular disease. In juvenile foveal dystrophies the G-ERG helps to differentiate the various types. The significance of the M-ERG is rather limited, since its height depends on the cone density in the stimulated area. As a result a lower response may be due to a disturbance within the macular area or to an excentric fixation; a normal response mostly means a good macula.

REFERENCES

ARDEN, G.B. & BANKES, J.L.K.: Foveal electroretinogram as a clinical test. *Brit. J. Ophthal.* 50: *740* (1966).

ASHER, H.: The electroretinogram of the blind spot. *J. Physiol. (Lond.)* 112: *40* P (1951).

BRINDLEY, G.S. & WESTHEIMER, G.: The spatial properties of the human electroretinogram. *J. Physiol. (Lond.)* 179: *518-537* (1965).

414

DEUTMAN, A.F.: Electro-oculography in families with vitelliform dystrophy of the fovea. *Arch. Ophthal.* 81: *305-316* (1969).

DEUTMAN, A.F.: The hereditary dystrophies of the posterior pole of the eye. Thesis Rotterdam. Assen, Van Gorcum, 1971.

FRANCOIS, J., ROUCK, A. de. & FERNANDEZ-SASSO, D.: Electrooculography in vitelliform degeneration of the macula. *Arch. Ophthal.* 77: *726-733* (1976).

FRANCOIS, J., ROUCK, A. de., CAMBIE, A. & ZANEN, A.: L'électrodiagnostic des affections rétiniennes; Rapport Société Belge d'Ophthalmologique 1974. Paris, Masson, 1974.

JACOBSON, J.H.: Clinical electroretinography. Springfield, Thomas, 1961.

JAYLE, G.-E., BOYER, R.-L. & SARACCO, J.-B.: L'électrorétinographie; tome second; Rapport Société Française d'Ophtalmologie 1964. Paris, Masson, 1965.

LITH, G.H.M. VAN. & HENKES, H.E.: The local electric response of the central retinal area. In: Advances in electrophysiology and -pathology of the visual system; Proc. 6th Iscerg Symp., Erfurt 1967; ed. by E. SCHMÖGER, p. 163-170. Leipzig, Thieme, 1968.

LITH, G.H.M. VAN. & HENKES, H.E.: The relationship between ERG and VER. *Ophthal. Res.* 1: *40-47* (1970).

LITH, G.H.M. VAN.: The combined use of the macular electroretinogram (M-ERG) and the visually evoked responses (VER). *Ophthalmologica* 162: *208-212* (1971).

LITH, G.H.M. VAN., MEININGER, J. & MARLE, G.W. VAN.: Electrophysiological equipment for total and local retinal stimulation. In: 10th Iscerg Symposium, Los Angeles 1972; ed. by J.T. Pearlman. *Docum. Ophthal. Proc. Ser.* 2: *213-218* (1973).

LITH, G.H.M. VAN. & DEUTMAN, A.F.: Elektro-Ophthalmologie der juvenilen hereditären Maculadegenerationen. Berichte 73. Zusammenk. Deutsche Ophthal. Gesellschaft, Heidelberg 1973, p. *108-115.* München, Bergmann, 1975.

OGUCHI, Y., KOORNSTRA-LUNT, S.F., LITH, G.H.M. VAN & WITZIER, A.: Electro-ophthalmology in senile macular degenerations. Published in this issue.

PADMOS, P. & NORREN, D.V. VAN.: The vector-voltmeter as a tool to measure electroretinogram spectral sensitivity and dark adaptation. *Invest. Ophthal.* 11: *783-788* (1972).

PERDRIEL, G.: Explorations fonctionelles et électrophysiologiques au cours de dégénerescences maculaires séniles. *Arch. Ophthal. (Paris)* 29: *877-880* (1969).

PETERSON, H.: The normal B-potential in the single flash clinical electroretinogram; a computer technique study of the interference of sex and age. Acta Ophthal., suppl. 99. Copenhagen, Munksgaard, 1968.

THALER, A., HEILIG, P. & SLEZAK, H.: Elektroretinogramm und Elektrookulogramm bei juveniler Retinoschisis. *Klin. Mbl. Augenheilk.* 163: *699-703* (1973).